Visual Histology

Visual Histology

DAVID T. MORAN, Ph.D.
Associate Professor
Departments of Cellular and Structural Biology and Otolaryngology
University of Colorado School of Medicine
Denver, Colorado

J. CARTER ROWLEY, III, B.S.
Researcher V
Departments of Cellular and Structural Biology and Otolaryngology
University of Colorado School of Medicine
Denver, Colorado

LEA & FEBIGER 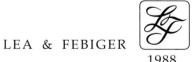 PHILADELPHIA
1988

Lea & Febiger
600 South Washington Square
Philadelphia, Pa. 19106-4198
U.S.A.
(215) 922-1330

Library of Congress Cataloging-in-Publication Data
Moran, David T.
    Visual histology.

    Includes bibliographies and index.
    1. Histology—Atlases.   I. Rowley, J. Carter.
II. Title.   [DNLM: 1. Histology—atlases.
QS 517 M829v]
QM557.M63 1988   611'.018   87-3835
ISBN 0-8121-1062-5

PRINTED IN THE UNITED STATES OF AMERICA
Print Number: 5 4 3 2 1

Dedication

THIS BOOK is dedicated to the cells and tissues it describes; to the Master Builder who oversaw, and oversees, their creation and evolution; and to Professor Keith Roberts Porter, who taught us how to look at, study, photograph, and, best of all, appreciate the elegant cells and tissues of which we ourselves are made.

Preface

FORTUNATELY, for students and professors alike, the learning of histology, or microanatomy, can be simple and enjoyable. This atlas grew out of a general principle of learning: that anything is simple once you understand it. We have found that histology is very simple to understand once you learn how to see the material. Histology is a visual art that, somewhat ironically, is based on the study of structures that cannot be seen. In order to study microanatomy, then, we need optical aids. The major optical instrument available to the student is the light microscope. Wondrous though the light microscope is, however, it has one serious shortcoming: it does not show cell boundaries, because each cell is surrounded by a structure called the cell membrane that lies beyond the resolving power of the light microscope.

This severe limitation of the light microscope can cause considerable confusion in the laboratory portion of a microanatomy course, because students using the microscope for the first time are unable to tell where one cell ends and another begins. How can the student be expected to study the microscopic anatomy of cells and tissues if he or she cannot see the size and shape of the fundamental unit of structure—the cell?

This atlas came into being to solve that problem. Fortunately, another kind of microscope, the transmission electron microscope, can clearly resolve cell membranes, even at low magnification—well within the magnification range of the light microscope. Unfortunately, electron microscopes are too expensive to buy and maintain for general student use. Although many superb photographs taken with the electron microscope are available, most of these are taken at high magnification, beyond the range of the students' light microscopes, and novices find it difficult to make the perceptual leap from what they see at low magnification by light microscopy to the high-magnification images of tissues available in the literature.

To address this problem, we have assembled a collection of light and electron micrographs of the same tissues in which the electron micrographs are taken at low magnification. In many cases, we show matched pairs of light and electron micrographs of serial "thick" and "thin" sections of the same tissue block, photographed at the same magnification and described with identical labels. We have found the use of matched light and electron micrographs of the same tissue to be an extremely effective teaching tool that allows students to learn the material rapidly. With practice, students develop a kind of "x-ray vision," formerly the province of experienced research electron microscopists, with which they can mentally superimpose images observed by low-magnification electron microscopy onto the fuzzy images seen with the light microscope. This allows students to accurately identify structures that formerly were "invisible" to them by light microscopy.

We firmly believe in the saying, "A picture is worth a thousand words." Consequently, we have supplied each plate of pictures with a text description of about a thousand words. The atlas is organized to maximize ease of use and speed of learning. First, it is subdivided into 20 major chapters that correspond to 20 major areas of study—starting with cells, moving into tissues, and progressing into organs. Where necessary, each chapter starts off with an overview that gives perspective to the specific images that are to follow. Next, a series of plates is presented. Each plate has a one-page description that allows the reader to look back and forth between text and micrograph with no irksome page-turning. The important structures on each plate are labeled, and the labels are identified in the figure legend and used in the text.

We fully realize that, although histology is a visual art, we need to use descriptive anatomic terms when talking about the material. Since the study of microanatomy may be the student's first foray into the formidable world of anatomic terminology—whether the student is an undergraduate, a medical student, a dental student, a graduate student, a nursing student, or simply a curious person who wants to understand his or her own inner workings—the terminology can be bewildering. To that end, we have italicized every key word as it is encountered for the first time in the atlas and have written a complete glossary, placed at the end of the book, that gives a succinct working definition of each term.

Throughout this atlas, we have used human and primate material wherever possible. In certain cases, where a very small organ was required (each of our tissue samples had to be small enough to fit into a 1-mm-wide slot in an electron microscope specimen grid) we chose to use a small mammal, since primate organs tend to be rather large. In other cases, when our fixation of primate material did not meet our high standard of tissue preservation, we chose available mammalian material rather than take a monkey's life for a particular photograph. Wherever possible we used animals whose lives were to be terminated during the course of biomedical research.

This atlas is not a comprehensive treatment of the subject matter. To make it so would have made the book very expensive. We are aware of the increasing strain on the student's pocketbook and intend this atlas to be affordable, which means its length must be limited. We have, nevertheless, attempted to offer a strategic sampling of key tissues and organs that should give the student a strong foundation in visual histology and have presented a large number of photomicrographs. In a sense, this atlas is as much of an art book as it is a science book, for good science, done properly, is an art form. Also, the cells and tissues of which we are made are intrinsically of great aesthetic beauty; for in their creation, form has followed function.

Tilloo Cay, Abaco, Bahamas
Denver, Colorado, U.S.A.

DAVID T. MORAN
J. CARTER ROWLEY, III

Acknowledgments

THERE are a number of people we wish to thank who have helped create this atlas. Dr. Keith Porter offered much-needed encouragement at the onset of the project and generously supplied Figure A in Plate 10–4. Cecile Duray-Bito did a superb job with the drawings that appear in the overviews, and was a great pleasure to work with. Pam Eller and Kathy Ferguson were both extremely helpful in many phases of materials preparation. Drs. Nolan Rucker and James Stevens generously offered their veterinary skills in obtaining primate tissues. Dr. Bruce Jafek kindly supplied us with tissues from the nose and ear for our chapter on the senses; Drs. Cedric Raine, Stephen Roper, and Thomas Mehalick were extremely helpful in providing tissues for the chapter on nerves when our own fixations fell short of the mark. Dr. Stanley Gould also helped by supplying fresh surgical specimens for the chapter on the female reproductive system.

Shelley Rowley offered much-needed encouragement and support throughout the entire project. Dr. Kimberly Janes was a great help; being a student of medicine at the time this was written, she offered most valuable and incisive critiques of the manuscript, and was able to present us with the "student's-eye view" that helped us to maintain our focus. Jack Rowley generously provided, in addition to encouragement, the tranquil setting in which much of the thinking and writing for this book were done. In addition, we thank Ron Metusalem and the Tilloo Cay Foundation for Biological Research for their generous support throughout this project. Finally, we are most grateful to our publishers, Lea & Febiger, for their faith in us, their encouragement, their cooperation, and their patience—which, it seems, has no bounds.

Contents

1

Cells

Overview

This is a book about cells and tissues. Its primary objective is to build a series of visual three-dimensional images of the cells and tissues that make up the human body. This particular chapter, headed by the all-encompassing title "cells," is intended to prepare you to recognize and understand the images of cells and tissues, photographed by light and electron microscopy, that are presented in this atlas.

The number and variety of cells within every person is tremendous. Fortunately, the Herculean task of visualizing the complexity of the very cells of which we are made is greatly simplified when you realize that many cells, despite their dramatic differences in structure and function, are really more alike than not: they are variations on a theme. And what is that theme? Simply this: *cells are designed to generate order out of chaos.*

We are surrounded by chaos. Biologists are wont to refer to chaos as *entropy*—the concept, described in the second law of thermodynamics, that everything tends toward disorder. Entropy pervades our lives. Clean clothes, for example, don't happen on their own. The act of wearing and using clothes soils them. Does the pile of dirty clothes that results from a week's hard use suddenly appear in pristine form, washed, folded, and stacked in neat piles in your dresser drawers come Monday morning? Of course not. You painstakingly gather the

heap of soiled clothes at the end of the week, put them in the washer, dry them, press them, fold them, carry them to the dresser, sort them, and put them neatly away. All of which takes *energy.* It takes energy to generate order out of chaos.

In the example given above, we are dealing with several pairs of pants or skirts, blouses or shirts, a few assorted undergarments, and some socks—maybe 50 items in a busy week. A "typical" mammalian cell has about ten billion protein molecules to look after. Since everything tends toward disorder, and numbers compound the problem exponentially, the entropic possibilities faced by a cell during the course of its daily life are bewildering. How do cells deal with entropy? How do they generate such exquisite order in the face of potential molecular chaos? In microanatomic terms, cells accomplish order by means of beautifully bioengineered components that, at the expense of considerable amounts of energy, see that the right molecules get in the right places at the right times. All of which is a formidable logistic problem. How do cells do it?

That is, in large part, what this book is all about. A look at the microscopic anatomy of the cell can help us to understand how cells generate order from chaos and, by so doing, achieve that most precious quality—life. When you look at a cell with the light microscope, the first thing you are likely to see is the *nucleus*—a large, round, dark-staining body that contains the genetic material. In many cells, the nucleus appears to be suspended in a small sea of *cytoplasm,* a pale-staining matrix that often contains small, blurry objects visible only when stained. The cytoplasm is surrounded by an outer limiting membrane called the *cell membrane* (also *plasmalemma* or *plasma membrane*). Unfortunately, the cell membrane, which measures only 80 Å wide, is much too small to be seen with the light microscope (whose limit of resolution is 2000 Å). This inability is a source of confusion to beginning students of microanatomy; if you can't see a cell's boundaries, you can't see where one cell ends and another begins. What you often see under the light microscope, then, is a gaggle of purple nuclei in a field of amorphous material. What can that tell about the organization of cells and tissues? How does that provide any insight into the ways in which cells generate order from chaos?

Enter the electron microscope. The electron microscope, which has the ability to resolve very small (2.5-Å) objects, has allowed us to see that the cytoplasm is not a field of amorphous material at all, but rather a highly organized system of organelles and inclusions. Once you see a number of electron images of a particular cell, you will rapidly recognize that kind of cell, much as you learn to recognize a particular make of automobile among a spate of others on a busy highway. This kind of sight-recognition not only allows you to distinguish specific cells in electron images, it allows you to mentally superimpose what you've seen in the electron microscope upon similar cells when you look at them with the light microscope. In the following chapters, you will look at a variety of cells as seen with the light microscope and with the electron microscope at similar magnifications. By carefully comparing the light and electron images of the very same cells, you will develop a kind of "x-ray vision" that will allow you to skillfully interpret light-microscopic images that once looked like little more than a group of nuclei in a fuzzy field.

It is first helpful to look at the kinds of structures you're likely to see within cells. In order to build up a "visual vocabulary" of cell components, this overview contains two illustrations: a drawing of a "typical" mammalian cell (Figure 1-1) and a low-magnification electron micrograph of a cell from the monkey pancreas (Figure 1-2). By referring to the image of specific structures in both the drawing and the electron micrograph as they are discussed, you can develop a good mental picture that will provide a basis for recognition of these same structures as they are encountered throughout the atlas.

Starting with the outside of the cell, the first structure is the cell membrane. Called by a number of names, including the plasma membrane, plasmalemma, and outer limiting membrane, the cell membrane is crucial to a cell's function because it is the interface between the outside world and the inside of the cell; the cell membrane lies between the order within the cell and the potential disorder without.

The composition of the membrane surrounding a particular cell can vary dramatically from region to region. In addition, the cell membranes surrounding different kinds of cells can be different from one another. Referring to "the cell membrane" as a unit can be misleading because doing so implies that the cell membrane is a single entity. This erroneous notion of the homogeneity of the cell membrane is unfortunately reinforced by images generated by transmission electron microscopy of sectioned material. The electron images of a variety of cellular membranes look quite similar.

A "typical" cell membrane, for example, is shown in the electron micrograph in Figure 1-2. This illustration is a relatively low magnification electron micrograph of a cell from the pancreas of the squirrel monkey. If you look at the region indicated by the arrow, you will see a pair of dark lines where two cells are adjacent. These dark lines represent the cell membranes of two neighboring cells. At higher magnification, as shown in the inset, each cell membrane looks like a set of railroad tracks: that is, each cell membrane looks like two electron-dense lines separated by a clear interspace. This appearance led to the name the *unit membrane,* which refers to the electron image presented by the cell membrane and the membranes that surround the cytoplasmic *organelles* when viewed in cross-section by conventional transmission electron microscopy. The uniform appearance of the membranes surrounding the cell and its organelles is misleading. Mem-

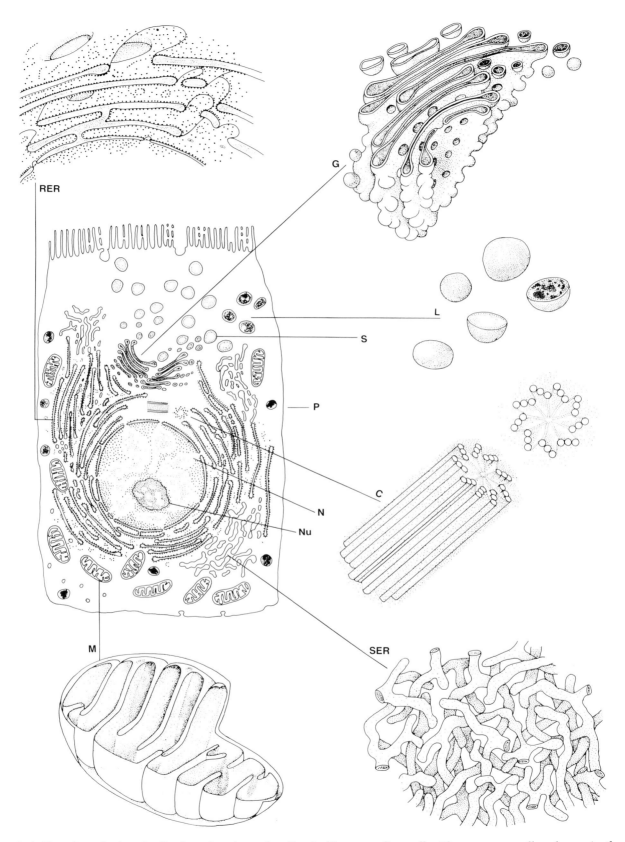

FIG. 1–1. Drawing of a longitudinal section through a "typical" mammalian cell with some organelles shown in three-dimensional view. C, centriole; G, Golgi apparatus; L, lysosomes; M, mitochondrion; N, nucleus; Nu, nucleolus; P, plasma membrane; RER, rough endoplasmic reticulum; S, secretory granule; SER, smooth endoplasmic reticulum.

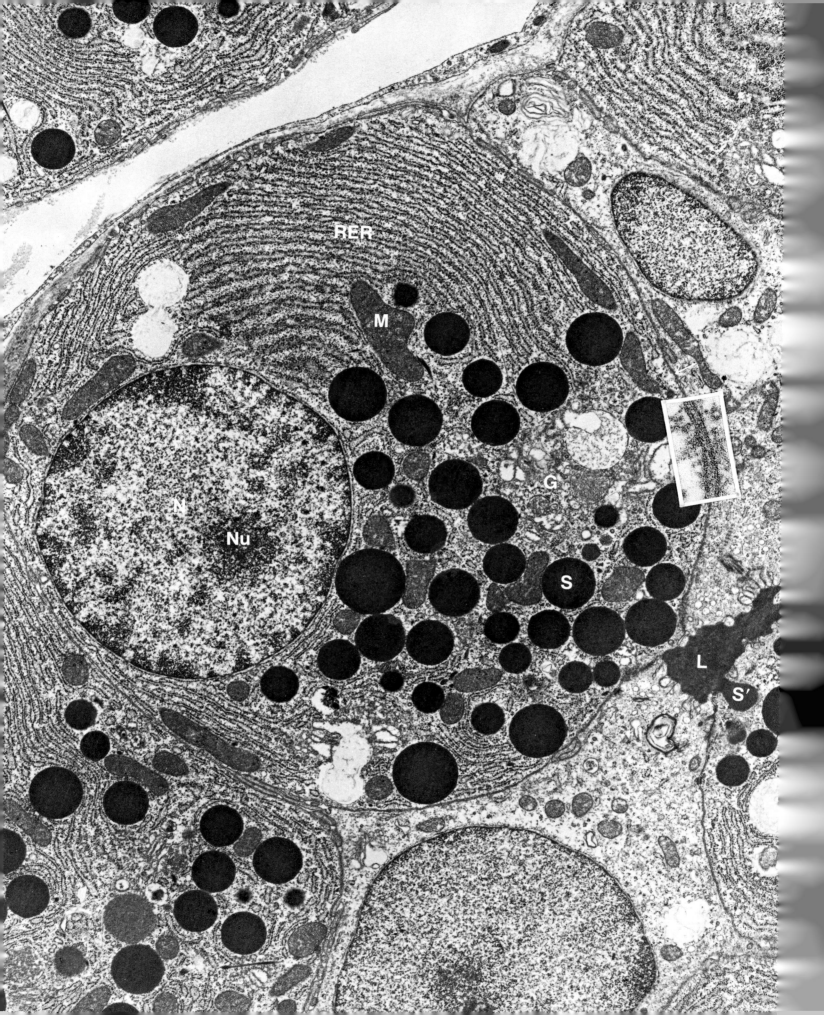

branes vary tremendously in structure and function. To be sure, membranes share many similarities in fundamental organization; they are bimolecular lipid leaflets that contain proteins. But the lipids and the proteins can vary considerably in composition, assume a variety of configurations, and perform a variety of functions. The membranes in the myelin sheaths surrounding the axons of nerves, for example, are effective electrical insulators, whereas the cell membranes of proximal tubule cells of the kidney are highly efficient ion pumps.

Looking back at the diagram (Figure 1-1) and electron micrograph (Figure 1-2), the cell is seen to contain a number of organelles that are surrounded by membranes. These organelles include *mitochondria* (M), the *rough endoplasmic reticulum* (RER), the *smooth endoplasmic reticulum* (SER), the *Golgi apparatus* (G), *secretory granules* (S), *lysosomes* (L), and the nucleus (N). Why are so many organelles surrounded by membranes? Different parts of the cell must perform different functions, and membranes provide a superb means for compartmentalization within the cell. Membrane-limited organelles may be thought of as compartments that can move about from one region of the cell to another. In addition, each cell contains on the order of ten billion protein molecules. Many of these proteins are enzymes that catalyze biochemical reactions, which depend upon surface contact between the participants in the reaction. Membranes not only provide a tremendous amplification of surface area within the cell, they contain specific enzymes. The specificity of molecular interactions that occur in enzymatically catalyzed biochemical reactions, then, can be greatly enhanced by the presence of membranes within cells.

Mitochondria

The mitochondrion provides an excellent example of an organelle that uses membranes to perform exquisite biochemical maneuvers. Often—and quite appropriately—referred to as "the power plant of the cell," the mitochondrion contains two sets of membranes: an *outer membrane,* which defines the outer limits of the organelle, and an *inner membrane,* which is folded into little baffles called *cristae.* Mitochondria produce ATP, the chemical energy "currency" of the cell, in large quantities. Cells with high energy requirements usually have many mitochondria. Cells with very high energy requirements usually have mitochondria that contain many cristae. The membranes of the cristae contain arrays of enzymes associated with oxidative phosphorylation, one of the essential phases of ATP production. Increasing the number of mitochondrial cristae vastly amplifies the amount of membrane surface available for the enzymes involved in the process of oxidative phosphorylation.

The Endoplasmic Reticulum

The endoplasmic reticulum comes in two morphologically distinct varieties: rough and smooth. The rough-surfaced endoplasmic reticulum, usually called the rough endoplasmic reticulum or the rough ER, consists of a series of interconnected, flattened, membrane-limited sacs (called *cisternae*) in which the membranes are encrusted with *ribosomes.* Ribosomes, which have the electron-microscopic appearance of small dense dots, are the sites of protein assembly in cells. Consequently, the rough ER, being a system of membranes and attached ribosomes, participates in the synthesis and concentration of proteins.

The smooth endoplasmic reticulum, which lacks ribosomes, is quite different. It is organized into a system of interconnected tubules and is associated with a variety of functions such as glycogen metabolism, steroid synthesis, and enzymatic detoxification of noxious substances. Ultimately, the rough and smooth ER are physically interconnected and should be thought of as different manifestations of a common system of intercellular membranes.

FIG. 1–2. Electron micrograph of a thin section taken through an exocrine cell of the monkey pancreas. G, Golgi apparatus; L, lumen of acinus; M, mitochondrion; N, nucleus, Nu, nucleolus; RER, rough endoplasmic reticulum; S, secretory granule; S', secretory granule pouring its contents into lumen of acinus; arrow, pair of plasma membranes of two adjacent cells. 12,000 X. Inset: high-magnification electron micrograph of region indicated by arrow in which two plasma membranes, running parallel to one another, are cut in cross section; micrograph shows the trilaminar appearance of each of the two plasma membranes. 129,000 X

The Golgi Apparatus

The Golgi apparatus, named after a turn-of-the-century Italian anatomist who had a tremendous impact on biology, is a complex system of membrane-limited sacs and vesicles that is concerned with the modification and packaging of proteins and protein-polysaccharide complexes. Often working in concert with the rough ER, the Golgi apparatus receives material elaborated by the rough ER, chemically modifies it with enzymes in the Golgi membranes, and concentrates and packages the new product within membrane-limited vesicles called secretory granules. In addition, the Golgi can package proteins into membrane-limited vesicles, such as lysosomes, for use within the cell itself.

Lysosomes

Lysosomes are membrane-limited organelles that contain a broad spectrum of vicious hydrolytic enzymes capable of breaking down everything from nucleic acids to proteins to fats. Originally called "suicide bags" because early cell biologists surmised the cell could open its lysosomes, release their contents, and rapidly dissolve itself when "its number was up," lysosomes serve a variety of essential functions. For one thing, cells use lysosomes to dispose of worn-out organelles. In addition, specialized cells such as macrophages use lysosomes in the intracellular destruction of ingested foreign materials such as bacteria. Other cells, such as endocrine cells of the pituitary gland, use lysosomes to digest excess product synthesized by the cell that is not needed at the time.

The Nucleus

The nucleus, which contains the genetic material, is surrounded by a double membrane continuous with the endoplasmic reticulum. Consequently, the membranes surrounding the nucleus, called the *nuclear envelope,* represent a perinuclear cisterna of the endoplasmic reticulum. The nuclear envelope is perforated by *nuclear pores,* small openings that permit the vital exchange of materials between nucleus and cytoplasm. The nucleus contains the *chromosomes*—discrete units of DNA, the genetic material, complexed with protein—visible only when the cell is in the midst of *mitosis,* or cell division. At other times, the chromosomes are less condensed, and their strands are woven into an indecipherable tangle within the nucleoplasm called *chromatin.* When the chromatin is somewhat condensed, meaning that the genetic material is not unwound and thus is not available for "translation" of the genetic code into messenger RNA (which later dictates the sequence of amino acids that are strung together to make protein), the chromatin stains darkly. This clumped, nontranscriptionally active chromatin is called *heterochromatin.* Transcriptionally active chromatin, which takes little stain and thus looks pale, is called *euchromatin.* A glance at the nucleus, then, can determine whether a given cell is likely to be active in the transcription of messenger RNA. If it is pale and has a great deal of euchromatin, it probably is active; if it stains darkly and has a great deal of heterochromatin, it probably is not.

Within the nucleus lies the *nucleolus.* The nucleolus, a dark-staining body that contains an amorphous part and a fibrillar component, is the site where the components of ribosomes are synthesized.

The membrane-limited organelles briefly described above, and others as well, will be encountered frequently in the atlas. A number of other cytoplasmic components that are not enveloped by membranes should be mentioned in this overview.

Microtubules

Microtubules, as the name suggests, are tiny tubules that have an electron-dense wall and a clear center. Measuring only 240 Å in diameter, microtubules have a number of important functions. They form the spindle fibers of the mitotic spindle. In addition, they are present in the *axoneme* found in the shaft of the cilium and flagellum. Furthermore, they perform a number of supporting, or *cytoskeletal,* functions.

Centrioles

Centrioles are small cylinders, consisting of nine radially disposed "triplets" of microtubules and associated dense material, that are often found in the region called the cell center.

Centrioles migrate to the poles of the mitotic spindle in animal cells. In addition, they are found at the base of the cilium, where they are called *basal bodies.*

Microfilaments

Microfilaments, like microtubules, are extremely important parts of the cytoskeletal apparatus of cells. Microfilaments contain the protein *actin* and are often associated with cytoplasmic movements and regional shortening of the cell. Microfilaments, being quite small (around 50 Å in diameter), often associate in groups, or bundles, in parallel array.

Cilia and Microvilli

Cilia and *microvilli* are both specializations of the cell surface. Cilia are extremely interesting in that they are motile. The ciliary shaft is specialized in such a way that the cilium can bend in an organized fashion. Groups of cilia can coordinate their beats in a wavelike manner and move material along the surface of the cell. Microvilli, also extensions of the cell surface, are quite different from cilia. Each microvillus is a fingerlike extension of the cell membrane that is supported by a core of actin filaments. Microvilli increase the area of the cell surface available for absorption. Microvilli are plentiful in regions such as the intestine or the kidney where mass transport of material in and out of the cell is required.

Many structures in the cytoplasm that have not been emphasized in this overview will be encountered in the chapters of this atlas. By now, however, you will be familiar enough with the major "cast of characters" found within the typical cell to be able to begin study of cells and tissues.

Plate 1–1

The Pancreatic Acinar Cell: A Protein Factory

In our study of cells, we begin with a truly remarkable cell, the *pancreatic acinar cell*—a cell that is highly specialized for the assembly and packaging of proteins for export. Proteins are macromolecules made of amino acids. Pancreatic acinar cells take up amino acids from the blood and assemble them into *enzymes,* which are proteins. Among the enzymes manufactured by pancreatic acinar cells are amylase (which digests carbohydrates), trypsin (which digests proteins), and lipase (which digests fats).

The subcellular components used by the pancreatic acinar cell to synthesize, package, and release proteins for export are illustrated by electron microscopy in the plate at right. Each pyramid-shaped acinar cell, like all cells, is surrounded by a plasma membrane (arrows). A large, round nucleus (N) with a prominent nucleolus (Nu) is found near the base of the cell. Much of the cytoplasm of the cell is filled with rough endoplasmic reticulum (RER). The rough ER consists of an extensive series of flattened, membrane-limited sacs, or cisternae. The outer surface of these cisternae is encrusted with thousands of ribosomes, tiny ribonucleoprotein particles that serve as sites of protein assembly. Numerous mitochondria (M) are evident in the cytoplasm as well. These mitochondria provide chemical energy, in the form of ATP, necessary for the biosynthesis of macromolecules that takes place in the pancreatic acinar cell.

A glance at the electron micrograph at right will reveal that the apex of the cell looks different from the base of the cell. The apical pole of the cell is crammed with membrane-limited, electron-dense inclusions called *zymogen granules* (Z). Zymogen granules contain the protein to be exported from the cell; that is, they contain the pancreatic enzymes that will be poured out of the cell and into the *lumen* (L) of the acinus. (The acinus is a ball-shaped group of acinar cells clustered about a central hole, or lumen, that leads to a duct that will convey the secretions out of the pancreas and into the duodenum of the small intestine, where the secretions assist in the digestion of food). Among the zymogen granules is the Golgi apparatus (G), which consists of a series of flattened, membrane-limited sacs and vesicles. No ribosomes are found on Golgi membranes.

The structural polarization evident within the pancreatic acinar cell—that is, the marked difference between the apical and basal regions, or poles, of the cell—is an extremely important feature, for it underlies the functional polarization that makes this type of cell such an efficient protein factory. Raw materials in the form of amino acids in the circulating blood are delivered by capillaries to the base of the cell. These amino acids, the building blocks of protein, are transported across the plasma membrane and into the cell itself. Once within the cytoplasm, the amino acids make contact with the tremendous surface area of the rough endoplasmic reticulum. The ribosomes on the outer surface of the rough ER, in concert with appropriate messenger RNA and transfer RNA molecules, facilitate the assembly of amino acids into proteins. The newly synthesized protein molecules are then released within the cisternae of the RER. Small ribosome-free vesicles called *transfer vesicles* bud off from the RER in the region of the Golgi apparatus. Transfer vesicles fuse with the Golgi membranes and empty their proteinaceous contents into the Golgi. The Golgi apparatus then modifies—and packages—the newly formed enzymes into membrane-limited vesicles that fuse to form the conspicuous zymogen granules. Under appropriate conditions of nervous or hormonal stimulation, the pancreatic acinar cell discharges its content of zymogen granules into the lumen of the acinus, then prepares itself for another cycle of synthesis, storage, and release of digestive enzymes.

Electron micrograph of acinar cells from the pancreas of the squirrel monkey. G, Golgi apparatus; L, lumen of acinus; M, mitochondrion; N, nucleus of acinar cell; Nu, nucleolus; RER, rough endoplasmic reticulum; Z, zymogen granules; arrows, plasma membranes of adjoining acinar cells. 11,000 X

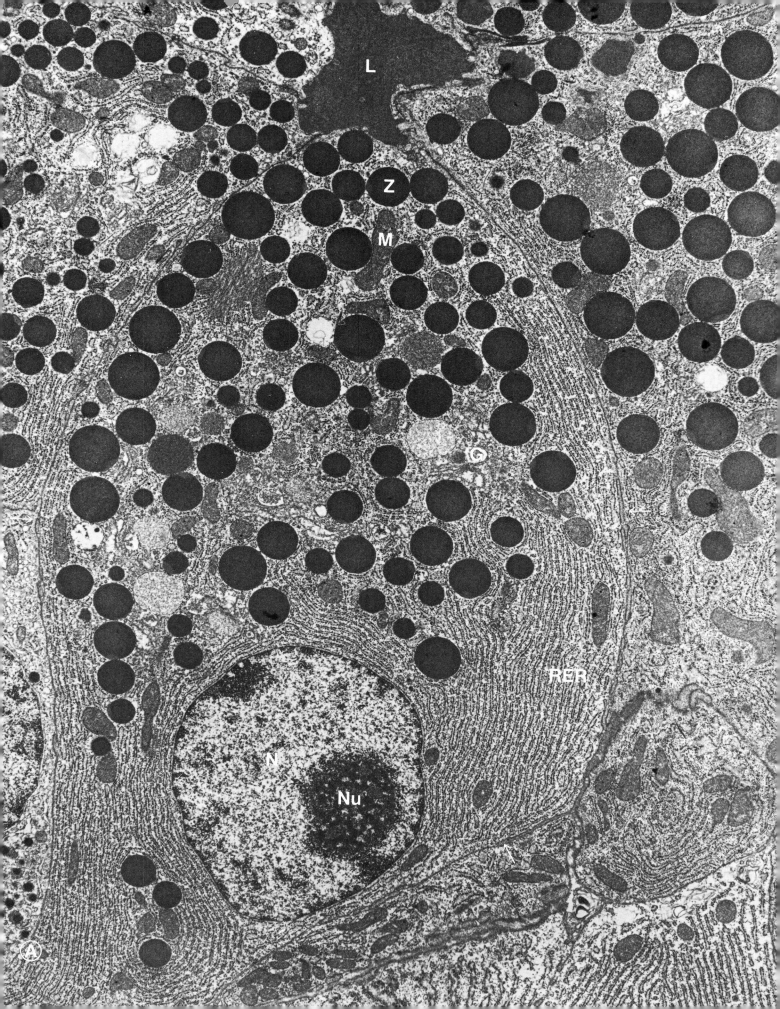

Plate 1–2

The Paneth Cell: A Glycoprotein Factory

Paneth cells are large cells, situated within the recesses of the intestinal glands, that possess prominent gylcoprotein-containing secretory granules. Although they were discovered over a century ago, the precise function of Paneth cells is not known. What is known, however, is that the large secretory granules found in the apical cytoplasm of Paneth cells contain the antibacterial enzyme *lysozyme.* It is also known that the Paneth cells of rodents can phagocytose and degrade intestinal microorganisms with their lysosomal apparatus. Consequently, it is generally believed that Paneth cells may contribute to the regulation of intestinal flora. Whatever their function in the intestine, their structure suggests that they are different from other intestinal cells. They are long-lived, are not known to undergo mitosis, and are instantly recognizable with the light and electron microscope by virtue of their large, unique, glycoprotein-packed secretory granules.

Figure A, a low-magnification electron micrograph, reveals the major ultrastructural features of a Paneth cell within the intestine. Like the pancreatic acinar cell depicted in Plate 1–1, the Paneth cell is pyramidal. The pyramid configuration is adopted by many secretory cells and serves them well. They need a large surface area at the base of the cell to take in raw materials, and a large volume of basal cytoplasm to contain the mass of rough endoplasmic reticulum associated with the synthesis of proteins for export. Once the proteins are synthesized and condensed into tightly packed secretory granules, the cell product—now at the apical pole—requires little volume to house it and can be accommodated at the narrow vertex of the pyramid. Such pyramidal cells can then be conveniently arranged around a common lumen into which their secretions can be poured. In the Paneth cell in Figure A, for example, the nucleus (N), with its prominent nucleolus (Nu), sits at the broad base of the cell (arrow). The basal cytoplasm is tightly packed with parallel stacks of flattened cisternae of the rough endoplasmic reticulum (RER). A prominent Golgi apparatus (G) is evident in the vicinity of the large secretory granules (S).

Figure B shows the striking structural and functional spatial relationship between the rough ER, Golgi apparatus (G), and secretory granules (also called secretory vesicles) (S). Here, the cisternae of the RER bud off periodically to give rise to transfer vesicles (T), which are tiny membrane-limited vesicles filled with secretory product generated by the rough endoplasmic reticulum that carry material to the Golgi for further processing and packaging into secretory vesicles (S′). The transfer vesicles enter the Golgi at its convex face, or *forming face.* Within the Golgi, complex sugars are added to the protein molecules by enzymes on the Golgi membranes. The resultant glycoproteins are released from the Golgi at its concave face, or *secretory face.* There, the glycoprotein-laden vesicles, commonly called *condensing vacuoles,* have a coarse, dense, granular matrix (arrowhead). The condensing vacuoles fuse to form secretory granules. In this image, an individual secretory granule (S′) has been captured at an early stage in its formation. In addition, several mature secretory granules (S) are evident.

Figure A. Low-magnification electron micrograph of a Paneth cell from the mouse. CT, connective tissue of the lamina propria; G, Golgi apparatus; L, lysosome; M, mitochondrion; N, nucleus; Nu, nucleolus; RER, rough endoplasmic reticulum; S, secretory granule; arrow, base of Paneth cell. 9,000 X

Figure B. Electron micrograph of secretory region in the apical cytoplasm of a Paneth cell. G, Golgi apparatus; L, lysosome; RER, rough endoplasmic reticulum; S, secretory granule; S′, secretory granule forming from condensing vacuoles of the Golgi; T, transfer vesicle at forming face of Golgi; arrowhead, condensing vacuole at secretory face of Golgi. 25,000 X

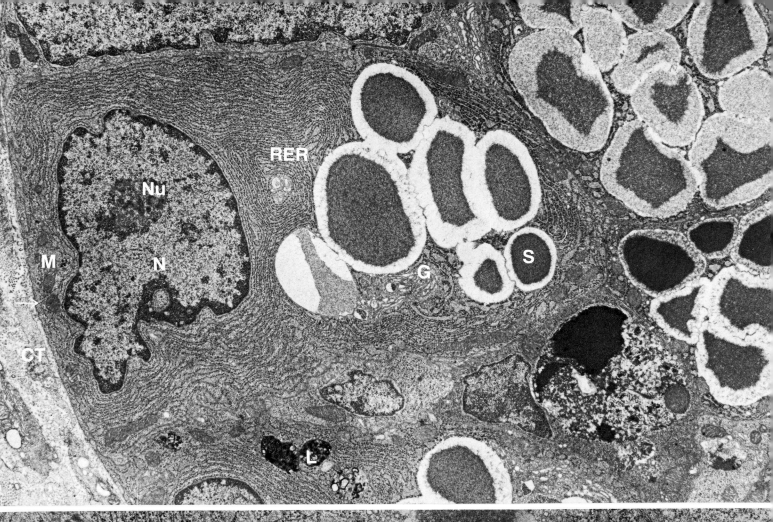

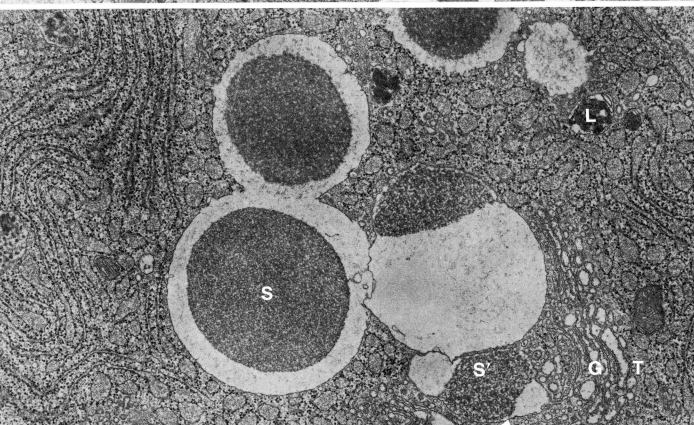

Plate 1–3

The Goblet Cell: A Mucus Factory

The epithelium lining the intestine contains many goblet cells. The primary function of the goblet cell is to secrete *mucus*, a slippery, viscous substance, rich in mucopolysaccharides, that serves to protect and lubricate the lining of the intestine. It comes as no great surprise that goblet cells were so named because they resemble goblets; they usually have a broad apex and a narrow base. As shown in Plates 1–1 and 1–2, most secretory cells engaged in the elaboration of proteins for export are shaped like pyramids: they have broad bases and narrow cell apexes. Given that the goblet cell is a secretory cell, one might wonder why it is organized in the opposite way, like an inverted pyramid with a broad apex and a narrow base.

The answer lies in the nature of its secretory product. The goblet cell makes enormous quantities of mucus, and mucus is highly hydrated. Consequently, the secretory product of the goblet cell occupies a much greater volume in the apical pole of the cell than, say, the zymogen granules occupy in the apical pole of the pancreatic acinar cell. A little enzyme goes a long way; a little mucus doesn't. Hence, while the secretory product of the pancreatic acinar cell, which is in concentrated form and has a low water content, can be packaged in a small space, the mucus elaborated by the goblet cell cannot.

The plate at right is a low-magnification electron micrograph of a goblet cell from the ileum of the small intestine. The goblet cell, readily recognized by its large complement of mucus droplets (MD), is flanked on either side by intestinal absorptive cells (A) with a radically different structure. The absorptive cells have many microvilli (mv)—tiny fingerlike projections of the plasma membrane supported by cores of actin filaments—projecting from the cell surface. The microvilli at the left side of the figure are cut in longitudinal section; others, at the right side, are cut nearly in cross section (*). Goblet cells, too, normally have some microvilli. When the cells begin to release mucus droplets, as the cell at right is doing, the microvilli are lost, and the membrane-limited mucus droplets are released into the lumen of the intestine (L).

The mucus droplets are elaborated by a system of intracellular organelles that are quite similar to those illustrated earlier within the pancreatic acinar cell and the Paneth cell. Protein synthesis occurs on the many ribosomes that adorn the surface of the rough endoplasmic reticulum (RER). The newly synthesized proteins, along with some attached sugars, are released into the lumen of the rough endoplasmic reticulum. From there, they are passed into the Golgi apparatus, wherein the proteins are modified and more sugars are added. At the secretory face of the Golgi, condensing vacuoles containing the freshly made mucus fuse (arrow) and form the large membrane-limited mucus droplets. The mucus droplets accumulate in the apical cytoplasm, and are packed so tightly that the remainder of the cytoplasm—and the nucleus (N)—are shoved aside and forced to occupy a relatively small space at the base (and along the sides) of the cell. When viewed with the light microscope, the mucus droplets of a goblet cell are usually conspicuous; the cytoplasm, however, is not, and the nucleus is often barely visible as a dense, flattened body at the base of the cell.

Electron micrograph of a longitudinal section through a goblet cell from the ileum of the small intestine. A, columnar absorptive cells that flank the goblet cell; G, Golgi apparatus; L, lumen of intestine; MD, mucus droplets; MV, microvilli cut in longitudinal section; N, nucleus of goblet cell; RER, rough endoplasmic reticulum; *, microvilli cut in near cross section; arrow, condensing vacuoles fusing to form mucus droplet. 15,000 X

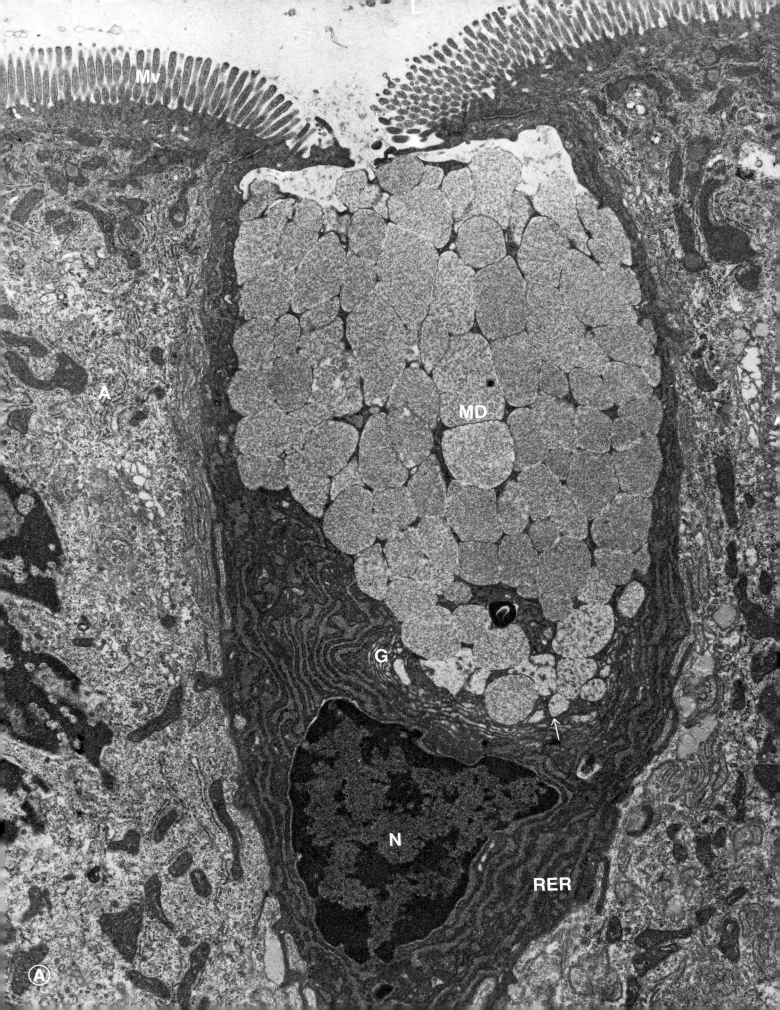

Plate 1–4

The Ovarian Endocrine Cell: A Steroid Factory

The cells we have examined so far—the pancreatic acinar cell, the Paneth cell, and the goblet cell—all actively synthesize proteins, protein-carbohydrate complexes, or both. The subject of Plate 1–4, an endocrine cell from the ovary, is quite different: this cell synthesizes and secretes *steroid hormones.* Steroid hormones, constructed from the *cholesterol* molecule, are more akin to fats than to proteins or polysaccharides. Possessed of a 17-carbon, 4-ring system, steroid hormones—of which there are many kinds in the body—are made by cells using cholesterol as starting material.

Since the ovarian endocrine cell makes a product different biochemically from the products of the cells examined thus far, one would correctly predict that the ovarian endocrine cell's microanatomy would be different as well. In Plate 1–4, this cell, shaped like a long, slender football, is found in the theca interna of a growing follicle in the ovary, where it secretes a steroid hormone that is a precursor of the female sex hormone, *estrogen.* The cell is not filled with stacks of rough ER; instead, its cytoplasm contains an abundance of the smooth endoplasmic reticulum (SER). As described in the overview of this chapter, the smooth ER consists of a series of branched, interconnected, membrane-limited tubules. The smooth ER, so named because its membranes are ribosome free (hence "smooth"), contains many enzymes necessary for cholesterol biosynthesis. Consequently, cells that make cholesterol, steroids or both usually have a well-developed smooth ER. The cytoplasm of the cell in Figure A contains many large, spherical, electron-lucent lipid droplets (L). These lipid droplets are filled with cholesterol, the precursor of the steroid hormones made by the cell. In addition, the cell has many large, strange-looking mitochondria (M). These mi-

tochondria, like those of most steroid-secreting cells, have vesicular or tubular cristae. These mitochondria possess an enzyme that participates in the conversion of cholesterol to steroid hormones. The relationship between the special arrangement of the mitochondrial inner membranes and steroidogenesis, however, is unknown.

The ovarian endocrine cell, then, has three ultrastructural features that are pronounced in and characteristic of steroid-secreting cells: a well-developed smooth endoplasmic reticulum, large mitochondria with tubular cristae, and an abundance of lipid droplets in the cytoplasm.

The nucleus (N) of the ovarian endocrine cell looks different from the nuclei we have seen thus far because the nucleus at right has been caught in tangential section; that is, the knife grazed the edge of the nucleus instead of passing through its center. (A nucleus cut in cross section [N'] is evident in another cell at the bottom of the plate). The tangential section through the nucleus reveals the structure of *nuclear pores* (arrowhead). The nucleus, as you recall from the overview, is surrounded by the nuclear envelope, which consists of two sets of membranes that are continuous with the endoplasmic reticulum. At intervals around its perimeter, the nuclear envelope is perforated by openings, the nuclear pores, that facilitate exchange of materials between the nucleus and the cytoplasm. A cross sectioned nuclear pore is encircled in the nucleus (N') in the cell at the bottom of the figure.

Several red blood cells, or *erythrocytes* (E), are evident in the capillary that runs right next to the ovarian endocrine cells. Endocrine organs, which release their product into the bloodstream, are almost invariably endowed with a rich supply of capillaries.

Longitudinal section through a steroid-secreting endocrine cell in the theca interna of a growing follicle in the ovary. E, erythrocyte; L, lipid droplet; M, mitochondrion; N, tangentially sectioned nucleus; N', nucleus cut in cross section; SER, smooth endoplasmic reticulum; arrow, free ribosomes in clusters (polysomes); arrowhead, tangentially sectioned nuclear pore; circle, cross sectioned nuclear pore. 13,200 X

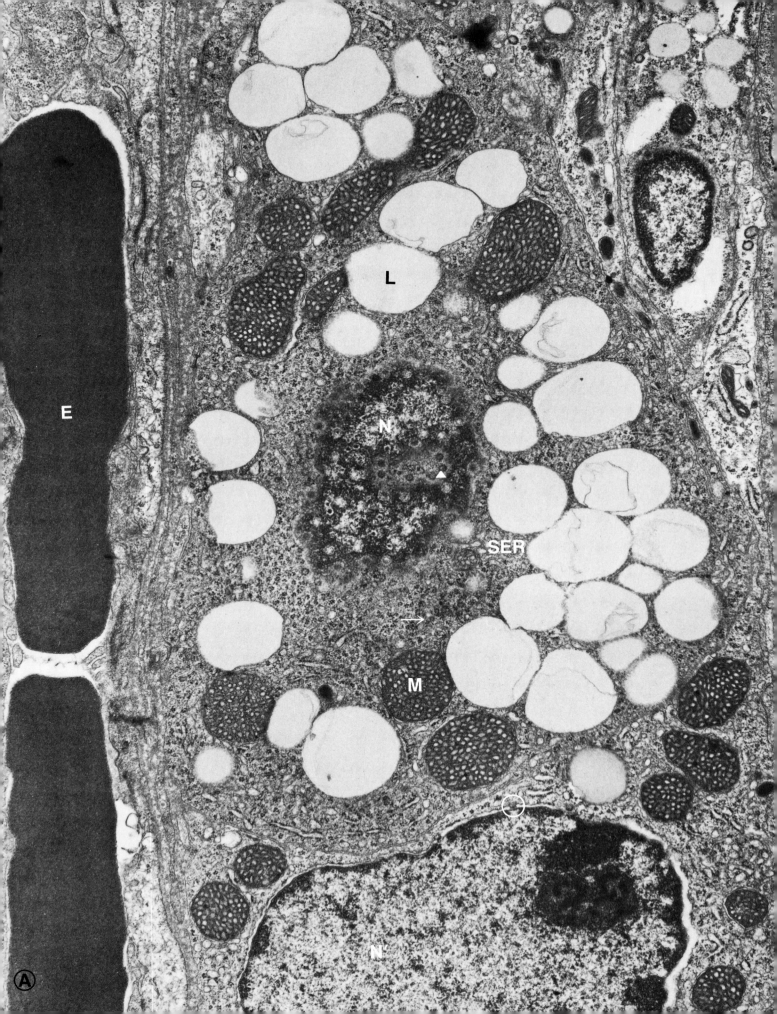

Plate 1–5

The Osteocyte: A Quiescent Cell

Thus far, we have investigated the ultrastructure of cells that are engaged in the large-scale production of macromolecules. Although somewhat different from one another in fine structure, all of these cells share several common characteristics; they are large cells possessing an extensive cytoplasm equipped with a wide array of organelles related to the biosynthesis and storage of secretory products. The osteocyte illustrated at right, however, is strikingly different from the cells depicted previously in this chapter. Seen here as a small cell in a large field of bone (B), the osteocyte (O), which sits in the center of the field, looks unremarkable. The most conspicuous feature is the round nucleus (N), which consists mostly of heterochromatin (*).

Heterochromatin, which represents dense aggregates of DNA and protein that stain darkly, is made up of portions of chromosomes that are coiled and not transcriptionally active; that is, they are not engaged in the transcription of messenger RNA from the genetic material, DNA. Cells with large amounts of heterochromatin are usually relatively inactive in terms of protein synthesis, and this osteocyte is no exception. In the metabolic heyday of this osteocyte, when it was young and vigorous, the cell had an extensive cytoplasm, packed with ribosome-studded cisternae of the rough endoplasmic reticulum and replete with stacks of Golgi membranes. At that time, the cell, then called an *osteoblast*, produced prodigious amounts of *collagen*, a fibrous protein that makes up the bulk of the connective tissue in the body, and provides the framework for the mineralized matrix of bone. The osteoblast laid down collagen until it painted itself into a corner and encased itself in the very product of its own secretory activity. Once imprisoned in calcified bone matrix (B), the cell disassembled most of its organelles, resorbed the better part of its own cytoplasm, and went into retirement, assuming the shrunken form of the osteocyte in Plate 1–5. The osteocyte, now but a shade of its former self, lies within a *lacuna* (L). The entire lacuna was once filled with the turgid cytoplasm of the active osteoblast. Now, the lacuna is crossed by only a few strands of cytoplasm. These strands of cytoplasm (arrows), called *osteocytic processes*, pass through tiny channels in the bone matrix called *canaliculi* (C). The osteocyte processes provide the living link between neighboring osteocytes and nearby capillaries that permit the osteocytes to receive the few nutrients they need to carry on their quiescent life, during which they serve to maintain bone.

Mature osteocytes, although dormant, are necessary to keep bone alive. In addition, they stand at the ready to be recalled into active service should the need arise. In times of low blood calcium, they can generate an active cytoplasm and resorb needed calcium from bone. In addition, they can serve to rebuild bone lost from injury or disease. The osteocyte at right, however, is doing no such thing; it is a dormant cell, and its structure betrays its biosynthetic quiescence.

Cross section taken from compact bone in the femur of the squirrel monkey showing an osteocyte sitting in a field of bone. B, calcified bone matrix; C, canaliculus; L, lacuna; N, nucleus of osteocyte; O, cytoplasm of osteocyte; arrow, cytoplasmic extension of osteocyte (osteocyte process); *, heterochromatin. 13,200 X

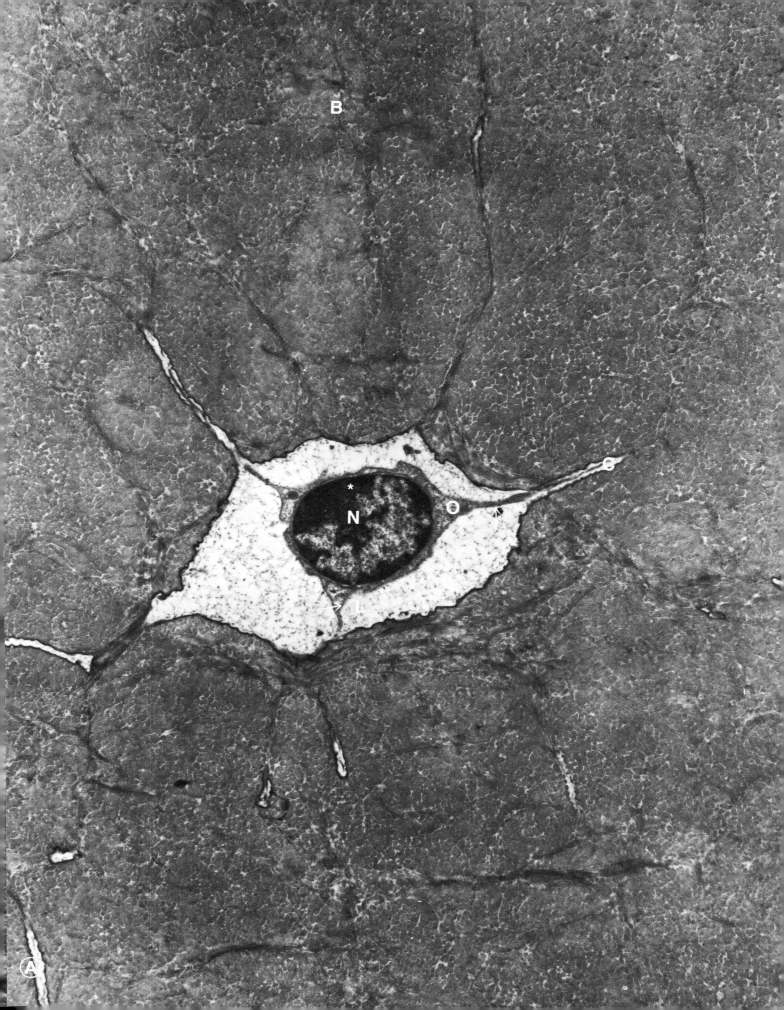

Plate 1–7

Stages In The Life Of A Cell: The Lymphocyte And The Plasma Cell

The cells that we have observed up to this point have been mature cells. Although it is tempting to think that these cells, frozen in time by electron microscopy were always as they appear today, it simply is not so. Cells, like the very people they compose, have cycles of life and may adopt quite different structures to suit their stage of life at any given time.

The cells illustrated at right look quite different from one another. Figure A depicts a lymphocyte in the circulating blood; Figure B displays a plasma cell in the connective tissue.

The lymphocyte (L) in Figure A is a small, round cell. Its nucleus (N), which contains a prominent nucleolus (Nu), occupies most of the space in the cell. The scanty cytoplasm contains a few mitochondria (M), a small Golgi stack (G), some free ribosomes, and a well-developed centriole (arrow). The centriole, which contains a well-organized array of three triplets of microtubules in its core, is shown at higher magnification in the inset. (Centrioles are found at the poles of the mitotic spindle of dividing animal cells, provide the basal bodies found at the bases of motile cilia, and often—as in the lymphocyte shown here—occupy the cell center in interphase cells). The lymphocyte, flanked on one side by an erythrocyte (E), is in close contact with the capillary wall (C).

The plasma cell (P) shown in Figure B is dramatically different from the lymphocyte. The plasma cell produces *antibodies,* immunoglobulins that combine with foreign antigens and, in so doing, provide the first line of defense in the immune response. This particular plasma cell was found in the loose connective tissue of the lamina propria of the small intestine. In this electron image, it occupies a position between another plasma cell (P') and a small nerve bundle (NB). The cell membrane of the plasma cell is in close contact with connective tissue fibrils (CT). Its cytoplasm contains an extremely well developed system of rough endoplasmic reticulum (RER). Numerous mitochondria (M) are present. A prominent Golgi stack (G) sits atop the large nucleus (N). All of these ultrastructural features underline the fact that the plasma cell is active in the biosynthesis of proteins for export, proteins that take the form of antibodies.

Based on the relationship between structure and function in cells, the plasma cell appears to be a cell of high metabolic activity engaged in intense protein synthesis, whereas the lymphocyte does not. These cells that look so different from one another, however, are actually different forms of the same cell. Certain kinds of lymphocytes, called B-lymphocytes, represent the immature form of plasma cells. The B-lymphocyte is, in a sense, the transport form of the plasma cell. B-lymphocytes do not perform their functions in the bloodstream; they are not really blood cells at all, but connective tissue cells that simply use the bloodstream to get from their birthplace in the bone marrow or lymphoid tissues to their ultimate destination in the connective tissues. Under appropriate conditions, the B-lymphocyte will leave the circulation, enter the connective tissues, and develop into a mature, full-blown, antibody-producing plasma cell such as the one shown in Figure B.

Figure A. Electron micrograph of a lymphocyte in a capillary in the lung of the macaque. C, capillary wall; E, erythrocyte; G, Golgi apparatus; L, lymphocyte; M, mitochondrion; N, nucleus; Nu, nucleolus; arrow, centriole. 16,800 X (Inset of centriole, 60,500 X)

Figure B. Electron micrograph of a plasma cell in the lamina propria of the intestine. CT, connective tissue fibrils; G, Golgi apparatus; M, mitochondrion; N, nucleus; NB, nerve bundle; P, plasma cell; P', adjacent plasma cell; RER, rough endoplasmic reticulum. 15,000 X

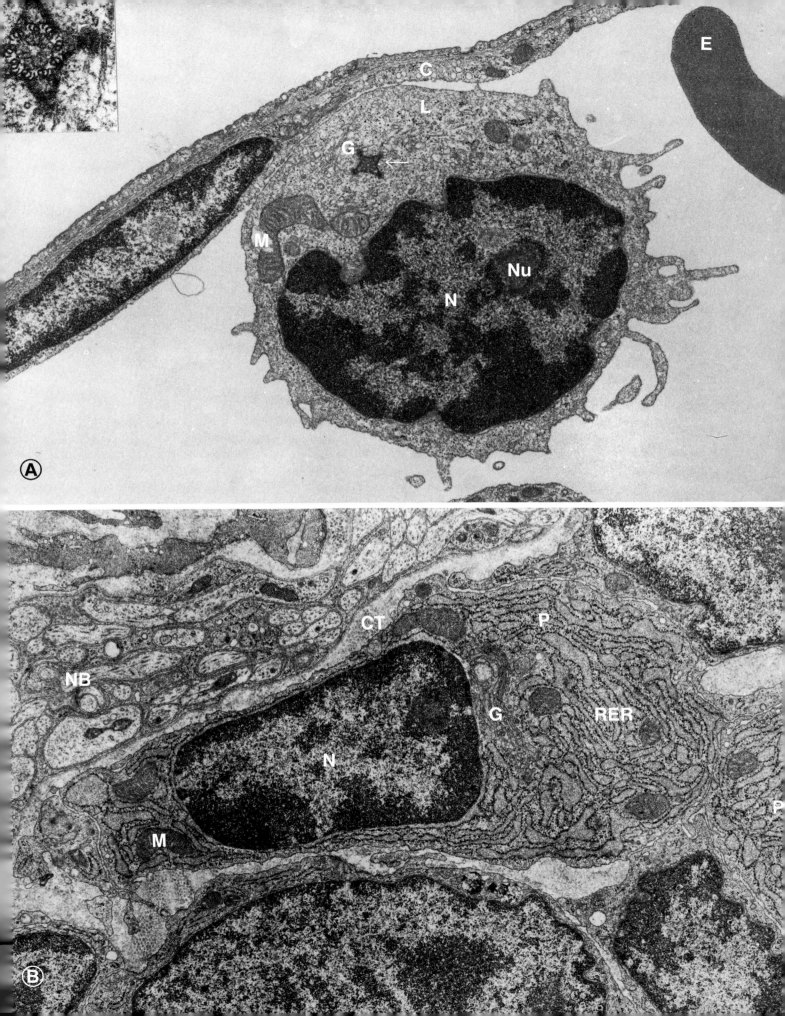

Plate 1–8

The Ciliated Cell: Specializations Of The Cell Surface

The cell surface, as described in the overview to this chapter, is an interface between the cell and its surroundings. In many ways, a cell is akin to a sessile organism; it is at the mercy of its environment. As a result, many cells have evolved intricate modifications of the cell surface that interacts with their immediate environment. Many of these modifications exist at the molecular level and cannot be seen. Other modifications of the cell surface, such as cilia and microvilli, are complex, highly efficient structures that are not only visible by light and electron microscopy, but also present in sufficient numbers to be available for experimental investigation.

The nasal cavity is lined by tissue that is directly exposed to the atmosphere. It produces copious amounts of mucus that serves to lubricate the surface of the nasal cavity, prevent it from drying out, and entrap foreign particles present in the air. To prevent chronic congestion, the mucus must be removed as fast as it is produced, by either swallowing or expectorating. To facilitate removal, the conductive airways of the respiratory system are equipped with motile cilia, whose coordinated beating moves the blanket of mucus upwards toward the mouth. The plate is an electron micrograph of a ciliated cell within the epithelium of the human nasal cavity. The tall, columnar cells have prominent nuclei (N) at the basal pole of the cell and a conspicuous Golgi apparatus (G) in the center. Clusters of mitochondria (M) fill the apical pole of the cell. These mitochondria are well positioned to produce ATP as an energy source for the motile cilia nearby. Cilia (C) project upward from the cell surface into the nasal cavity (NC), in which they move the layer of mucus (removed during tissue preparation) toward the oral cavity. Each cilium, actually a mechanochemical engine fueled by ATP, inserts into a basal body (B), a centriole-like structure that sits just beneath the cell surface. The ciliary shaft, a small structure measuring 0.2 μm in diameter, is stabilized by a somewhat stiff axoneme.

When seen in longitudinal section at low magnification, as in Plate 1–8, the axoneme appears as a set of dense lines that run parallel to the ciliary long axis. When cut in cross section and viewed on end at high magnification, as in the inset, the ciliary axoneme presents a striking and distinct ultrastructure. The plasma membrane, here displaying its typical trilaminar "railroad-track" image, covers the outside of the cilium. Within the space enclosed by the plasma membrane lies the axoneme, which has the "9 + 2" arrangement of microtubules typical of motile cilia. Nine outer doublets of microtubules, arranged in a ring just inside the plasma membrane, surround a central pair of microtubules in the core of the axoneme. Close inspection of the image will reveal that several electron-dense "arms" extend from each outer doublet toward its neighbor in a clockwise direction. These structures, called *dynein arms* (arrow, inset), provide the force for ciliary movement. Movement of the arms causes adjacent outer doublets to slide past one another. This sliding is restrained by a set of radial spokes (arrowhead, inset), not clearly shown here, that extend from the central pair to the outer doublets. The restraining force of the radial spokes, when set against the active sliding of adjacent doublets generated by the dynein arms, transduces the sliding movement into a bending movement—the very bending movement associated with the active stroke of the motile cilium. The coordinated beating of the cilia of the respiratory epithelium moves the blanket of mucus along the surface of the nasal cavity at an astonishingly rapid rate.

Electron micrograph of a longitudinal section through the epithelium lining the human nasal cavity. B, basal body; C, cilium; D, degenerating cell; G, Golgi apparatus; M, mitochondrion; N, nucleus; NC, nasal cavity. 11,500 X
Inset: Cross section through motile cilium from the same epithelium. Arrow, dynein arm; arrowhead, radial spoke. 131,000 X

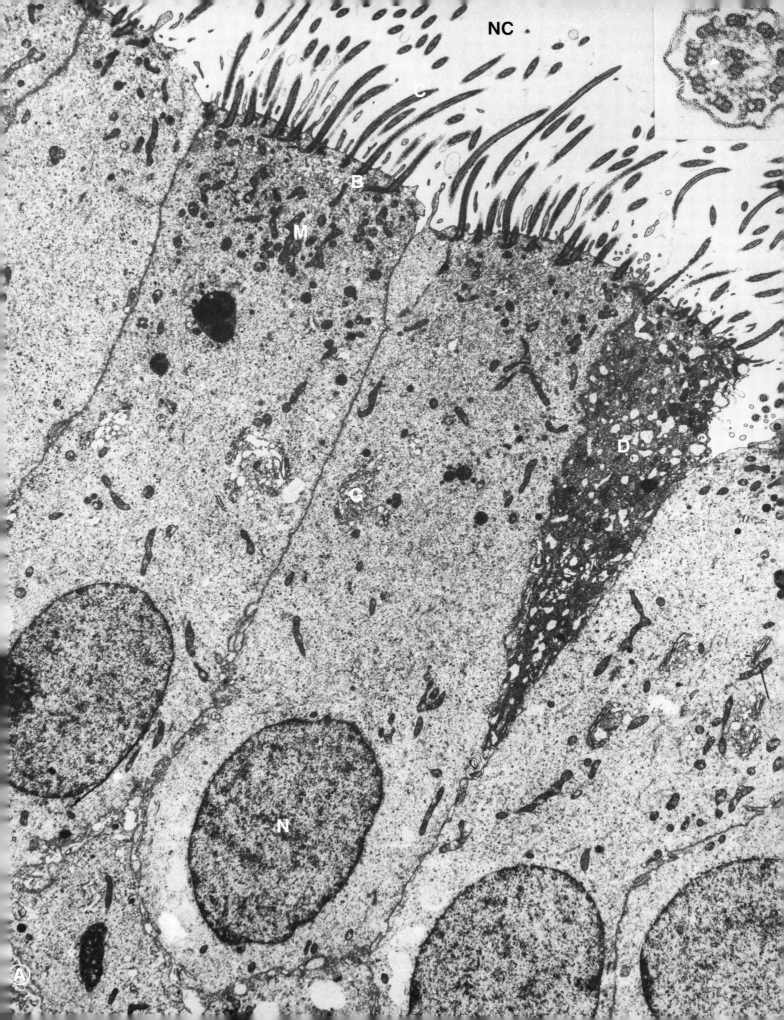

2

Epithelia

Overview

Having introduced cells, we move now to tissues—groups of cells and their products that perform specific functions. The classic tissues—epithelia, nerve, muscle, and connective tissue—are combined to make up the major organs that, taken together, form the organism known as the human body.

The first class of tissue we shall consider is the *epithelium.* Epithelia cover the body and line the inner and outer surfaces of organs. Although they are supported by connective tissue, they contain none; although they are underlain by capillaries, epithelia are avascular.

Epithelia are organized in a variety of ways, and their spatial organization both permits and reflects their functions. Epithelial nomenclature is straightforward, usually employing two or three words for each descriptive term. The first word tells whether the tissue is made of one cell layer (simple) or of more layers (stratified). The second word describes the shape of the uppermost layer of cells, be they *squamous, cuboidal,* or *columnar.* The third word, if any, describes the way in which the uppermost cells are specialized. Some epithelia are specialized by bearing cilia; others, by being filled with the water-resistant protein keratin. The integument, for example, is covered by a stratified squamous keratinized epithelium. This name indicates that skin consists of several cell layers, the uppermost cells of which are flat and filled with keratin.

Because form follows function in biologic systems—a recurring theme in the study of microanatomy—epithelia adopt specific forms in order to perform specific functions. Given that epithelia are surfaces, one can, as a simple exercise in armchair bioengineering, list the possible functions a biological surface *can* perform, design a cellular surface capable of performing each function, and generate the actual epithelial classes that organs *do* have in the human body.

Among these functions is the ability of a cellular surface to selectively transport substances across itself. In addition, it can elaborate and secrete materials; conversely, it can absorb materials from its surroundings. Furthermore, a biologic surface can protect its contents from water loss, physical damage, and the like; and it can move materials along itself. These functions differ from one another and call for a variety of cellular designs. In the lungs, where gas exchange occurs, and in capillaries, which supply nutrients and gases to all cells of the body, rapid transport of materials is essential. These organs need a single thin layer of flat cells—a simple squamous epithelium. Active transport of materials, on the other hand, requires more metabolic machinery, necessitating a single layer of cells with more bulk to house the cytoplasmic organelles that do the work. Consequently, simple cuboidal epithelia often constitute surfaces such as those in the kidney that actively transport molecules and ions against a concentration gradient. Secretory surfaces, too, require large cells that contain the cytoplasmic machinery required to synthesize and package proteins, glycoproteins, and other macromolecules for export. Consequently, most secretory surfaces consist of a single layer of large cells— either a simple cuboidal or simple columnar epithelium. The same holds true for absorptive epithelia; they need space to house the organelles required to process materials taken up into the cell.

Protective surfaces, however, face a different set of problems. They must place a layer of tough, waterproof, expendable cells at the epithelial surface and provide for their periodic replacement. This requirement calls for a stratified squamous epithelium, in which flattened surface cells *(squames)* are periodically shed and replaced by mitotic activity and differentiation of other underlying cells.

These and several other examples of the ways in which form follows function in epithelia are depicted and described in this chapter.

Plate 2–1

Simple Squamous Epithelium: The Lung

As mentioned in the overview, epithelia are cellular linings or coverings. Of these, perhaps none are thinner or more delicate than the simple squamous epithelia that line the lungs and capillaries. Figures A and B are a matched pair of light and electron micrographs of serial sections taken through the monkey lung that clearly show the super-thin nature of the epithelia that line the alveoli of the lungs and the capillaries that course through them.

The lung is designed to move material across its borders rapidly. In an average day of rest, a person's lungs exchange some 550 L (138 gal; 17 ft³) of oxygen and carbon dioxide between blood and the atmosphere. This extremely rapid and efficient gas exchange is facilitated by the design of the thin, gossamer-like epithelium lining the lung's airspaces, or alveoli, and their associated capillaries.

Both alveolus and capillary are lined by a single layer of flat cells that provide an excellent example of simple squamous epithelium. Figures A and B at right are light and electron micrographs of sections taken through an *interalveolar septum*—a wall separating two adjacent alveoli—in the lung of the macaque. Here, the air-filled alveolar spaces (A) lie above and below the interalveolar septum itself (S). The lung, of course, is highly vascular, and many capillaries (C) supply the interalveolar septum with blood. Although details of its construction are not evident by light microscopy (Figure A), the extreme flatness of the interalveolar septum's simple squamous epithelia is nevertheless apparent. The barrier interposed between blood and air can be as thin as 0.15μm, approaching the limit of resolution of the light microscope. When the area enclosed within the circle is viewed by electron microscopy, as in Figure B, one can see that the wall of the septum is actually two cell layers thick—each layer consisting of the simple squamous epithelium lining the alveolus and the simple squamous epithelium lining the adjacent capillary. This construction is evident in the area indicated by the arrow. Here, the two epithelia have pulled apart and are seen to be separated by an artifactual space in which splayed connective tissue fibrils (CT) are evident. The prominent nucleus (N) helps to identify the capillary endothelial cell to which it belongs.

The epithelial cells that line capillaries are routinely referred to as *endothelial* cells, and the capillary epithelium is called an *endothelium*—a term reserved for the layer of flat cells lining blood vessels, lymph vessels, and other cavities. A structure called the *basement membrane* underlies the capillary endothelium as with all epithelia. The basement membrane varies in thickness. In some epithelia it is visible by light microscopy. When viewed with the electron microscope, the basement membrane is seen to consist of a thin, amorphous feltwork, some 500 to 800 Å thick, called the *basal lamina,* closely associated with small bundles of reticular fibers embedded in a protein-polysaccharide ground substance. As its name suggests, the basement membrane always covers the bottom of an epithelium and separates the epithelium from the structures that it overlies.

Figures A and B. Matched pair of light and electron micrographs of nearly serial sections taken through the lung of the macaque. A, alveolar space; B, (Figure B only) basement membrane; C, capillary; CT, connective tissue fibrils (Figure B only); E, erythrocyte; N, nucleus of capillary endothelial cell; S, interalveolar septum; 1, alveolar epithelium; 2, capillary epithelium (endothelium); circle, attenuated region of interalveolar septum; arrow, artifactual separation of alveolar and capillary epithelia. Figure A, 2,000 X; Figure B, 8,500 X

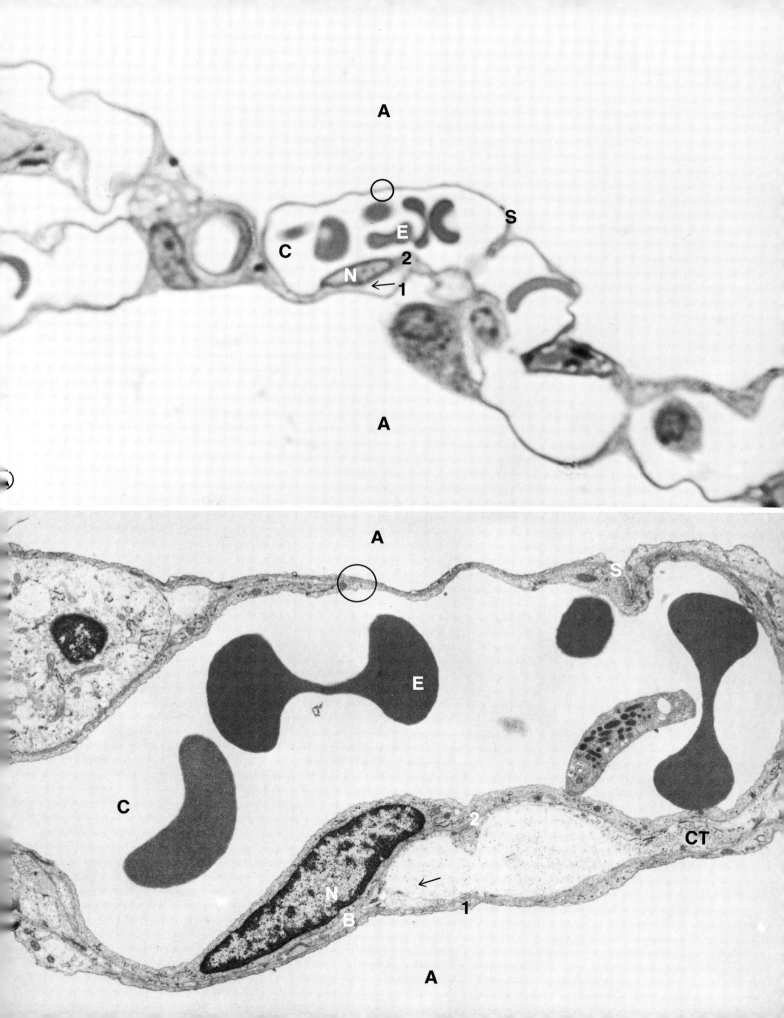

Plate 2–2

Simple Cuboidal Epithelium: The Thyroid Gland

As mentioned in the overview, cells engaged in the active biosynthesis or degradation of macromolecules are frequently cuboidal. An epithelium composed of a single layer of such cells, called a simple cuboidal epithelium, is easy to recognize in histological preparations.

Figure A at right is a high-magnification light micrograph of a section taken through the thyroid gland; Figure B is a low-magnification electron micrograph of a corresponding region within the same tissue sample. The thyroid gland, described in Chapter 19, consists of a collection of individual functional units called *follicles.* Each follicle is a spherical structure consisting of a central mass of colloidal material (CO) surrounded by a simple cuboidal epithelium (E). The epithelial cells elaborate and secrete the colloid, which contains, among other things, thyroglobulin—thyroid hormone complexed with a carrier protein.

The thyroid gland is an endocrine organ. The hormone it produces, delivered directly into the bloodstream, is borne by the blood to target tissues located at some distance from the organ itself. The thyroid gland is unique among endocrine organs in that it stores large quantities of hormone prior to the hormone's release into the general circulation. This capacity for storage may have developed in part because thyroid hormone molecules contain the element iodine; since iodine is not always present in the mammalian diet, the ability to manufacture excess hormone when iodine is available and to store it for use in times of dietary iodine deficiency may have conferred a selective advantage upon animals equipped to do so.

The mechanism of release of thyroid hormone is unusual. When called upon by the hypothalamus to release hormone, the simple cuboidal epithelium of the thyroid gland follicles actively takes up tiny droplets of colloid from the follicular interior by *pinocytosis.* Once thyroglobulin is within the cytoplasm, the hormone itself—usually diiodothyronine or triiodothyronine—is enzymatically cleaved from the carrier protein and released from the basal pole of the cell. Once free in extracellular space, the hormone diffuses rapidly into the capillaries within the rich vascular bed that underlies the epithelium.

From the discussion above it is evident that the cuboidal cells of the thyroid follicle are active in the biosynthesis and degradation of macromolecules. Figure B at right shows that this activity is manifest in the cytoplasmic organization of the cells. Around the centrally located nuclei (N), for example, are profiles of many mitochondria (M) and cisternae of the rough endoplasmic reticulum (RER). The endoplasmic reticulum is active in the synthesis of materials that are packaged within the numerous secretory vesicles (V) that populate the apical pole of the cell. The apical cell surface bears small, finger-like projections called microvilli (arrow) that amplify the area of the cell membrane available for the exchange of materials in and out of the cell.

Most of the cell components lie close to or beneath the limit of resolution of the light microscope and thus are difficult to detect in Figure A. Although the nuclei (N) are evident by light microscopy, the secretory vesicles (V) and mitochondria (M) appear only as fuzzy areas of increased density embedded in an amorphous cytoplasm. One can learn to identify structures barely visible at the level of the light microscope by carefully comparing light micrographs, such as that in Figure A, with electron micrographs of corresponding areas, such as that in Figure B.

Figures A and B. Light and electron micrographs of the simple cuboidal epithelium that lines follicles within the thyroid gland. Parts of two adjacent follicles, each with its own epithelium, are shown. CO, colloid; E, epithelium; M, mitochondrion; N, nucleus of epithelial cell; RER, rough endoplasmic reticulum (Figure B only); V, secretory vesicle; arrow, small microvilli (Figure B only). Figure A, 4,750 X; Figure B, 7,900 X

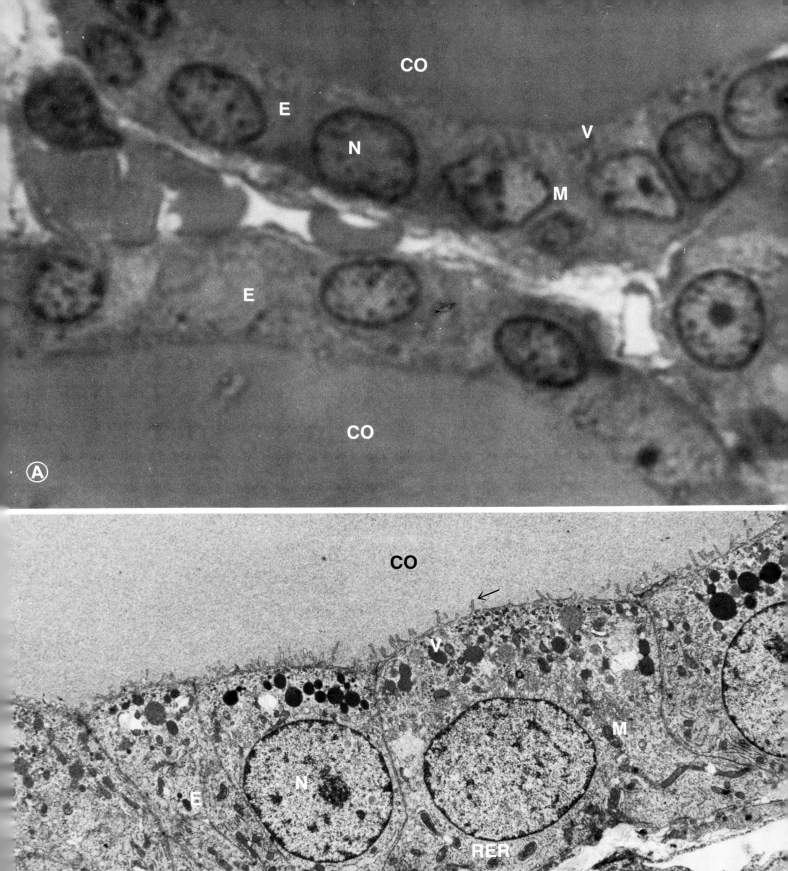

Plate 2–3

Simple Columnar Epithelium: The Intestine

A simple columnar epithelium consists of a single layer of cells in which each cell is taller than it is wide. Considerable variation exists between the height-to-width ratios of cells in different kinds of simple columnar epithelia; consequently, some are described as "low columnar" and others as "high columnar." Unfortunately, the specificity of terminology is limited. In many cases, low columnar and high cuboidal epithelia are difficult to distinguish from one another.

Figures A and B at right are a matched pair of light and electron micrographs of serial thick (1μm) and thin (800 Å) sections taken through the first segment of the small intestine, the duodenum. Here, the intestinal surface is thrown into folds called *villi* that greatly increase the area of intestinal surface available for absorption of ingested nutrients. In the figures at right, a portion of a villus (V) that projects into the intestinal lumen (L) has been cut in longitudinal section. The outer surface of the villus, exposed to the lumen and its contents, is lined by a simple columnar epithelium (EP) that rests upon the *lamina propria* (LP). The lamina propria is a thin core of loose connective tissue that lends structural support to the villus. The dotted line marks the boundary where the basement membrane of the epithelium makes contact with the lamina propria.

The primary function of the epithelium covering the duodenum is the absorption of digested food. Consequently, these epithelial cells are endowed with surface specializations that facilitate transport of nutrients from the lumen of the gut into the cell. Furthermore, the cell possesses a system of cytoplasmic organelles capable of breaking down absorbed materials into molecular components suitable for delivery into the circulatory system which then distributes the components to the body. In Figures A and B, the lumenal surface of the intestine is modified to form a *brush border* (BB). Also called the *striated border,* the brush border is composed of thousands of tiny, finger-like microvilli (MV) that provide each cell with a thirtyfold increase in surface area. Beneath the brush border, the apical portion of the lateral surfaces of the cells maintains contact with one another by *junctional complexes* (arrows) that appear, at low magnification, as dense dots. The junctional complex, consisting of a *tight junction* (zonula occludens), an *intermediate junction* (zonula adherens), and a *desmosome* (macula adherens), serves to bind the cells together and prevent direct diffusion of materials from the lumen of the intestine into the intercellular spaces.

At their apical poles, the columnar absorptive cells of the epithelium contain numerous vesicles, mitochondria (M), and elements of the rough endoplasmic reticulum (RER). Above the nuclei, dilated cisternae of the Golgi apparatus (G, Figure B) are present. In a section cut at right angles to the epithelial surface, as in Figure A, the nuclei (N) are aligned in a single row in the middle of the epithelium; the simple columnar nature of the epithelium is apparent. Unfortunately, sections are frequently not cut at the ideal angle, and the microscopist is faced with that major histological problem—misleading images produced by the plane of section. Were the intestinal epithelium cut in an oblique plane of section, it would appear to contain more than one layer of nuclei, lending a false appearance of stratification to the epithelium. Fortunately, with experience, you will learn to differentiate between true stratified columnar epithelia (which are rare) and obliquely sectioned simple columnar epithelia (which are common).

Figures A and B. Matched pair of light and electron micrographs of serial sections taken through the simple columnar epithelium of the duodenum. BB, brush border; EP, epithelium; G, Golgi apparatus (Figure B only); L, lumen; LP, lamina propria (Figure A only); M, mitochondria (Figure B only); N, nuclei; MV, microvilli; RER, rough endoplasmic reticulum (Figure B only); V, villus (Figure A only); arrow, junctional complex; dotted line, border between epithelium and lamina propria. Figure A, 4,000 X; Figure B, 4,300 X

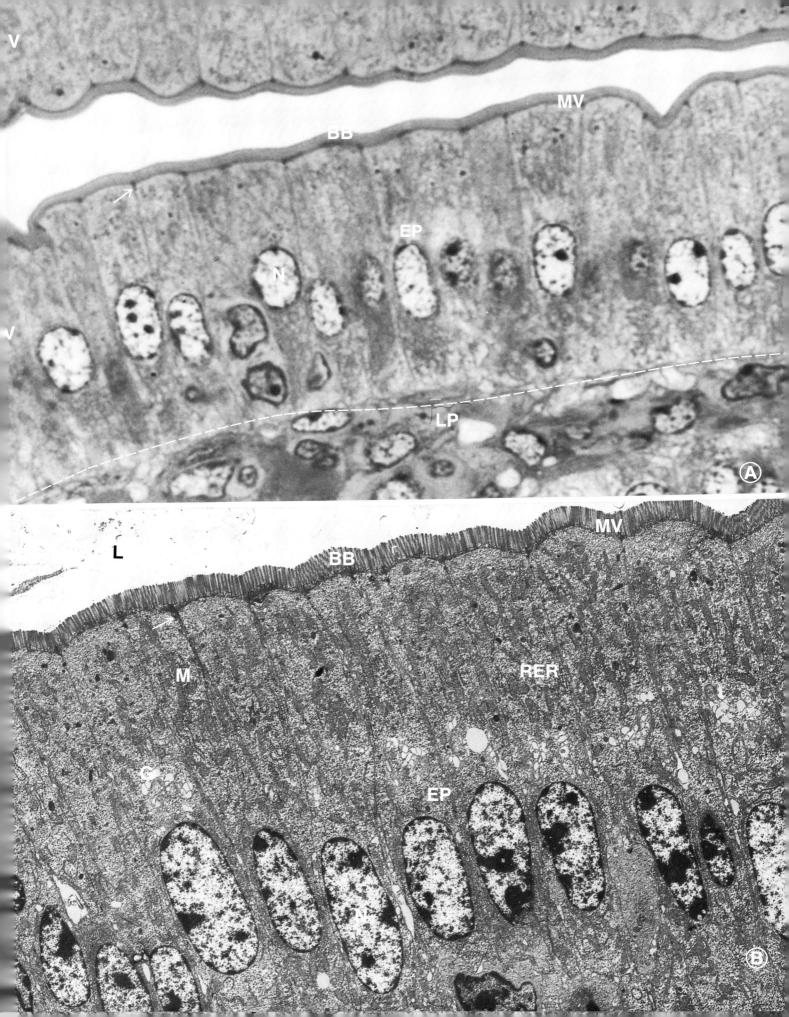

Plate 2–5

Pseudostratified Columnar Epithelium: The Trachea

Thus far, we have examined simple epithelia, which consist of a single layer of cells, and a stratified epithelium, which consists of several layers of cells. Now we come to a pseudostratified epithelium—one that looks stratified but is not. A pseudostratified epithelium actually consists of one layer of cells in which each cell makes direct contact with the basement membrane.

A single layer of cells can give the false appearance of stratification because in a pseudostratified epithelium, several different cell types, different in height, sit side by side. Their nuclei frequently lie at different levels, and some cells do not reach the epithelial surface. This arrangement is shown clearly in Figures A and B at right—a matched pair of light and electron micrographs of the pseudostratified columnar epithelium that lines the trachea of the monkey. Here, the apical surface of the epithelium contacts the tracheal lumen (L); the basal surface rests upon a very well developed and conspicuous basement membrane (BM). The tracheal epithelium contains three cell types: ciliated cells (C), goblet cells (G), and basal cells (B). The nuclei of these different kinds of cells all lie at different levels, lending a false appearance of stratification to the epithelium. The nuclei of the ciliated cells (N1), for example, lie in the middle of the epithelium, whereas the goblet cells' nuclei (N2) are pushed down to the base of the cell. The nuclei of the basal cells (N3) lie right next to the basement membrane (BM). Why are the cells of the tracheal epithelium arranged in this manner?

The primary function of the trachea is to carry air, large volumes of it every day, from the mouth to the lungs and back out again. Since raw atmospheric air is unsuitable for admission to the lungs, the epithelium of the trachea, along with that of the nasal cavity, must moisten the air, trap airborne particles and bacteria taken in with every breath, and then get rid of the entrapped particles. During all of these operations, the tracheal epithelium must protect itself from drying out. The tracheal epithelium accomplishes these tasks by covering itself with a moving layer of viscous, highly hydrated *mucus.*The sticky mucus traps airborne particles the way flypaper collects flies. All the while, it is protecting the cells beneath from desiccation and is actively moistening the inhaled air. The mucus needs to be replaced frequently by the goblet cells. After the mucus is secreted and established on the epithelial surface by the goblet cells, it must be moved up to the mouth to be swallowed or expectorated. This task is accomplished by the ciliated epithelial cells, whose cilia (arrow) beat in a highly coordinated, wavelike fashion (called the *metachronal wave*) with their active strokes directed toward the oral cavity. During the course of life, the ciliated cells and goblet cells of the pseudostratified columnar epithelium of the trachea occasionally need to be replaced. Replacements are provided by mitotic activity of the basal cells that lie close to the basement membrane.

Figures A and B. Matched pair of light and electron micrographs of serial sections taken through the trachea of the macaque. B, basal cells; BM, basement membrane; C, ciliated cell; G, goblet cell: L, lumen of trachea; N1, nucleus of ciliated cell; N2, nucleus of goblet cell; N3, nucleus of basal cell; arrow, cilia that project from surface of ciliated cell. Figure A, 1,750 X; Figure B, 1,750 X

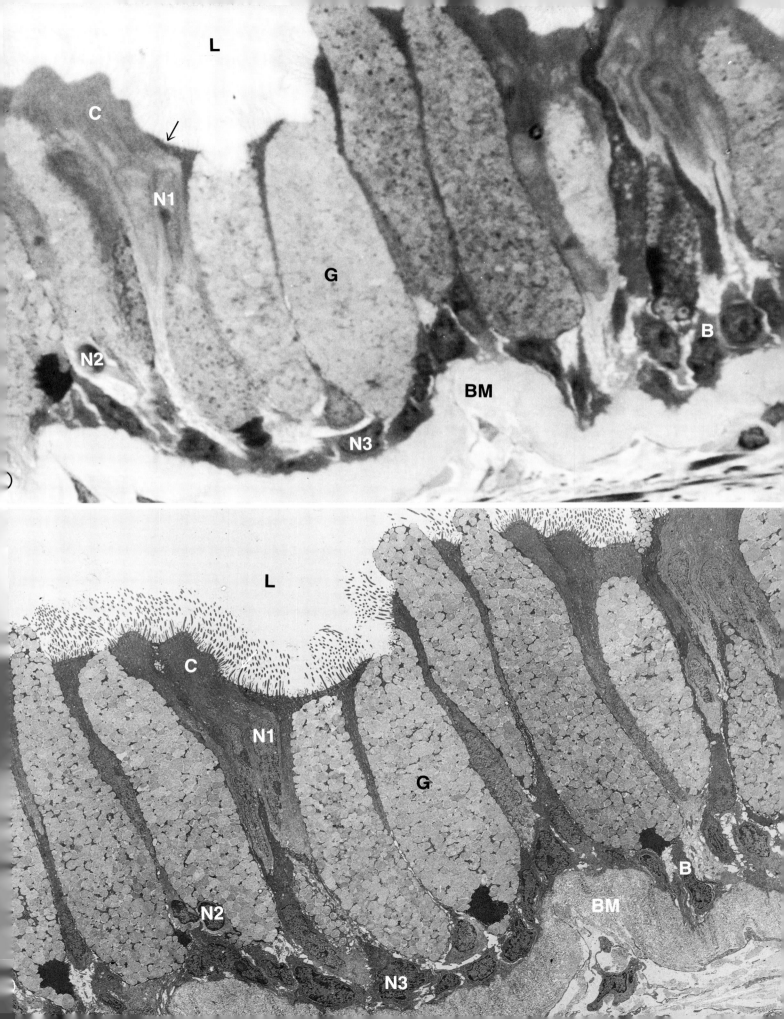

3

Connective Tissue

Overview

As human beings, we are often quick to forget that we are organisms—groups of organs held together in such a way that we can walk, talk, live, love, and study microanatomy. We can perform all of these highly specialized functions because our various organs are held together in precisely the right spatial arrangements. The key words here are *"held together"*; we are held together by groups of extremely efficient and carefully designed cells and tissues collectively called *connective tissue.*

There are several kinds of connective tissue. All are variations on a common theme, in that they are combinations of cells and extracellular fibers and fluids that are strong, resilient, and capable of repairing themselves. In this chapter, we will examine the various kinds of cells, fibers, and fluids that make up the connective tissues of the human body.

The most common type of cell found in connective tissue is the *fibroblast.* A cell that can adopt many shapes, depending on its activity, the fibroblast produces the two major classes of extracellular material found in connective tissue: *fibers* and *ground substance.* Fibers are strands of proteinaceous macromolecules that make connective tissues strong, resilient, and elastic; ground substance is a complex, viscous fluid that makes up the *matrix* in which the fibers and cells are embedded.

The three main types of fibers in connective tissue are *collagenous fibers, reticular fibers,* and *elastic fibers.* Of these, collagenous fibers are the strongest and also the most common. While the strength and durability of leather is well established, few realize that leather consists of interwoven collagenous fibers—fibers that originate from the dermis of the skin of large mammals. Strong though leather is, the collagenous fibers from which it is made are even stronger in the living animal. Collagenous fibers possess a formidable tensile strength; they can withstand pulling forces of up to 300 kg/cm^2 without rupturing. Under those conditions, the collagenous fibers will stretch very little—3% at most. The properties of collagenous fibers are derived from the fibrous protein *collagen* from which they are assembled.

Because collagenous fibers stretch so little and connective tissue so often needs to be elastic, the elastic fiber has evolved. When stretched, an elastic fiber can return to its original length. Elastic fibers, which are also made by fibroblasts, have two components—a fibrous core and an amorphous covering. The amorphous covering, made of the protein *elastin,* is thought to be responsible for the capacity of elastic fibers to recoil after being stretched. It is no accident, then, that connective tissues subjected to deformation often contain both kinds of fibers, collagenous fibers for strength and elastic fibers for elasticity. Perhaps the best-known example of this kind of connective tissue is found in the wall of the aorta, which with every beat of the heart must stretch to withstand tremendous hydrostatic forces and then instantly recover its original shape when those forces are reduced.

The third class of connective tissue fiber, the reticular fiber, is apt to confuse beginning students of microanatomy. Before the advent of electron microscopy, histologists had identified a class of connective tissue that consisted of fine fibers, thinner than collagenous fibers, that had special staining qualities. These fibers, often distributed in a spiderweb or "reticular" fashion, were called reticular fibers after their configuration. They are common to organs of the immune system, in which they form the connective tissue framework for the spleen and lymph nodes. More recently, electron microscopists have shown that reticular fibers are actually made of collagen fibrils. (A *fibril* is a tiny structure, visible by electron microscopy but too small to be seen by light microscopy. Many fibrils, when packed together, make up a fiber). Within a given reticular fiber, the collagen fibrils that compose its core are covered by a glycoprotein coat that resembles material of the basement membrane. In organs such as the spleen and lymph node, the reticular fibers are surrounded by thin cytoplasmic extensions of reticular cells—cells, quite similar (perhaps identical) to fibroblasts, that are thought to elaborate the reticular fibers. In ordinary histologic preparations not specially stained to detect them, reticular fibers are impossible to distinguish from collagenous fibers.

Connective tissue has been classified into several categories based on the manner of packing of the fibers and the ratio of cells to fibers. Connective tissue that features many densely packed fibers going in many different directions is known as *dense irregular connective tissue.* Found in such places as the dermis of the skin and the submucosa of the gut, dense connective tissue is well suited to binding epithelial sheets to underlying tissues.

Connective tissues that are subjected to the exertion of heavy forces in one direction, such as the forces that pull on tendons and ligaments, are quite different. They have densely packed collagenous fibers oriented parallel to one another. This type of connective tissue,

known as *dense regular connective tissue,* has many fibers and relatively few cells. The paucity of cells, most of which are fibroblasts, may account for the slow healing of torn tendons.

Connective tissue in which there are relatively few fibers and lots of cells is *loose connective tissue.* Found in such places as the lamina propria of the gut, loose connective tissue is composed of fibers that run in many directions and form an open, watery, cellular meshwork. Loose connective tissue often contains collagenous fibers, elastic fibers, and reticular fibers woven together in a variety of ways.

Connective tissue cells are varied. Most abundant is the fibroblast, which seems to be capable of secreting all of the types of fibers. *Mesenchyme cells,* too, are abundant. Mesenchyme is embryonic connective tissue; mesenchyme cells, therefore, are embryonic connective tissue cells. Despite their embryonic nature, mesenchyme cells persist in the connective tissues of the adult. Similar in appearance to undifferentiated fibroblasts, these mesenchyme cells are capable of developing into whatever type of connective tissue cell is required at the moment. They are thought to be multipotent and can differentiate into fibroblasts, cartilage cells, bone cells, and, on occasion, smooth muscle cells.

In addition to mesenchyme cells, *macrophages* and *mast cells* are widely distributed throughout connective tissue. Macrophages are large cells filled with enzyme-packed lysosomes that can phagocytose (i.e., engulf and digest) unwanted foreign particles and cellular debris. Mast cells, however, are different. Filled with conspicuous large granules containing heparin and histamine, mast cells can "degranulate"—often in response to injury—and release heparin, which slows blood clotting, and histamine, which increases capillary permeability. In this manner, mast cells participate in the inflammatory response; they promote the flow of blood out of the bloodstream and into tissue spaces, where blood cells and antibodies can fight infection.

Chapter 4 will describe the various types of cells found in circulating blood—the so-called red blood cells, or erythrocytes, and the white blood cells, or leukocytes. The white blood cells include, among others, lymphocytes, monocytes, neutrophils, and eosinophils. These so-called white blood cells are actually connective tissue cells; they perform their function in the connective tissues of the body, not in the blood. The bloodstream simply serves to transport them from their point of origin (usually in the bone marrow, lymph nodes, or spleen) to their ultimate destination in the connective tissues. Consequently, microscopic examination of connective tissue often reveals the presence of lymphocytes, monocytes (which are im-mature macrophages), neutrophils (which are phagocytes), and eosinophils (which phagocytose antigen-antibody complexes). In addition, cells called *plasma cells* are frequent inhabitants of loose connective tissue. Plasma cells, derived from a class of lymphocyte called the B-lymphocytes, are large cells filled with many cisternae of the rough endoplasmic reticulum that manufacture and release antibodies that bind to antigens in the course of the immune response.

Plate 3–1

Dense Irregular Connective Tissue

Plate 3–2

Dense Regular Connective Tissue: The Tendon

The function of the tendon is to provide a link between muscle and bone and to cause the bone to move when the muscle contracts. The simplicity of tendon function is reflected in its straightforward microanatomy. Tendons and related ligaments, which hold bones together, are made of dense regular connective tissue that consists of a small population of fibroblasts in a field of parallel collagenous fibers.

Figures A, B, and C at right illustrate the fundamental microanatomy of dense regular connective tissue. Figure A is light micrograph of a longitudinal section through a monkey tendon. The image appears as a series of dark, parallel streaks in a pale, amorphous background. The dark, parallel streaks are actually fibroblasts (F), or parts of fibroblasts, cut in longitudinal section. The pale, amorphous background consists of hundreds of tightly packed collagenous fibrils (C), all oriented parallel to one another and to the long axis of the tendon itself.

The microanatomy of the dense regular connective tissue of the tendon is more readily apparent when viewed by electron microscopy. Figure B is an electron micrograph of a longitudinal section through the same tendon shown in Figure A. Here, a lone fibroblast (F) is visible, sandwiched between the parallel, densely packed collagenous fibers (C) it has laid down around itself. Fibroblasts in tendons tend to be flat, and this one has been sectioned at right angles to its broad axis. Consequently, it appears quite long and extremely thin and seems to have very little cytoplasm. The most prominent feature of this fibroblast is the long, dark nucleus (N). Its large complement of condensed chromatin suggests that the cell is relatively quiescent; that is, it is not producing large amounts of collagen. The cytoplasm is spread out in a thin envelope around the nucleus. Immediately around the perimeter of the cell lie collagen fibrils that, on close inspection, display the periodic cross-banding pattern so characteristic of collagen.

The fibrillar nature of the collagen is immediately evident in Figure C, an electron micrograph of a cross section through a tendon. Here again, as in Figure B, we see a single fibroblast (F) surrounded by a field of collagen fibrils (C). In this figure the fibrils, having been cut in cross section and viewed on end, have a distinct punctate appearance. As a result, the image shows a lone fibroblast's nucleus amidst thousands of more or less evenly spaced dots. The dots, each of which represents a single collagen fibril, are of relatively uniform size, measuring about 1300 Å in cross-sectional diameter. In the region just beneath the nucleus, a stray, wavy collagen fibril has been cut in longitudinal section along part of its length (arrow); its cross-striations are visible even at this relatively low magnification.

Figure A. Light micrograph of a longitudinal section through a tendon from the finger of the squirrel monkey. C, collagenous fibers; F, fibroblast. 500 X

Figure B. Electron micrograph of a longitudinal section through the same tendon shown in Figure A. C, collagen fibrils; F, fibroblast; N, nucleus of fibroblast. 11,400 X

Figure C. Electron micrograph of a cross section through the same tendon photographed in Figures A and B. C, collagen fibrils; F, fibroblast; N, nucleus of fibroblast; arrow, part of collagen fibril cut in longitudinal section. 13,000 X

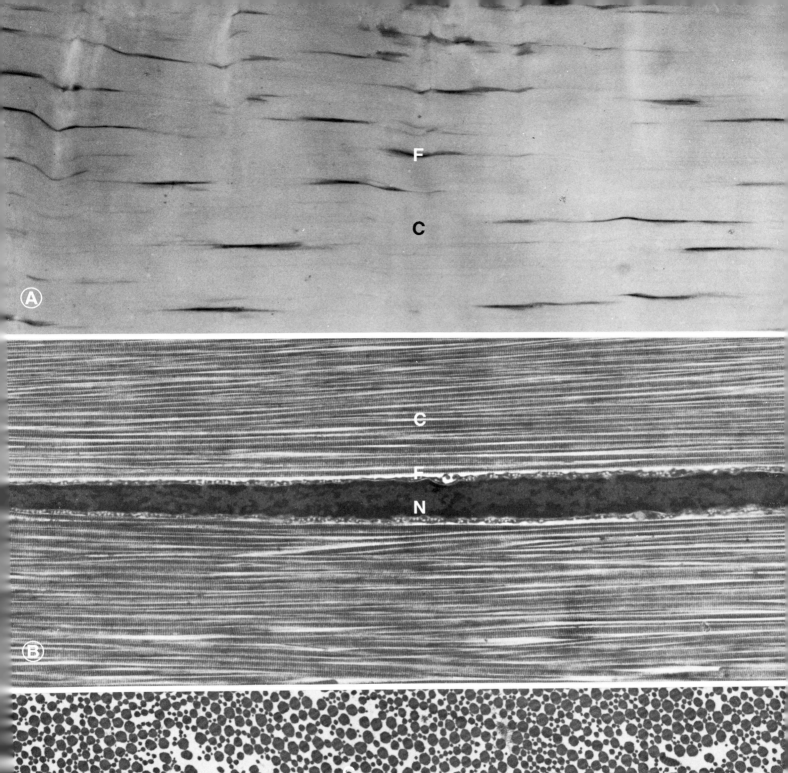

A

B

C

Plate 3–3

Reticular Fibers:
The Framework Of The Spleen

As described in the overview, connective tissue may contain any (or all) of three kinds of fibers; collagenous fibers, reticular fibers, and elastic fibers. Of these, reticular fibers are perhaps the most difficult to envision. Reticular fibers often coexist with collagenous fibers in the same connective tissue and are impossible to identify with the light microscope unless special stains, such as silver stains, are used.

Although widely distributed throughout the connective tissues of the body, reticular fibers perform a crucial function in establishing the connective tissue framework of tissues and organs associated with the immune system. The spleen and lymph nodes, for example, are two organs of a somewhat "mushy" consistency that would melt into a puddle were they not held together by a spiderweb-like framework of reticular fibers. Figures A and B at right are electron micrographs that depict a reticular fiber caught in cross section as it passes through (and supports) the so-called red pulp of the spleen.

The reticular fiber (arrow) consists of three components. First, the core of the fiber contains a number of individual collagen fibrils (C) that are presumed to be similar to those found in collagenous fibers. Here, they appear as a series of electron-dense dots, much as they did in the cross sectioned tendon described earlier in this chapter. Second, the collagen fibrils within the reticular fiber are closely associated with some dense, amorphous material (A) that resembles the amorphous component of the basement membrane. Third, both the collagen fibrils and the associated dense, amorphous material are surrounded by a thin cytoplasmic extension (R) of a reticular cell. (The reticular cell, often called a *reticulocyte,* elaborates reticular fibers).

One of the most dramatic features differentiating reticular fibers from collagen fibers is that collagen fibers are "naked" fibers, unlike reticular fibers, which are surrounded by thin envelopes of cytoplasm from reticular cells. This difference raises a question about the functional significance of the cellular covering of reticular fibers. If the primary role of reticular fibers is structural support, why are they not, like collagenous fibers, naked fibers? The answer to that question is unknown at present. It is interesting to speculate that, because reticular fibers are found throughout tissues and organs of the immune system, perhaps the presence of a reticular cell wrapping on the outside of the reticular fiber has some functional significance related to the workings of the immune system. It is well known, for example, that cell membranes have many specific receptors on their surfaces. This fact is particularly true of cells of the immune system, which rely on highly specific surface-to-surface interactions with cells and antigens in the normal course of their lives. In organs of the immune system, the reticular fibers provide a framework to which cells of the immune system are attached. Covering that framework with a cell membrane—the cell membrane of the reticular cell, in this case—provides a receptor-rich surface that facilitates the function of the immune cells that attach to that framework. In Figures A and B, a lymphocyte (L), located at the upper left corner of each micrograph, sits so that its outer limiting membrane is closely apposed against the cell membrane of the reticular cell (*), thus establishing a large surface area of contact between the two cells.

Figures A and B. Electron micrographs of a reticular fiber from the red pulp of the spleen of the macaque cut in cross section. A, amorphous material associated with collagen fibrils; C, collagen fibrils; E, erythrocyte in red pulp of spleen; L, lymphocyte; R, cytoplasmic extension of reticular cell; arrow, reticular fiber; (*) close contact between cell membranes of lymphocyte (L) and reticular cell (R). Figure A, 18,000 X; Figure B, 44,000 X

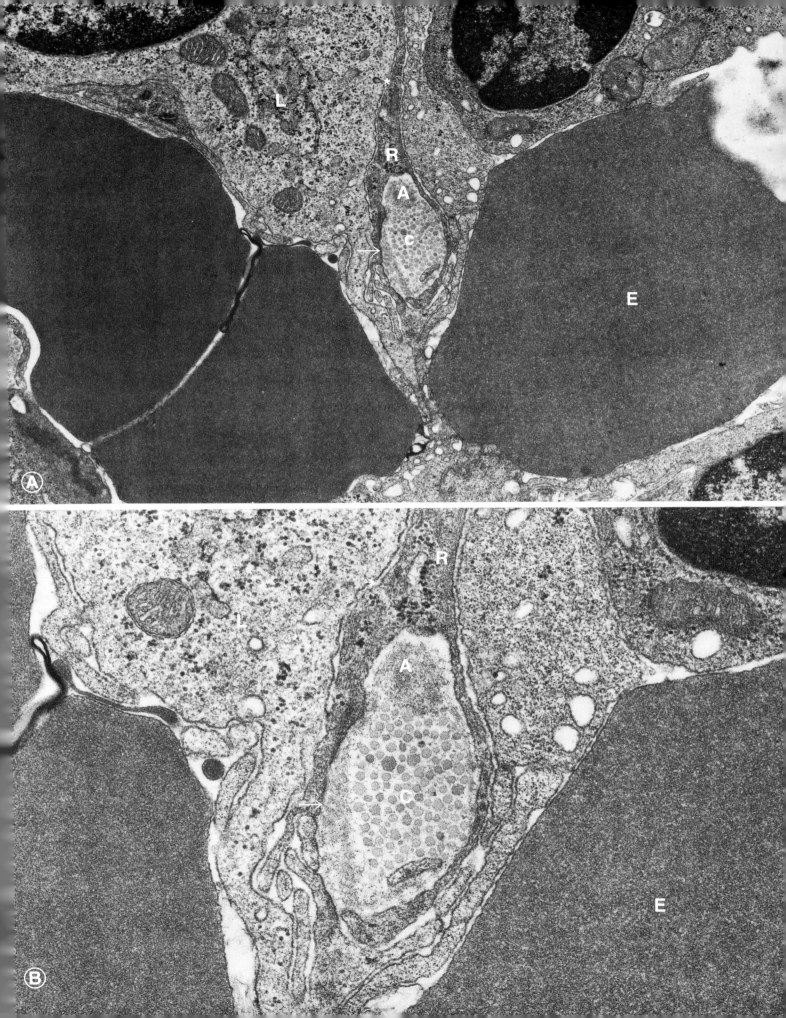

Plate 3–4

Fibroblasts, Mast Cells, And Macrophages

Connective tissue consists of a mixed population of cells embedded in an extensive extracellular matrix of fibers and ground substance. The cells found in connective tissue are of many types, including fibroblasts, mast cells, macrophages, plasma cells, and all the cells usually known as white blood cells—i.e., lymphocytes, monocytes, neutrophils, and eosinophils. The white blood cells, which are actually connective tissue cells, will be described in Chapter 4. Here, we will concentrate on three other connective tissue cell types of considerable importance: fibroblasts, mast cells, and macrophages.

In Figure A, the electron microscope reveals several fibroblasts. Fibroblasts typically have large, centrally located, football-shaped nuclei (N). The nucleus has a peripheral ring of densely stained heterochromatin (*) and a prominent nucleolus (Nu). Out in the cytoplasm and near the nucleus lies a well-developed Golgi complex (G) closely affiliated with abundant cisternae of the rough endoplasmic reticulum (RER). Taken together, these organelles produce and release molecular precursors of collagen fibrils as well as the amorphous ground substance in which the collagen fibrils (C) come to be embedded.

In addition to fibroblasts, mast cells are often evident in sections of connective tissue. Usually located near blood vessels, mast cells—one of which is illustrated by electron microscopy in Figure B—are large cells of irregular shape. The most prominent feature of the mast cell, aside from the nucleus (N), is its large content of electron-dense granules (G) that occupy the bulk of the cytoplasm. These granules contain heparin, an anticoagulant, and histamine, which increases capillary permeability. When released from the mast cell, these substances promote the flow of blood from small vessels into connective tissue spaces at sites of infection or injury, thereby facilitating the process of inflammation essential for proper healing.

Connective tissue also contains a large number of highly specialized macrophages, which are large cells capable of phagocytosis. During the process of phagocytosis, a macrophage will detect unwanted material such as bacteria and cellular debris, send out a pseudopodial extension of its cytoplasm, and engulf the foreign matter. The engulfed matter, drawn into the macrophage's own cell body, is subsequently digested by enzymes contained within the macrophage's many lysosomes. Figures C and D at right are electron micrographs that depict macrophages in action. In Figure C, a macrophage (M) is shown engulfing and digesting an aged red blood cell (E) that has escaped from the leaky, blood-bearing sinusoids of the spleen. Here, the nucleus (N) of the macrophage is visible, as is the bulk of its cell body. The lysosomes (L) that carry the lethal digestive enzymes are abundant. This macrophage has squeezed itself between the reticular fibers (R) that form the connective tissue framework of the spleen. When the macrophage has finished digesting the erythrocyte, it will recycle its components for further use. Bilirubin will go to the liver to be incorporated into bile, and hemosiderin will go back to the bone marrow to serve as a source of iron for new, growing erythrocytes.

In Figure D, another macrophage is seen as it engulfs a dying neutrophil. The neutrophil (NP), which is quite large, nearly fills the field. The only portions of the macrophage visible here are part of its cell body and the pseudopodial extensions (PE) with which it embraces the neutrophil.

Figure A. Fibroblasts in loose connective tissue. C, collagen fibrils; G, Golgi complex; N, nucleus; Nu, nucleolus; RER, rough endoplasmic reticulum; *, peripheral ring of heterochromatin. 12,000 X

Figure B. Mast cell from the lamina propria of the human tongue. CT, connective tissue; G, electron-dense cytoplasmic granules; N, nucleus of mast cell. 7,000 X

Figure C. Macrophage engulfing erythrocyte in monkey spleen. E, erythrocyte; L, lysosome; M, macrophage; N, nucleus; R, reticular fibers. 9,000 X

Figure D. Macrophage engulfing neutrophil in monkey spleen. M, macrophage; NP, neutrophil; PE, pseudopodial extension of macrophage. 13,500 X

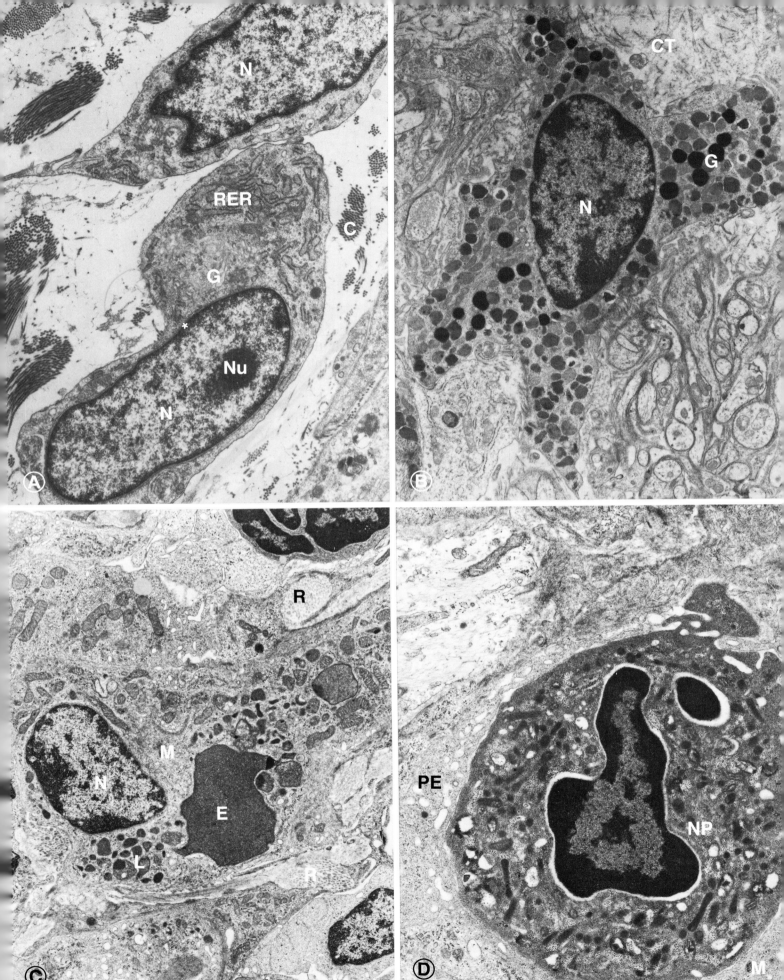

Blood

Overview

Human beings are exquisitely constructed communities of cells held together by a network of connective tissues. For a human being to live, the cells must live. To do so, each cell must exchange gases with the atmosphere, receive nutrients, and dispose of its waste products. Many cells are deeply hidden in nearly inaccessible recesses. Such cells receive the stuff of life from *blood*.

Blood, carried by the circulatory system, transports vital gases and nutrients to every cell of the body and then transports toxic wastes away to the kidneys and liver for disposal. Cells are faced with formidable logistic problems, solved largely by the circulatory system and the fluid that courses through it. Local lack of blood-flow leads to certain and swift cell death. Immediate and devastating dangers are posed by stroke, coronary artery occlusion, and similar disorders of the blood-vascular system.

Blood may be thought of as a kind of liquid connective tissue. In addition to coursing through your vessels, blood permeates the extravascular connective tissue spaces between all cells, tissues, and organs; it is in the extravascular, intercellular spaces that much of its work is done. Blood consists of two major parts each quite different from the other: a liquid phase, the *plasma*, and a mixed population of cells, the *formed elements* of the blood. Blood plasma is an extremely complex fluid, containing among other things, proteins, fats, sugars, hormones, nitrogenous wastes, antibodies, and salts, most of which are invisible by conventional light and electron microscopy. This chapter focuses on the formed elements of the blood—the cells and platelets most frequently observed in the general circulation.

The formed elements of the blood, shown in Figure 4-1, include red blood cells, called erythrocytes, white blood cells, called leukocytes, and platelets. Platelets are a class unto themselves. Active in the process of clot formation, they are fragments of enormous cells call *megakaryocytes.*

Red blood cells are the most familiar of the formed elements and are the most numerous of the circulating blood cells. Filled with hemoglobin and concerned with oxygen transport, erythrocytes give the blood its characteristic red color. White blood cells, which differ radically from red blood cells, tend to be the most frequently misunderstood of the formed elements. Confusion commonly results from the fact that, although leukocytes are called blood cells, they really are not blood cells at all, but connective tissue cells. Leukocytes are found in blood samples because they use the circulatory system as a means of transportation from their birthplace to their functional station in the connective tissues. White blood cells are primarily concerned with fighting infection; they destroy

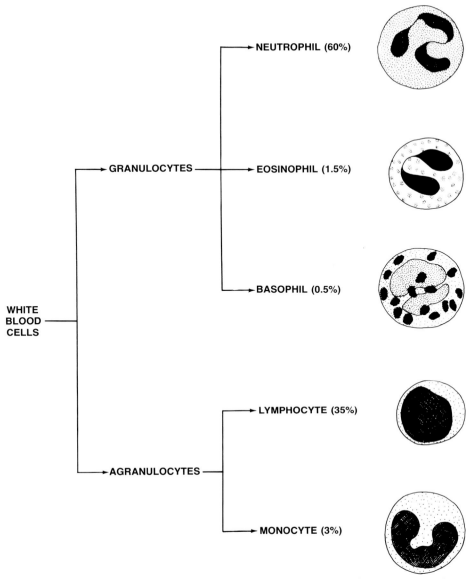

FIG. 4–1. Classes of white blood cells showing their appearance and frequency of occurrence in human blood smears.

invasive microorganisms and foreign antigens. The relative population of leukocytes, which can reflect the status of one's health, is usually determined by blood samples taken in the clinic because white blood cells use blood to carry them to their destinations and because, of all tissues, blood is the easiest on which to perform biopsy. The five morphologically distinct types of white blood cells are *neutrophils, eosinophils, basophils, lymphocytes,* and *monocytes.* There are two major categories of white blood cells; those that have intracellular granules (the *granulocytes*) and those that do not (the *agranulocytes*). The granulocytes include the neutrophils, eosinophils, and basophils; the agranulocytes include the lymphocytes and monocytes. The classes of blood cells are represented diagrammatically in Figure 4–1. The light and electron microscopy of red and white blood cells is illustrated in the following plates of this chapter.

Plate 4–1

The Red Blood Cell

Red blood cells (erythrocytes) carry oxygen. The red blood cell, which is dedicated to the performance of that single function, provides an excellent example of the intimate interrelationship between structure and function.

The unique shape of the red blood cell is best appreciated when viewed by scanning electron microscopy. Figure A is a striking scanning electron micrograph that catches a white blood cell (L) in the act of phagocytosing an erythrocyte (E). In this micrograph, the shape of the erythrocyte is a biconcave disk—a three-dimensional structure that, in some ways, resembles an automobile tire wrapped up in a plastic bag. This peculiar shape, central to the proper functioning of the erythrocyte, must fulfill three functional requirements that seem somewhat at odds with one another. First, the red cell must bind and hold all the oxygen it can. This requirement means it must maximize its contained volume of hemoglobin, the oxygen-binding protein. Second, it must accept oxygen in the lungs and give it up to other tissues quickly, which means the cell must have a large surface area to facilitate gas exchange. Third, the red blood cell must be flexible enough to squeeze through tiny, tortuous capillaries—some narrower than the width of a single erythrocyte—at very high speed. A biconcave disk will perform all of these functions.

In sectioned material, a red blood cell can present a number of different images, depending on the plane in which the cell is cut. In Figure B, a trans-mission electron micrograph of the lung, red cells are caught in a variety of planes of section as they wend their way through pulmonary capillaries. When cut in frontal section slightly off-center, they resemble doughnuts. When cut in perfect cross section, they look like figure eights. Some obliquely sectioned red cells look like scimitars; others, twisted as they round a tight bend in a capillary, resemble small sausages. Figure B illustrates another important characteristic of red blood cells: they exist in very high numbers. Between 40 and 50% of the volume of human blood is taken up by erythrocytes. Given that fact, the total number of red blood cells becomes staggering. There are, for example, on the order of 4.5 million red cells/mm^3 of blood. This translates to 4.5 billion red cells/cc^3 or 4.5 trillion red cells/L of blood. The average 150-lb person has a blood volume of 7 L, supporting (or rather supported by) a total population of 31.5 trillion red blood cells.

To maintain this tremendous population of red blood cells is no mean feat. Given that each erythrocyte has a life span of 120 days, bone marrow generates some 26 billion red blood cells every day, or 182 million every minute. During the time it took you to read this page, you have, for example, manufactured upwards of a half-billion red blood cells.

In addition to erythrocytes, blood contains white blood cells and platelets. The white blood cells are illustrated on the Plate 4–2.

Figure A. Scanning electron micrograph of a red blood cell being phagocytosed by a white blood cell. E, erythrocyte; L, leukocyte. (Micrograph courtesy of Dr. Keith R. Porter.) 9,000 X

Figure B. Transmission electron micrograph of blood cells circulating through capillaries in the lung of the macaque. AS, alveolar (air) space; C, capillary; E, erythrocyte; E', erythrocyte that escaped into air space during tissue preparation. 3,750 X

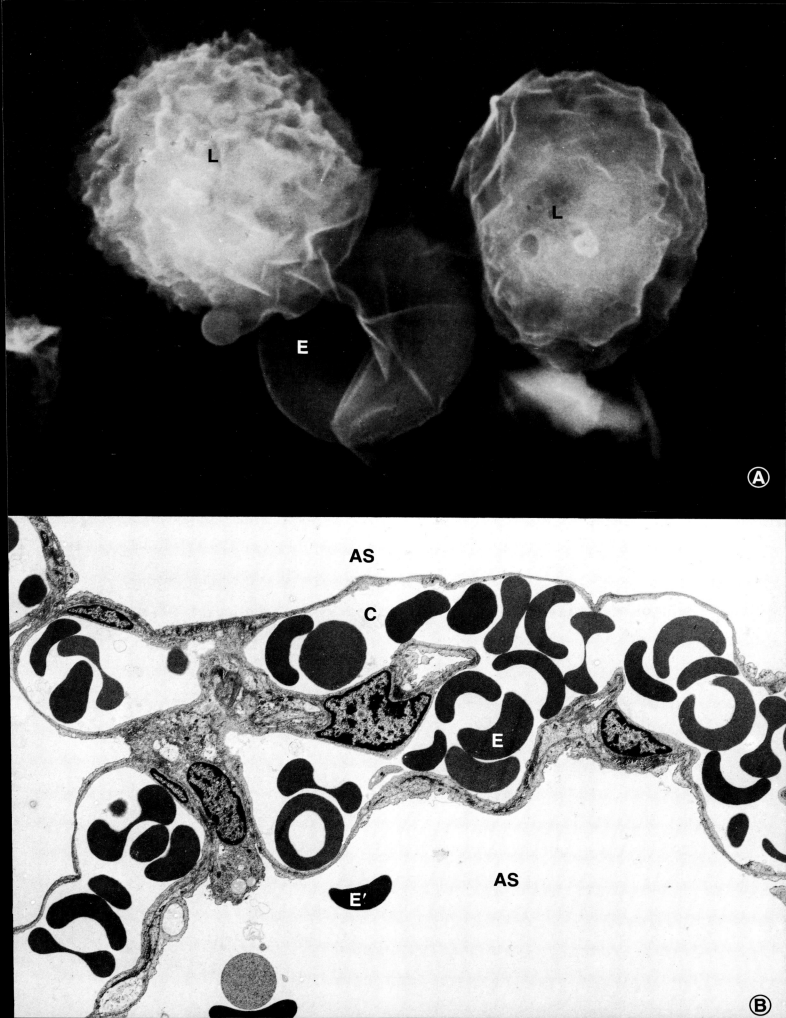

Plate 4–2

White Blood Cells: The Granulocytes

In the circulating blood, red blood cells outnumber white blood cells by a very wide margin. White cells are found in an average concentration of 7,000/mm³ of blood. For every 500 to 1,000 red cells observed there is only one white blood cell. This disparity occurs, in part, because white cells, being connective tissue cells, spend on the average only one day of their lifespan in the general circulation.

The three classes of granulocyte—the neutrophil, eosinophil, and basophil—are illustrated in Figures A through E at right. The granulocyte most commonly seen in circulating blood is the neutrophil (Figures A and B). Known by such names as *polymorphonuclear leukocyte, PMN*, or *poly*, the neutrophil has small cytoplasmic granules (G) and a complex, multilobed nucleus (N). The various names come from the images presented by neutrophils in blood smears, in which the granules take a neutral (purple) color with *Romanovsky's stains* and the complicated nucleus displays many shapes. Figure A shows a typical neutrophil in a light micrograph of a blood smear. Another neutrophil, this time fixed in situ in a capillary, is shown by electron microscopy in Figure B.

Chemotactically attracted to bacteria, neutrophils exit the general circulation at sites of infection or inflammation, whereupon they become actively phagocytic. Their granules become lysosomes, capable of enzymatically digesting a broad spectrum of macromolecules. Neutrophils often destroy themselves along with ingested foreign matter and aggregate to form pus.

Eosinophils, less common in the bloodstream than neutrophils, are primarily concerned with the phagocytosis of antigen-antibody complexes formed in the immune response. They perform their function in connective tissue, not blood, and frequently inhabit the lamina propria of the gut. In blood smears (Figure C), eosinophils are characterized by a dumbbell-shaped nucleus (N) and large, prominent, red (eosinophilic) granules (G). When viewed by electron microscopy, as in Figure D, these granules—called specific granules (G)—contain electron-dense crystals. The specific granules are thought to be lysosomes.

Basophils are the rarest of all granulocytes found in blood. Only 1 in 1,000 white blood cells is a basophil. A typical basophil in a blood smear is shown in Figure E. The basophil is a large cell filled with prominent blue (basophilic) granules (G). These large granules contain heparin, an anticoagulant, and histamine, which increases the permeability of capillary walls. Although the precise function of basophils is uncertain, it is generally thought that they leave the bloodstream, enter the connective tissues, and become mast cells. Mast cells, such as the one depicted by electron microscopy in Figure F, are connective tissue cells that, like basophils, contain large granules (G) filled with heparin and histamine. At sites of local injury or infection, mast cells degranulate and discharge their contents, which not only seem to cause capillaries to become leaky but also appear to impede blood clot formation.

Figure A. Light micrograph of neutrophil in human blood smear. G, granule; N, nucleus. 7,500 X

Figure B. Electron micrograph of neutrophil in capillary of monkey lung. G, granule (lysosome); L, lumen of capillary; N, nucleus. 10,000 X

Figure C. Light micrograph of eosinophil in human blood smear. G, granule; N, nucleus. 6,000 X

Figure D. Electron micrograph of eosinophil in capillary of monkey lung. C, capillary wall; G, specific granule; L, lumen of capillary; N, nucleus 8,600 X

Figure E. Light micrograph of basophil in human blood smear. G, granule. 8,000 X

Figure F. Electron micrograph of mast cell in human connective tissue. G, prominent cytoplasmic granules; N, nucleus. 8,000 X

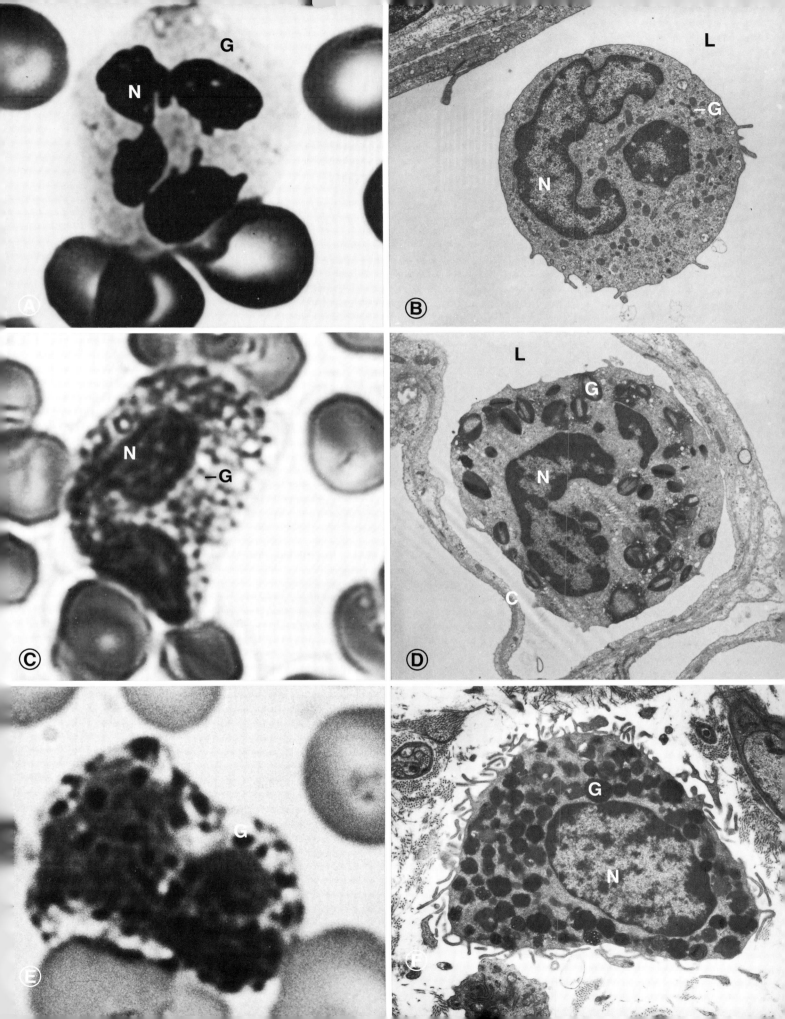

Plate 4–3

White Blood Cells: The Agranulocytes

The agranulocytes include lymphocytes and monocytes. Of these two classes of white blood cell, lymphocytes are far more common than monocytes. A typical blood smear shows ten lymphocytes for every monocyte. Like the granulocytes described earlier, the agranulocytes are connective tissue cells.

Lymphocytes are readily identifiable in the light microscope. As shown in Figure A, they are small, spherical cells with large, round nuclei (N). The nucleus occupies most of the volume of the cell, leaving only a thin crescent of cytoplasm (C) around part of the perimeter. These features facilitate the easy recognition of lymphocytes in electron micrographs. In Figure B, an electron micrograph of a blood-filled capillary, a lymphocyte is evident right next to the capillary wall (Ca). Here again, the nucleus (N) fills most of the cell, whereas the scanty cytoplasm contains a few mitochondria (M), a bit of endoplasmic reticulum, a Golgi complex (G), and a prominent centriole (arrow).

Monocytes, larger and scarcer than lymphocytes, are readily identifiable in blood smears by their lack of granules and a large, horseshoe-shaped nucleus (N) (Figures C and D). When monocytes leave the bloodstream, they enter the connective tissues to become macrophages, large cells that participate in the immune response and actively phagocytose unwanted foreign matter and cellular debris. Monocytes, then, may be thought of as the transport form of macrophages.

Although lymphocytes, too, participate in the immune response, they do so differently from monocytes. There are two classes of lymphocytes, not distinguishable by light microscopy: *T-lymphocytes*, derived from the *thymus*, and *B-lymphocytes*, born in the bone marrow. Although similar in appearance, T- and B-lymphocytes differ in function. While they both participate in the immune response and perform their functions outside of the bloodstream in the connective tissues, B-lymphocytes differentiate and mature to become plasma cells. Plasma cells manufacture and release antibodies, which are heavyweight proteins that bind to and inactivate foreign antigens, thereby defending the body from harmful bacteria, viruses, toxins, and the like.

Plasma cells have a distinct appearance. When viewed by light microscopy, as in Figure E, the plasma cell has a characteristic cartwheel nucleus (N) surrounded by a dense, highly basophilic cytoplasm (C). In Figure F, the electron microscope demonstrates the ultrastructure of the plasma cell. The cartwheel appearance of the nucleus is due to the presence of large, peripheral clumps of heterochromatin. The dense basophilia observed in the light microscope takes its origin in the abundant rough endoplasmic reticulum, whose parallel ribosome-studded cisternae pack the cytoplasm of the cell. The tremendous amount of rough endoplasmic reticulum, evident in the electron micrograph in Figure F, betrays the plasma cell's primary function: the production of protein, in the form of antibodies, for export.

Figure A. Light micrograph of lymphocyte in human blood smear. C, cytoplasm; E, erythrocyte; N, nucleus. 10,000 X

Figure B. Electron micrograph of lymphocyte in monkey lung capillary. Ca, capillary wall; E, erythrocyte; G, Golgi apparatus; M, mitochondrion; N, nucleus; arrow, centriole. 11,500 X

Figure C. Light micrograph of monocyte in human blood smear. E, erythrocyte; N, nucleus. 6,000 X

Figure D. Electron micrograph of monocyte in monkey lung capillary. Ca, capillary wall; M, mitochondrion; N, nucleus. 9,500 X

Figure E. Light micrograph of plasma cell in lamina propria of monkey intestine. C, cytoplasm; N, nucleus. 7,800 X

Figure F. Electron micrograph of plasma cell in lamina propria of monkey intestine. H, clumps of heterochromatin; M, mitochondrion; N, nucleus; RER, rough endoplasmic reticulum. 11,500 X

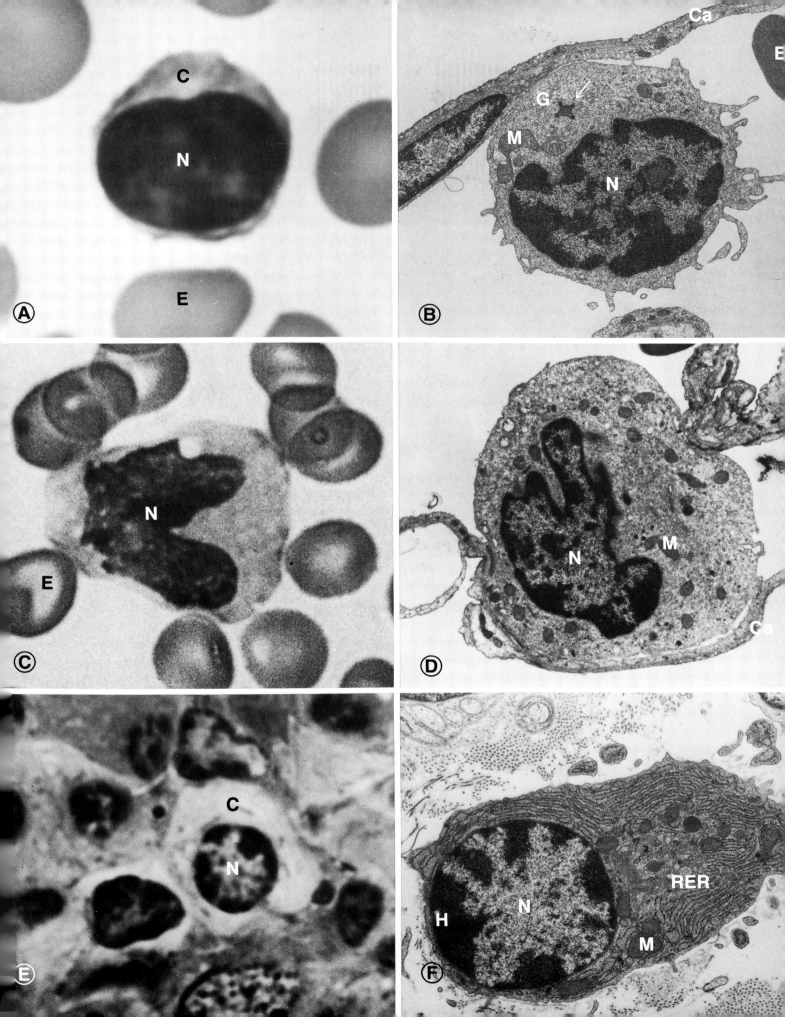

Cartilage

5

Plate 5–1

Hyaline Cartilage

Cartilage has three forms: *hyaline cartilage, elastic cartilage,* and *fibrocartilage.* Figures A and B at right are a matched pair of light and electron micrographs of serial sections that depict hyaline cartilage present in the trachea. Hyaline cartilage derives its name from the Greek word *hyalos,* which means glass. As its name suggests, hyaline cartilage is a smooth, glassy, translucent material that provides flexible skeletal support to the trachea, larynx, and ends of the ribs. It is also present at the epiphyseal plate of growing long bones and takes the form of articular cartilage in the joints where, lubricated by *synovial fluid,* its bearing surfaces are three times more slippery than an ice-ice interface.

Hyaline cartilage has unique and diverse characteristics. Like all cartilage, it is a specialized form of connective tissue that consists of cells and extracellular material. Cartilage cells, called **chondrocytes** (C), are embedded in an extracellular matrix (M), and it is the matrix that endows cartilage with its unique characteristics. As depicted at right, hyaline cartilage is covered by a tough, fibrous sheath of dense irregular connective tissue called the **perichondrium** (P). The perichondrium shown here contains a graded series of cells caught at different stages of development. The cells at the periphery of the perichondrium are flat fibroblasts (F) that, in time, differentiate to form the egg-shaped **chondroblasts** (CB), which in turn develop into round, mature chondrocytes. The chondrocytes, which often contain large lipid droplets (L), are responsible for the synthesis, secretion, and maintenance of the extracellular matrix. Should the chondrocytes die or become damaged, the cartilage matrix degenerates and can undergo calcification. Although the perichondrium can act as a source of new chondrocytes to a limited extent, cartilage does not regenerate well unless the animal is quite young.

The extracellular matrix of hyaline cartilage, located around and between the chondrocytes, is all-important and its structure, complex. The matrix contains a feltwork of randomly oriented collagen fibers that provide structural strength. These collagen fibers are embedded in an amorphous, gel-like **ground substance** endowed with two key properties. First, the ground substance binds to collagen; second, it has a tremendous affinity for water.

The ground substance is composed largely of **chondromucoprotein,** a copolymer of proteins and mucopolysaccharides secreted by chondrocytes. Like all cartilage, hyaline cartilage is avascular, and hence the diffusion of nutrients from the outer limits of the perichondrium into the core of the cartilage depends on the water-holding properties of its chondromucoprotein ground substance, since water facilitates diffusion. With aging, as the concentration of hydrophilic chondromucoprotein in the matrix surrounding a chondrocyte falls, so does its water content. Consequently, the rate of diffusion of nutrients to and metabolic wastes from the chondrocyte decreases rapidly, and the aging chondrocyte starves and dies. This process forms a vicious circle of degeneration, because the dead chondrocyte can no longer maintain its surrounding matrix, which may then undergo calcification and hinder diffusion of nutrients to nearby chondrocytes.

Because cartilage is avascular, many small arterioles (A) and capillaries (Ca) are closely associated with the perichondrium. In the micrographs at right, the myelinated axons of a small nerve (N) are present, as are several obliquely sectioned skeletal muscle fibers (MF). Several fat cells (FC), or adipocytes, laden with lipid, are scattered throughout the tissues beneath the cartilage.

Figures A and B. Matched set of light and electron micrographs of serial sections taken through the mouse trachea. A, arteriole; C, chondrocyte; Ca, capillary; CB, chondroblast; F, fibroblast; FC, fat cell; L, lipid droplet; M, matrix; MF, muscle fiber; N, nerve; P, perichondrium. Figure A, 1,250 X; Figure B, 1,250 X

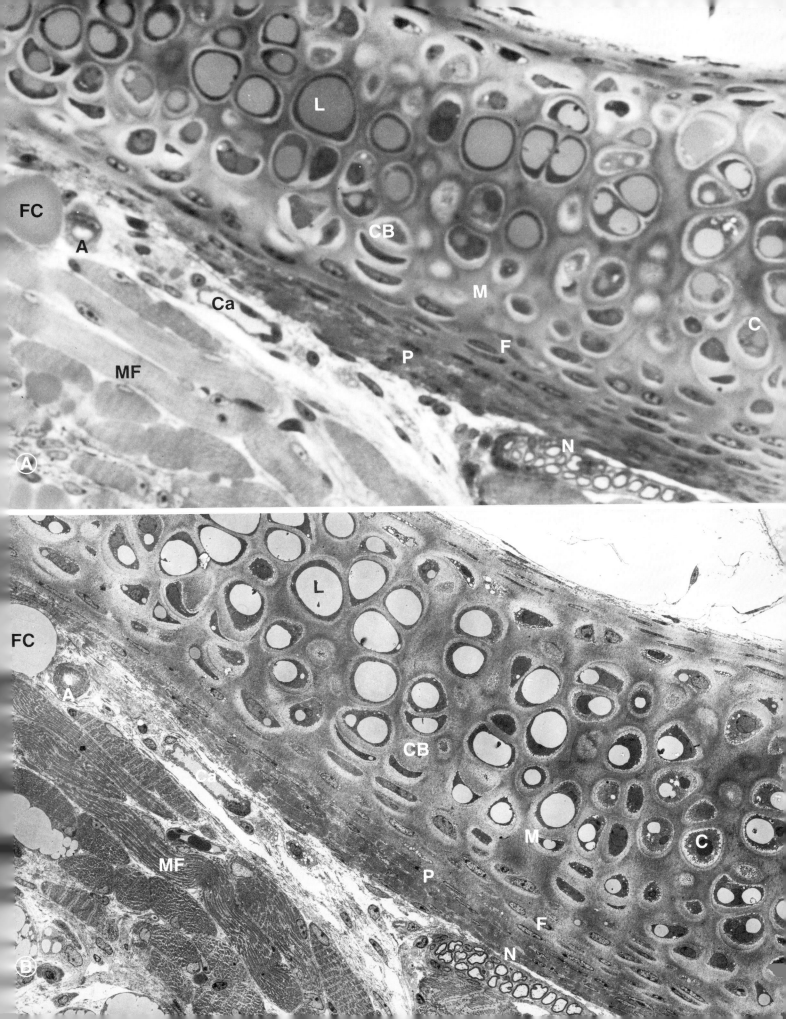

Plate 5–2

Elastic Cartilage And Fibrocartilage

In addition to hyaline cartilage, described in the previous plate, there are two other classes of cartilage: elastic cartilage (Figure A) and fibrocartilage (Figures B and C). Elastic cartilage is found in such places as the ear, the external auditory tube, and the eustachian tube. The matrix of elastic cartilage is criss-crossed by numerous branched elastic fibers rich in the protein elastin. These elastic fibers lend a high degree of flexibility and resilience to the matrix, endowing it with what polymer chemists call "memory." When bent, elastic cartilage will rapidly bounce back to its original form. Figure A is a low-magnification electron micrograph of a cross section cut through the external ear of the monkey. The outer margins of the cartilage, like those of hyaline cartilage, are defined by a fibrous perichondrium (P) made of dense connective tissue. The perichondrium contains collagen fibrils (CF), fibroblasts (F), and chondroblasts (CB). The mature chondrocytes (C) occupy spaces in the matrix (M) called lacunae. When viewed with the light microscope, elastic cartilage, if not specially stained to reveal the elastic fibers, looks very much like hyaline cartilage. Under the electron microscope, however, the elastic fibers are evident as clusters of electron-dense fibrils (arrows).

Although hyaline cartilage and elastic cartilage share many morphologic features, the third kind of cartilage, fibrocartilage, is unique. Its extracellular matrix has far more collagen and less chondromucoprotein than do the matrices of hyaline and elastic cartilage. In many ways, fibrocartilage resembles dense connective tissue. It lacks a true perichondrium, and often, as in the intervertebral disk, forms a structural and functional junction where cartilage and ligament meet. Figure B is a relatively high magnification light-microscopic image of a field of fibrocartilage in the intervertebral disk. Photographed here with the *Nomarski interference microscope*, the large collagen fibers (arrows) stand out in bold relief. The chondrocytes (C) look more like fibroblasts than cartilage cells, which is to be expected because their primary job is the biosynthesis of collagen. The chondrocytes are often fusiform, have dense cytoplasm, and frequently appear dark and retracted, indicating that they are probably inactive. The territorial matrix (arrowhead) immediately surrounding each chondrocyte contains tightly packed collagen fibers arranged in concentric circles around their cell of origin. Farther out in the interterritorial matrix, the collagen fibers (arrow) exhibit a more random orientation and are woven into a dense feltwork of great strength. Consequently, fibrocartilage is resistant to compression and is used to good advantage in such weight-bearing structures as the intervertebral disk.

An active fibrocartilage chondrocyte and its fibrous matrix are illustrated by electron microscopy in Figure C. Here, the cytoplasm is packed with ribosome-studded cisternae of the rough endoplasmic reticulum (RER), reflecting the cell's intense biosynthesis of protein for export. Many mitochondria (MC) are present to supply ATP for the cell's biosynthetic activities. The lobed nucleus (N) is outlined by a thick margin of heterochromatin (H), indicating that only a small portion of the cell's genome is transcriptionally active. The cell surface sends many fine filopodial processes (FP) into the matrix. The fibrous nature of the matrix is apparent in this electron micrograph.

Figure A. Electron micrograph of elastic cartilage from the ear. C, chondrocyte; CB, chondroblast; CF, collagen fibrils; F, fibroblast; M, matrix; P, perichondrium; arrows, elastic fibers. 1,100 X

Figure B. High-magnification light micrograph (Nomarski interference) of fibrocartilage from the monkey intervertebral disk. C, chondrocyte; arrow, collagen fibers; arrowhead, territorial matrix. 2,000 X

Figure C. Electron micrograph of chondrocyte within fibrocartilage of the monkey intervertebral disk. FP, filopodial process; H, heterochromatin; MC, mitochondrion; N, nucleus; RER, rough endoplasmic reticulum; arrow, collagen fibril. 7,300 X

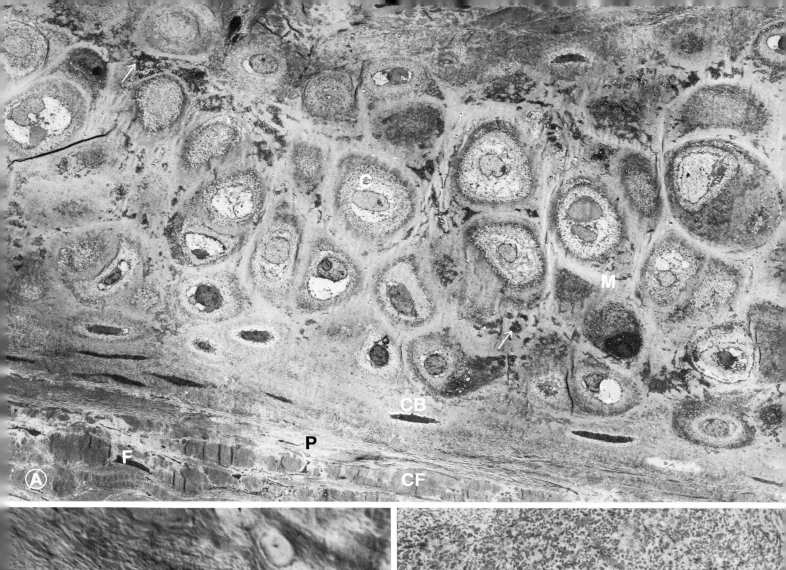

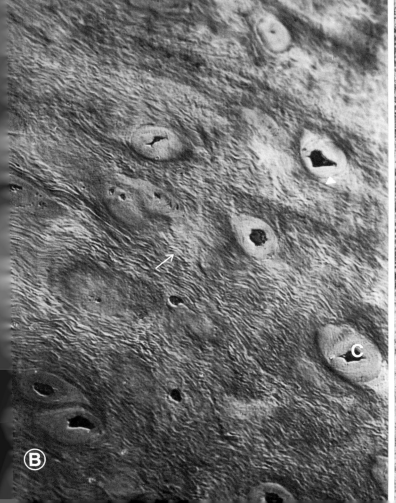

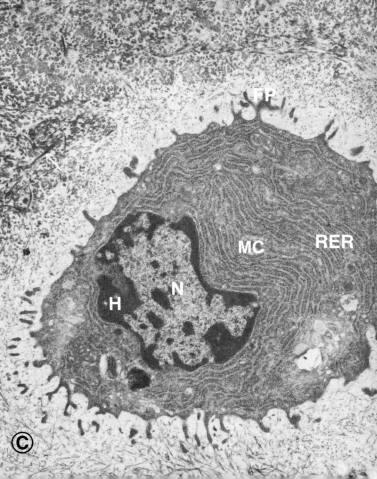

6

Bone

Overview

Bone is marvelous material. There are few substances, natural or man-made, that can match its durable combination of strength and flexibility. The femur of an adult athlete, for example, is so strong it can bear a vertical load of nearly 2000 lbs. Other bones, such as those in the middle ear, are so delicate they can transmit infinitesimally small sound vibrations so accurately that you can hear the exquisite overtones that issue forth from a Guarneri violin.

When tested against well-known man-made materials, bone fares extremely well. It is as strong as cast iron—it has the tensile strength of cast iron and can handle compressive loads as well as cast iron can—and yet is some 20 times more flexible; you can bend a bone 20 times more than a cast iron rod of similar size and shape before it will break. Although some new space-age materials—notably the carbon-fiber derivatives such as kevlar and graphite—can equal bone's strength and flexibility per unit of mass, none of these materials can repair itself as bone can.

Bone has the properties that suit it to be our mainframe in part because of the characteristics of the matrix. The unmineralized, organic bone matrix, called *osteoid,* consists mostly of collagenous fibers (95%) and associated amorphous ground substance (5%). The collagenous fibers of the osteoid seem to "seed" crystals of calcium salts, called ***hydroxyapatite crystals,*** which align themselves preferentially along the

collagen fibrils. Hence, mature bone consists of a framework of organic bone matrix that becomes heavily mineralized with carefully oriented crystals of hydroxyapatite.

Whereas hydroxyapatite gives hardness to bone, collagen is responsible for bone's flexibility. A whole bone, for example, immersed for some time in a decalcifying solution, will become completely decalcified; it will retain its shape and become extremely flexible.

Just as the materials of which bone is made are important, so also is the arrangement and orientation of those materials within the bone. Most long bones, for example, are basically hollow tubes. Hollow tubes are extremely strong, almost as strong as solid rods of the same material, and much lighter, because it is the wall of the tube (or rod) that plays the key role in resistance to strain, twist and compression. The walls of hollow long bones consist of ***compact bone***—bone that contains thousands of longitudinally oriented tiny tubes called ***osteons*** within it. Figure 6-1 is a drawing of a long bone, part of a femur that has been sawn in half along its length. The figure shows that a long bone has a dense wall of compact bone and a hollow core of ***spongy bone.*** The hollow core is traversed by bony plates (called ***trabeculae***) and spikes (called ***spicules***). These bony plates and spicules, made of spongy bone, are often aligned precisely along the lines of stress that pass through the bone with normal use. With

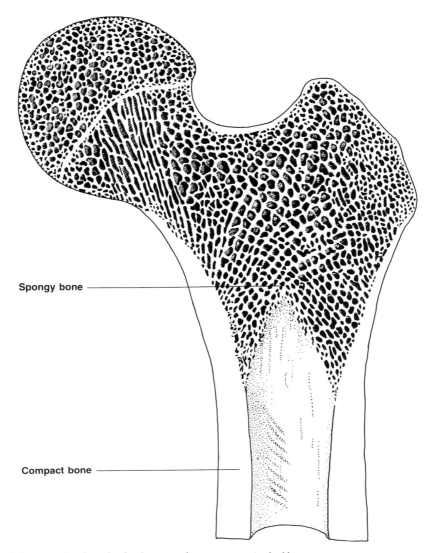

Spongy bone

Compact bone

FIG. 6–1. Drawing of the proximal end of a human femur sawn in half.

disuse, these trabeculae and spicules become disorganized.

The structural changes of spongy bone that accompany use and disuse point out one extremely important feature: bone remodels itself constantly. It has been calculated that every calcium ion in the skeleton is replaced at least once every 20 years. That bone is constantly being remodeled is beneficial to fracture repair. After detecting a break in its structure, bone immediately sets to work bridging the gap with new bone. This new bone, called *woven bone* or *callus,* is subsequently replaced with mature bone as remodeling continues. Bone's lability makes it suitable as a reservoir for minerals in general and for calcium in particular. Calcium

is an important ion in the biochemistry of cells, and the critical level of calcium ion in the blood that bathes those cells is maintained with the aid of the skeleton. In times of low blood calcium, bone gives up calcium to the blood. Conversely, in times of high blood calcium, bone may take up calcium and deposit it into its mineralized matrix.

Like all connective tissue, of which bone is a derivative, bone consists of a careful combination of cells and extracellular matrix. The extracellular matrix, as has been mentioned, consists of the organic component, or osteoid, and the mineral component, the hydroxyapatite crystals. The organic matrix is secreted by special cells called *osteoblasts.* Osteoblasts are akin to fibroblasts in that they secrete collagen and an associated amorphous ground substance. Unlike fibroblasts, however, they also secrete a substance that permits the collagen fibrils to become encrusted with crystals of hydroxyapatite. Once the osteoblasts are encased in mineralized matrix, they stop making osteoid and become known as *osteocytes.* Although osteocytes do not produce matrix, their presence is necessary to maintain bone in its living condition.

Just as some cells make bone, some cells destroy bone. These cells, called *osteoclasts,* are large, *multinucleate,* phagocytic cells that literally eat their way through bone and release its elements to the blood for further use elsewhere in the body. Working in concert, the osteoclasts, which chisel away at bone, and the osteoblasts, which lay it down, remodel bone during growth and adult life to maintain its most efficient size and shape.

Plate 6–1

Compact Bone: The Osteon

Plate 6–1

Compact Bone: The Osteon

As described in the Overview, there are two major classes of bone—compact bone and spongy bone. Compact bone, which is very strong and dense, forms the tough outer cortex of long bones. Spongy bone, as the name suggests, is loosely organized and consists of thin trabeculae that fill the marrow spaces in the hollow cores of long bones. This plate illustrates compact bone and its unit of structure, the osteon.

The osteon, also called the *Haversian system,* is an efficient structure. The osteon not only provides a model of the interrelationship between structure and function, but also demonstrates clearly how physical limitations of biological systems can govern the shape of the structures that evolve within those physical limits. One of the major limits that has imposed a certain geometry on compact bone involves diffusion. As mentioned in the chapter on cartilage, the cartilage cells, or chondrocytes, receive their nutrients by diffusion through the matrix. Bone cells, or osteocytes, cannot do that, simply because mineralized bone matrix is an effective diffusion barrier. Hence, whereas cartilage can be avascular, bone cannot.

The vascular component of bone, around which the osteon is organized, is shown in Figure A at right, a thick cross section through human compact bone that has been ground wafer-thin on an abrasive disk. The soft tissues are gone, leaving the mineralized bone matrix and the cavities and canals that, in life, contained the soft tissues. These cavities have been filled with India ink to provide contrast. The mineralized bone matrix appears grayish, and the cavities in which cells and soft tissues were situated are black. The center of the field is occupied by an osteon, whose outer limits are here traced by a dotted line.

Through the center of the osteon runs the *Haversian canal* (HC), a cylindric channel that contains one or more blood vessels. Because osteocytes must exchange metabolites with the general circulation to live and since mineralized bone matrix blocks diffusion, each osteocyte must exist close to a blood vessel. Consequently, osteocytes take station equidistant from the blood supply in concentric rings around the Haversian canal, as shown in Figure A. Here, the holes in which osteocytes sit, called lacunae (L), are filled with India ink and appear black. Close inspection of the light micrograph will reveal that each lacuna gives rise to a number of spiderweb-like projections called canaliculi (arrows). In living tissue, osteocytes send out thin cytoplasmic processes that pass through the canaliculi and touch one another. The osteoblastic processes from the innermost ring of osteocytes run centrally and contact the capillary in the Haversian canal. Consequently, metabolites can be exchanged between osteocytes and the bloodstream. Not only does this concentric arrangement of osteocytes around a central canal favor metabolite exchange, it also promotes an internal architecture of great strength. Tubes and cylinders are strong structures; it is no accident that engineers use them often in situations that call for structural strength combined with flexibility. The concentrically arranged osteocytes secrete cylindrical *lamellae* (layers) of bone around themselves. The lamellae, like the osteocytes themselves, are arranged in concentric layers. Furthermore, the lamellae contain organized arrays of collagen fibrils and mineralized matrix that vary in orientation from lamella to lamella, as do the overlapping, cross-grained layers in a sheet of plywood.

Although the structure of the osteon-filled compact bone appears rigid and permanent, it is not. Bone is constantly being remodeled during life; osteons are built, resorbed, and replaced. A mature osteon is outlined by the dotted line in the center of the field. Just to its left lie some interstitial lamellae (IL)—the remnants of an osteon that was resorbed to make way for a new one.

Ground cross section of human compact bone stained with India ink. HC, Haversian canal; IL, interstitial lamellae; L, lacuna; arrows, canaliculus; dotted line, perimeter of osteon. 700 X

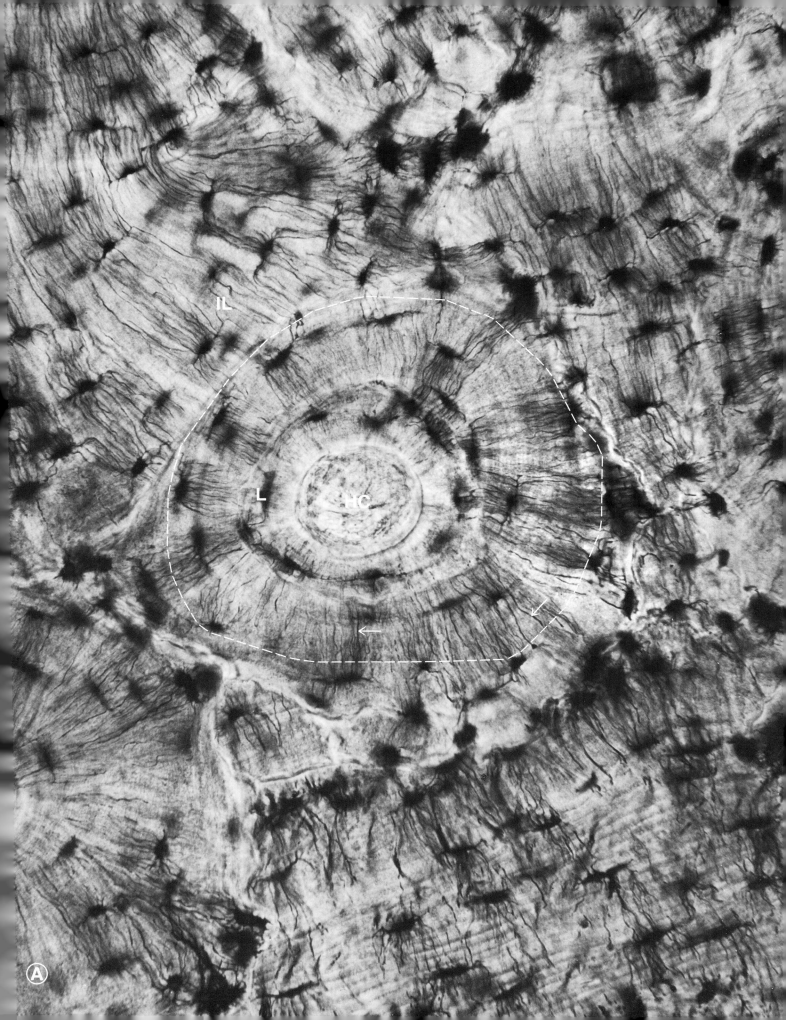

Plate 6–2

Bone: Remodeling And The Osteoclast

The osteon, illustrated by light microscopy in Plate 6-1, is the fundamental unit of structure of the compact bone found in the cortex of large long bones. Part of an osteon is shown at low magnification by electron microscopy in Figure A. Whereas all of the cellular elements of the osteon are absent from the section of ground bone shown in Plate 6–1, they are present and visible in Figure A at right. Here, the Haversian canal (HC) in the center of the osteon is lined by the thin endothelial cell of a single large capillary (C). Just outside the capillary but inside the bone (B) that surrounds the Haversian canal lie several mesenchymal cells (M), embryonic connective tissue cells that can develop into osteoblasts. One of the mesenchyme cells in the field has recently differentiated into an osteoblast (OB) that is actively secreting new bone matrix (∗). During the growth of bone, osteoblasts—large cuboidal cells that contain many cisternae of the rough endoplasmic reticulum—elaborate and secrete large quantities of osteoid. Osteoid consists mostly of collagen fibers associated with a small amount of amorphous ground substance. Shortly after osteoid is laid down by the osteoblast, the collagen fibrils within the osteoid "seed" crystals of calcium salts that mineralize the bone matrix and give it its characteristic hardness. Hydroxyapatite crystals appear in a mineralization front in the osteoid near the osteoblast. The mineralization front, evident in electron micrographs of growing bone, is indicated by an arrowhead in Figure A. In time, the mineralization front moves through the osteoid and surrounds the osteoblast. When the osteoblast is encased by mineralized matrix, it stops making osteoid, shrinks to a shade of its former self, and becomes an osteocyte. The osteocyte (O), one of which is shown sitting in its lacuna in Figure A, is connected with the blood supply (and with other osteocytes) by long, thin cytoplasmic extensions called osteocytic processes that pass through tiny channels, or canaliculi (arrows), in the mineralized bone matrix.

Paradoxically, as bone is being laid down in one place, it is often being removed from another. This phenomenon, essential to the continuous remodeling of bone, is shown clearly in Figure A. Here, an osteoblast is actively secreting osteoid that is becoming mineralized (arrowhead). While bone is being made near the center of the osteon, however, it is being destroyed at the periphery of the same osteon by a large phagocytic cell called an osteoclast (OC).

The osteoclast at the upper left corner of Figure A is shown at higher magnification in Figure B, in which part of the Haversian canal (HC) is at the bottom of the micrograph, surrounded by concentric lamellae of mineralized bone matrix (B). At the top of the micrograph, much of the osteon's bone is gone, and the region formerly occupied by bone is occupied by a very large osteoclast (OC). The osteoclast, which sits in a depression (arrowhead) called a *Howship's lacuna,* is a large, multinucleate cell; three of its nuclei (N1, N2, and N3) are visible in this thin section. Osteoclasts secrete *hydrolytic* enzymes that dissolve bone; the elements dissolved from the mineralized matrix are taken into the osteoclast's cytoplasm and released into the bloodstream. It is interesting to note that *parathyroid hormone* mobilizes osteoclasts. Consequently, bone resorption not only contributes to the remodeling of bone, but also serves to elevate blood calcium concentrations.

Figure A. Electron micrograph of an osteon in the femur of the squirrel monkey. B, bone; C, capillary; HC, Haversian canal; L, lamella; M, mesenchymal cell; O, osteocyte in lacuna; OB, osteoblast; OC, osteoclast; ∗, osteoid made by osteoblast; arrows, canaliculi containing osteocytic process; arrowhead, mineralization front. 3,500 X

Figure B. Enlarged photograph of osteoclast present in Figure A. B, bone; HC, Haversian canal; N1, N2, and N3, nuclei of osteoclast; OC, osteoclast; arrowhead, Howship's lacuna in which osteoclast sits. 5,200 X

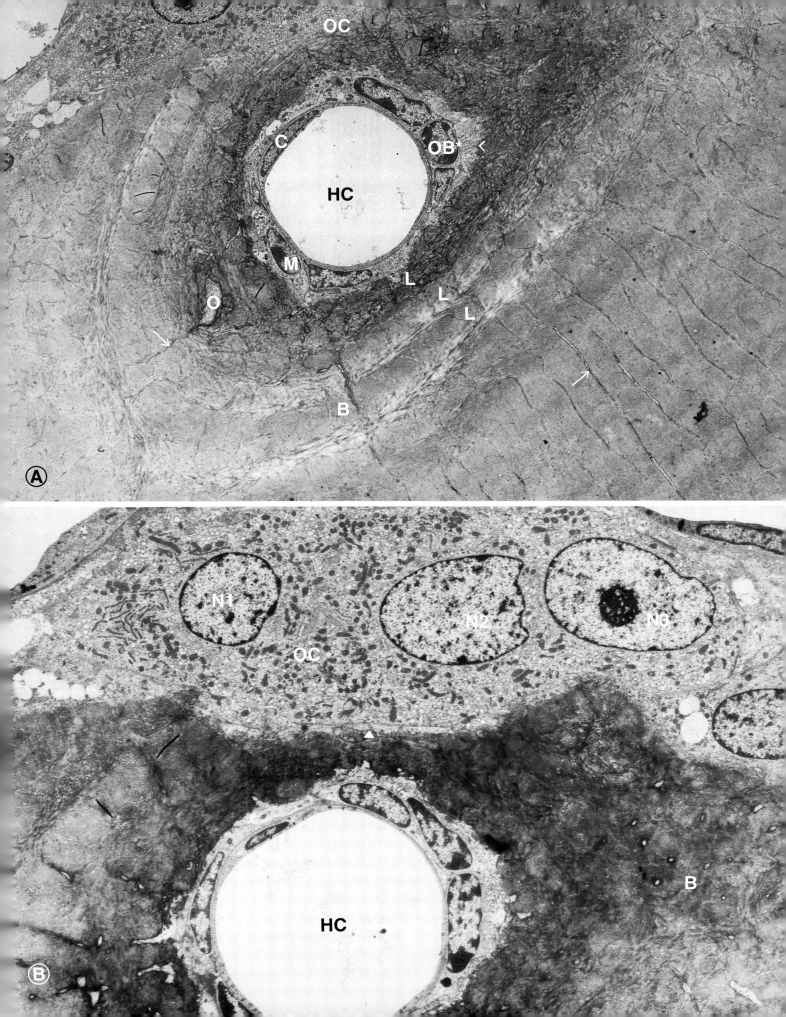

Plate 6–3

The Osteocyte

When osteoblasts stop secreting osteoid and become completely surrounded by mineralized bone matrix, they are known as osteocytes. Although osteocytes do not produce matrix, they seem to be essential for the maintenance of bone, and stand at the ready to act as osteoblasts once again should the need arise.

Figure A, an electron micrograph of a monkey femur, shows an osteocyte (O) sitting in its lacuna within a mass of mineralized bone matrix (B). The collagenous nature of bone is apparent at the perimeter of the lacuna (LC), where the characteristic cross-banded pattern of collagen (*) is visible in collagen fibrils oriented parallel to the plane of section. The ultrastructure of this osteocyte, like that of most osteocytes, suggests that it is an inactive, resting cell. Its centrally located nucleus (N) is filled with densely stained heterochromatin, indicating that most of the genetic material is supercoiled and not active in transcription of messenger RNA. The scanty cytoplasm is devoid of rough-surfaced endoplasmic reticulum, so prominent in the osteoblast, and the osteocyte has adopted a stellate shape. The cell body sends out many arms called osteocytic processes (OP) that tunnel through tiny canaliculi (arrows) in the mineralized bone matrix. It is through these osteocytic processes that the osteocyte takes in nutrients and sends out wastes. The processes from the osteocytes in the innermost lamellae of a given osteon extend into the Haversian canal and are available to exchange metabolites directly with the capillary (or capillaries) that course through the canal. The osteocytes at the periphery of the osteon, located some distance from the blood supply of the Haversian canal, send out osteocytic processes that make direct contact with osteocytic processes from other, more centrally located osteocytes. Presumably, metabolites are then transferred along the chain of osteocytes in a "bucket-brigade" fashion.

The cellular communication between osteocyte and capillary is shown clearly in Figure B. A Haversian canal (HC), shown at intermediate magnification, has two capillaries—a large, central capillary (C1) and a small, peripheral one (C2). Because the specimen shown here was fixed by intravascular perfusion, the blood cells have been washed out of the vessels and are not evident in the image. If you look at the periphery of the Haversian canal where the soft tissue meets the bone (arrowhead), you will see several places where osteocytic processes (OP) enter the connective tissue lining the canal itself (arrows). At that site, the canaliculus flares out like the mouth of a funnel. The osteocytic process seems to branch and sends out lateral extensions that form a ring around the perimeter of the canal, thereby greatly increasing the surface area of the cell available for metabolite exchange (see area near *).

Figure A. Osteocyte within osteon of monkey femur. B, mineralized bone matrix; LC, lacuna; N, nucleus; O, osteocyte; OP, osteocytic process; arrows, canaliculi; *, cross-banded collagen fibrils in bone matrix. 17,300 X

Figure B. Cross section through Haversian canal in monkey femur. C1, C2, capillaries; HC, Haversian canal; L, lamella of osteon; OP, osteocytic process; *, region where osteocytic process enters Haversian canal and branches; arrows, point of entry of osteocytic process into Haversian canal; arrowhead, perimeter of Haversian canal where soft tissue and osteoid meet mineralization front of bone matrix. 5,000 X

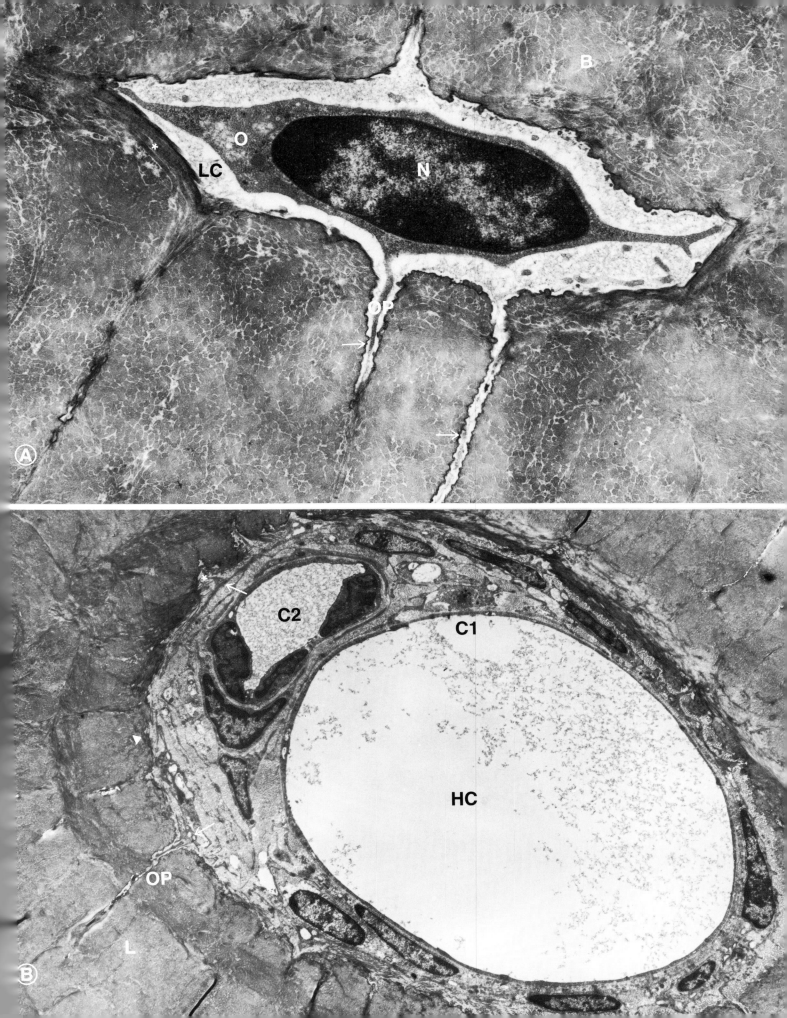

Plate 6–4

Bone Growth: The Osteon And Periosteum

Compact bone typically grows by apposition, which occurs by the secretion of material in successive layers, much as a mason lays a brick wall. Appositional growth occurs within osteons, which are the structural units located within thick regions of compact bone, and beneath the *periosteum,* a layer of dense connective tissue that covers the outside of compact bone.

Some imagination is needed to understand the way in which appositional growth occurs within the osteon. For example, in the Haversian system (or osteon) depicted in Figure A, the Haversian canal (HC) is in the center surrounded by several concentric lamellae of mineralized bone matrix, numbered L1, L2, L3, and L4. Of these, the outermost lamella, L4, is the oldest; the innermost lamella, L1, is the youngest. The innermost lamella, L1, was being laid down when the specimen was fixed. Consequently, several osteoblasts shown here—O and O'—were "caught in the act" while building a lamella. On the outside, these osteoblasts are surrounded by mineralized bone matrix (MB). On the inside, however, they are lined by osteoid (OS), which the osteoblasts have just secreted. Even at this low magnification, the collagenous fibers, of which osteoid is largely composed, are readily visible. These osteoblasts, then, have been photographed at a critical stage in their life cycle—a stage in which they are about to cease being osteoblasts, which actively secrete osteoid, and become osteocytes, which do not. When these cells become surrounded on all sides by mineralized bone matrix, they will be mature osteocytes—cells that maintain contact with soft tissue only by virtue of their osteocytic processes (arrows). Osteocytes become imprisoned in a penitentiary built of their own secretions.

One might wonder, knowing that mineralized bone matrix is hard and solid, how the outermost lamella, L4, got pushed out from the secretory osteoblasts of the Haversian canal. The answer is simple: it did not. When the osteon was young, its Haversian canal was huge, the same diameter as the outermost lamella. When the outermost lamella was formed, much as L1 is now being formed in Figure A, its osteocytes became surrounded by a ring of bone, the Haversian canal became smaller in diameter, and new osteoblasts differentiated from mesenchymal cells and made a smaller ring of bone, L3, just inside the oldest, outermost lamella. As successive layers of bone were laid down in this manner, one inside the other, the Haversian canal became smaller and smaller until it reached its present size as shown in Figure A. Whereas trees grow with the oldest annual rings in the center of the trunk, osteons grow in exactly the opposite way—their oldest lamellae are on the *outside.*

The appositional growth that occurs on the periosteum is much simpler to understand. The outer surface of most long bone is covered by periosteum, a tough membrane of dense connective tissue. The periosteum is to compact bone as the perichondrium is to cartilage. The periosteum (P), shown by electron microscopy in Figure B, contains collagenous fibers and connective tissue cells (CT). In addition, the inside of the periosteum—the side that abuts against the bone—contains osteoblasts (O). These osteoblasts secrete osteoid that becomes mineralized to form mineralized bone matrix (MB). As in the Haversian system, the osteoblasts, when encased within their own mineralized secretions, become osteocytes (OC). In this way, compact bone (B) increases in thickness at the periosteum.

Figure A. Cross section through developing osteon of monkey femur. B, bone; HC, Haversian canal; L1, L2, L3, and L4, lamellae of bone; MB, mineralized bone matrix; O, O', osteoblasts; OS, osteoid; arrows, osteocytic process. 4,800 X
Figure B. Electron micrograph of periosteum of mouse toe. B, bone; CT, connective tissue; MB, mineralized bone matrix; O, osteoblast; OC, osteocyte; P, periosteum. 2,800 X

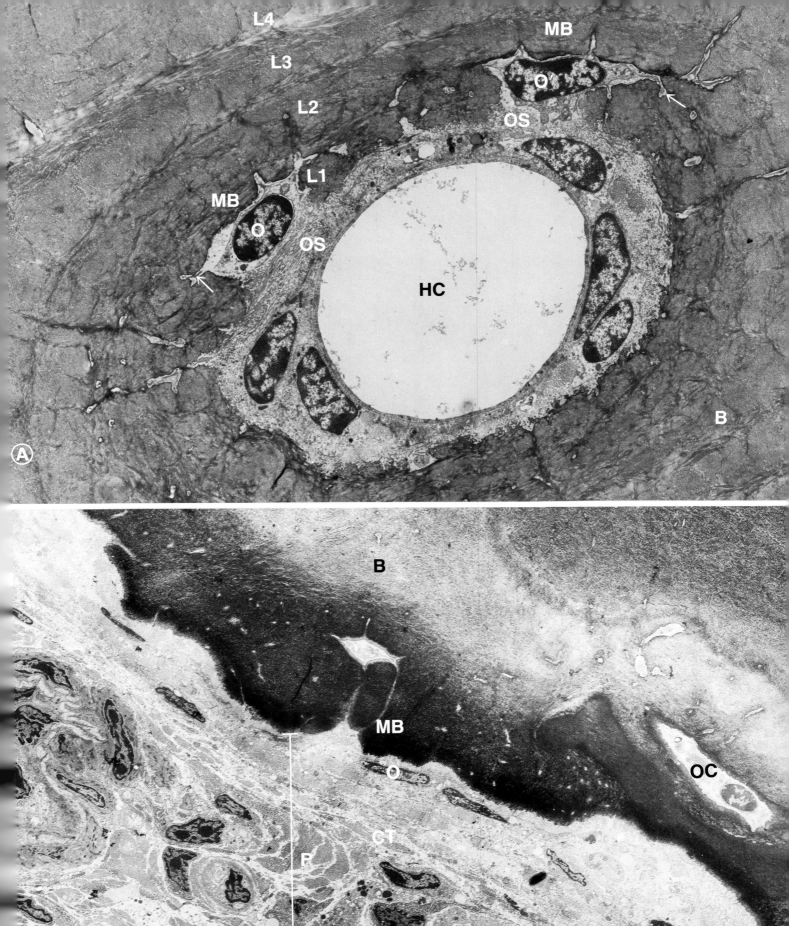

7

Muscle

Overview

The microanatomy of muscle is particularly fascinating in that the function of a muscle cell is clearly manifest in its ultrastructure. The most significant feature of a muscle cell, usually called a *muscle fiber,* is that it can change its shape rapidly, repeatedly, and predictably unlike most other cells in the body.

Cellular motility is one of the most extensively investigated phenomena in modern cell biology, and for good reason. Virtually all cells that have been studied display some capacity for movement, whether they move themselves in space, change their shape, or shuttle submicroscopic components about in their cytoplasm. What places muscle in a class by itself is that muscle cells have developed a tremendous hypertrophy of a macromolecular motile mechanism that is present, albeit on a smaller scale, in the majority of other somatic cells.

The three major histologic categories of muscle in the human body are *skeletal muscle, cardiac muscle,* and *smooth muscle.* Skeletal muscle, also called *striated muscle,* is innervated by motor nerves and is responsible for voluntary bodily movements. Cardiac muscle constitutes the bulk of the tissue of the heart and provides the contractile force that permits that organ to pump great volumes of blood with high speed and efficiency. Smooth muscle, innervated by the autonomic nervous system, provides the motive force for involuntary movements of organs such as the stomach, intestines, and blood vessels. Whereas skeletal and cardiac muscle

are somewhat similar in ultrastructure, smooth muscle is in a class by itself.

Skeletal muscle

Perhaps the most difficult concept in the microanatomic organization of skeletal muscle is the structural hierarchy of its components. Figure 7-1 demonstrates the architecture of skeletal muscle. Here, it is apparent that a whole muscle—a bicep, in this case—contains bundles of individual muscle fibers. Each muscle fiber is a discrete unit surrounded by its own plasma membrane. In muscle, the plasma membrane is often called the *sarcolemma.* By cellular standards, the skeletal muscle fiber is huge; it measures up to 0.1 mm (100 μm) in diameter and can reach many centimeters in length (Table 7-1). Each muscle fiber is a *syncytium*—one cell derived from many cells that came to be enveloped by a common plasma membrane.

Each individual muscle fiber is subdivided into many longitudinally oriented units called *myofibrils.* Each myofibril, in turn, is surrounded by a network of the smooth endoplas-

TABLE 7–1. *Typical Dimensions of Skeletal Muscle Fibers*

	LENGTH	WIDTH
Muscle fiber	1-30 cm	100 μm
Myofibril	1-30 cm	2 μm
Sarcomere (relaxed)	2.5 μm	2 μm
Sarcomere (contracted)	1.25 μm	2 μm

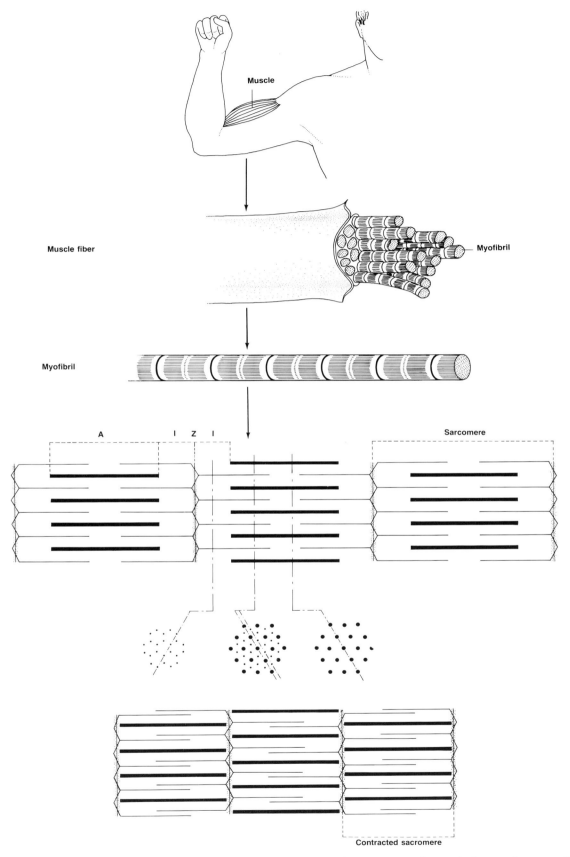

Fig. 7–1. Drawing of the microanatomy of muscle showing its levels of organization from whole muscle to myofilament.

mic reticulum called the *sarcoplasmic reticulum.* Each myofibril runs from one end of the muscle fiber to the other and is periodically subdivided along its length into contractile units called *sarcomeres.* Each sarcomere measures about 2.5 μm in length and consists of an orderly array of *actin* and *myosin filaments.* The actin and myosin filaments, called *myofilaments,* are carefully arranged so they can slide over one another during the process of muscle contraction. The ends of each sarcomere are capped by *Z-bands* (also called Z-lines or Z-disks). Actin filaments insert into the material of the Z-bands. Myosin filaments lie between the actin filaments and physically interact with them via tiny myosin cross-bridges—the ATPase-containing heads of the *heavy meromyosin* portion of the myosin molecule. Under appropriate conditions of neuronal stimulation, portions of the sarcoplasmic reticulum release calcium ions, which promote local hydrolysis of ATP, causing the myosin cross-bridges to move and thus forcing the actin filaments to slide over the myosin filaments. The actin filaments attached to the Z-bands at the opposite ends of the sarcomere draw the Z-bands close to one another, thus shortening the length of the sarcomere and of the muscle fiber itself.

Cardiac Muscle

Like skeletal muscle, cardiac muscle is made up of fibers composed of many parallel myofibrils. Each myofibril is constructed of a series of sacromeres aligned end to end along its length. Cardiac muscle fibers, however, are significantly different from skeletal muscle fibers in several important ways. First, cardiac muscle fibers are much smaller than skeletal muscle fibers and contain only 1 or 2 nuclei (as opposed to 100 to 1000 nuclei in a skeletal muscle fiber). Second, cardiac muscle fibers are branched. The branches of one cardiac muscle fiber attach to the branches of neighboring cardiac muscle fibers by highly specialized intercellular junctions called *intercalated disks.*

Smooth Muscle

Smooth muscle, as its name suggests, is devoid of the obvious striations observed in skeletal and cardiac muscle. Smooth muscle cells, or fibers, are small and mononucleate. Their contractile apparatus consists of actin and myosin filaments, but the myofilaments are not organized into sarcomeres; neither is the cytoplasm of smooth muscle fibers subdivided into myofibrils. Although the precise organization of the myofilaments (and hence the mechanism of contraction) is not yet fully understood in smooth muscle, it is certain that actin and myosin are present and do interact to effect significant changes in length of the smooth muscle fiber.

Plate 7–1

The Skeletal Muscle Fiber

Plate 7–1

The Skeletal Muscle Fiber

Human beings are capable of a wide range of movements, from the powerful movements of a weightlifter hoisting a barbell to the delicate finger movements of an eye surgeon performing a corneal transplant. Skeletal muscles power these voluntary movements. Whether the voluntary movements involve large muscles, like the thigh muscles of the weightlifter, or tiny muscles, like the finger muscles of the eye surgeon, the same unit of function, the skeletal muscle fiber, is responsible for voluntary movements. Taken together, all of the skeletal muscle fibers constitute approximately one half of a person's total body mass.

Each skeletal muscle fiber is actually a single cell—a huge, cylindric, multinucleate cell, quite different from any reviewed so far. Whereas most cells measure some 20 μm in diameter and have but a single nucleus, a typical skeletal muscle fiber may measure 100 μm in diameter and up to 30 cm in length and may contain several thousand nuclei. A single cell can be that large because of its genesis in the early embryo, in which each skeletal muscle fiber forms as a syncytium, a cell with many nuclei that is surrounded by a single plasma membrane.

The multinucleate nature of the muscle fiber takes its origin in early development, in which many embryonic muscle cells, called *myoblasts,* line up end to end to form long, thin *myotubes.* At a given time, the plasma membranes that separate adjacent myoblasts along the length of the tube fuse, and the cells become surrounded by a single membrane and thus take the form of a true syncytium.

Portions of several mature human skeletal muscle fibers, labeled F1 and F2, are illustrated in the matched pair of light and electron micrographs at right. Here, the perimeter of one muscle fiber (F2) is indicated by dotted lines. (Their ends, however, cannot be shown; skeletal muscle fibers, measuring several centimeters in length, are far too long to fit into one field of view.) The space between adjacent muscle fibers (arrow) is filled with a thin layer of connective tissue that envelops each muscle fiber. This connective tissue envelope, called the *endomysium,* surrounds the plasma membrane of the muscle cell, the sarcolemma. The sarcolemma is an excitable membrane; it can conduct electrical excitation, brought in by a nerve fiber, all over the surface of the muscle fiber. This conduction, as we shall see, is central to the control of the process of muscle contraction.

When viewed with the light microscope, as in Figure A, one of the most prominent features of skeletal muscle is manifest in the periodic striations along its length. The nature of these striations is clarified by electron microscopy in Figure B. The striations reflect the orderly arrangement of protein filaments called myofilaments that fill the cytoplasm of the muscle fiber. These myofilaments are composed largely of two proteins: actin and myosin. Traditionally—and erroneously—referred to as contractile proteins, actin and myosin are organized in a highly specific manner into contractile units, myofibrils. Myofibrils, in turn, are composed of units of function, sarcomeres. The structure and function of the sarcomere, described in the overview, is illustrated in Plate 7–2.

Most cells are capable of cytoplasmic movements of one sort or another. Many of these movements involve interactions between actin and myosin. In most cells, however, the actomyosin complexes are diffuse and do not form the most conspicuous part of the cell. In skeletal muscle, the reverse is true. A tremendous hypertrophy of the actomyosin system has taken place, and virtually all of the cytoplasmic volume is occupied by these contractile proteins. Even the nuclei (N), central and prominent in most cells, are pushed off to the side in skeletal muscle fibers. Mitochondria, however, are plentiful, and modifications of the endoplasmic reticulum are abundant. These will be shown at higher magnification later in this chapter.

Figures A and B. Matched pair of light and electron micrographs of serial longitudinal sections taken through the sternocleidomastoid muscles of the neck of an adult man. F1, F2, individual skeletal muscle fibers; N, peripherally located nucleus; dotted lines, perimeter of muscle fiber, F2; arrows, endomysium. Figure A, 2,350 X; Figure B, 2,800 X

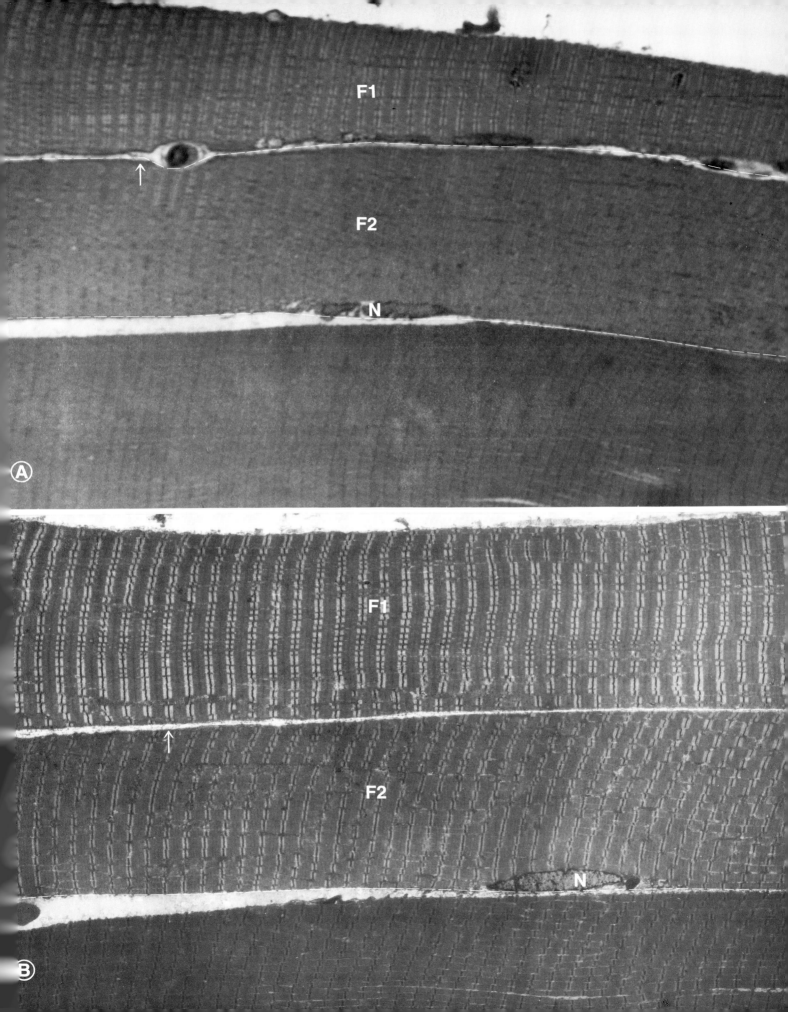

Plate 7–2

Skeletal Muscle: The Sarcomere

The sarcomere is the fundamental unit of contraction of the skeletal muscle fiber. In order to clearly understand the nature of the sarcomere, it is important first to understand the nature of the myofibril, in which the sarcomeres are aligned. A single skeletal muscle fiber consists of many myofibrils packed together in parallel, much like a jar filled with straws (Figure 7-1). Each long, thin, cylindric myofibril runs the entire length of the muscle fiber, separated from adjacent myofibrils by a system of membranes called the sarcoplasmic reticulum. A myofibril consists of a series of sarcomeres lined up end to end along the length of the myofibril. Figure A, a longitudinal section through a human skeletal muscle fiber, contains many myofibrils side by side; one myofibril is outlined by a dotted line. Many dark transverse Z-bands, which mark the ends of the sarcomeres, are arranged periodically along its length. Several sarcomeres are shown at high magnification in Figure B. Here, the Z-band (Z) appears as a somewhat amorphous, electron-dense structure. Next to the Z-band is the I-band (I), which contains actin filaments. Between the I-bands is the A-band (A), a dense region of the sarcomere that contains both actin and myosin filaments. (To get a better impression of the arrangement of actin and myosin filaments, see Figure C, a cross section through the A-band). In the center of the A-band is a somewhat less dense region called the H-zone. As shown in Figure 7-1, each sarcomere shortens during muscle contraction. This shortening is accomplished by the relative sliding of actin and myosin filaments over one another. When the actin filaments (in the I-band) and the myosin filaments (in the A-band) slide over one another, the Z-bands are drawn closer together, the sarcomere actively de-creases in length, and, as a result of collective sarcomere action, the whole muscle fiber shortens.

A sarcomere in a partially contracted state is shown in Figure D; note that the I-bands (I) have all but disappeared. A corduroy-like pattern is evident in the A-band (A). This pattern reflects the presence of cross-bridges between the thin actin filaments and the thick myosin filaments as they lie side by side in the A-band. These cross-bridges represent the movable part of the myosin molecules, which, in response to ATP, move back and forth in a ratchet-like fashion, producing the motive force for muscle contraction.

Two separate membrane systems are important in the control of muscle contraction: the sarcoplasmic reticulum and the *T-system.* As shown in Figure D, the terminal cisternae of the sarcoplasmic reticulum (SR) and a tubule of the T-system (T) are grouped together in a structure called the ***triad*** (dotted circle). Their structural grouping is functionally significant for several reasons. The terminal cisternae of the sarcoplasmic reticulum, which represent modifications of the smooth endoplasmic reticulum, can selectively take up and release calcium ion. Tubules of the T-system, which are invaginations of the sarcolemma (plasma membrane), can carry electrical excitation from the cell surface into the inner reaches of the muscle fiber. When a nerve stimulates a muscle, the electrical excitation travels inward along the T-system. The electron excitation causes the adjacent sarcoplasmic reticulum to release calcium, which triggers the process of muscle contraction by activating the ATPase on the myosin cross-bridges. ATP hydrolysis is followed by cross-bridge movement which, in turn, generates the force for muscle contraction.

Figure A. Longitudinal section through human skeletal muscle. N, nucleus of muscle fiber; Z, Z-band; dotted line, outline of single myofibril; brackets, limits of one sarcomere. 11,000 X

Figure B. Electron micrograph of sarcomeres within longitudinal section of relaxed human skeletal muscle. A, A-band; H, H-zone; I, I-band; M, mitochondrion; SR, sarcoplasmic reticulum; Z, Z-band. 35,500 X

Figure C. Cross section of myofibril of human skeletal muscle through A-band of sarcomere. A, A-band; SR, sarcoplasmic reticulum; dotted line, outline of single myofibril; arrow, "thick" (myosin) filament; arrowhead, "thin" (actin) filament. 84,000 X

Figure D. Longitudinal section through partially contracted sarcomere. A, A-band; I, shortened I-band; M, mitochondrion; SR, terminal cisterna of sarcoplasmic reticulum; T, tubule of T-system; Z, Z-band; dotted line encircles triad. 52,000 X

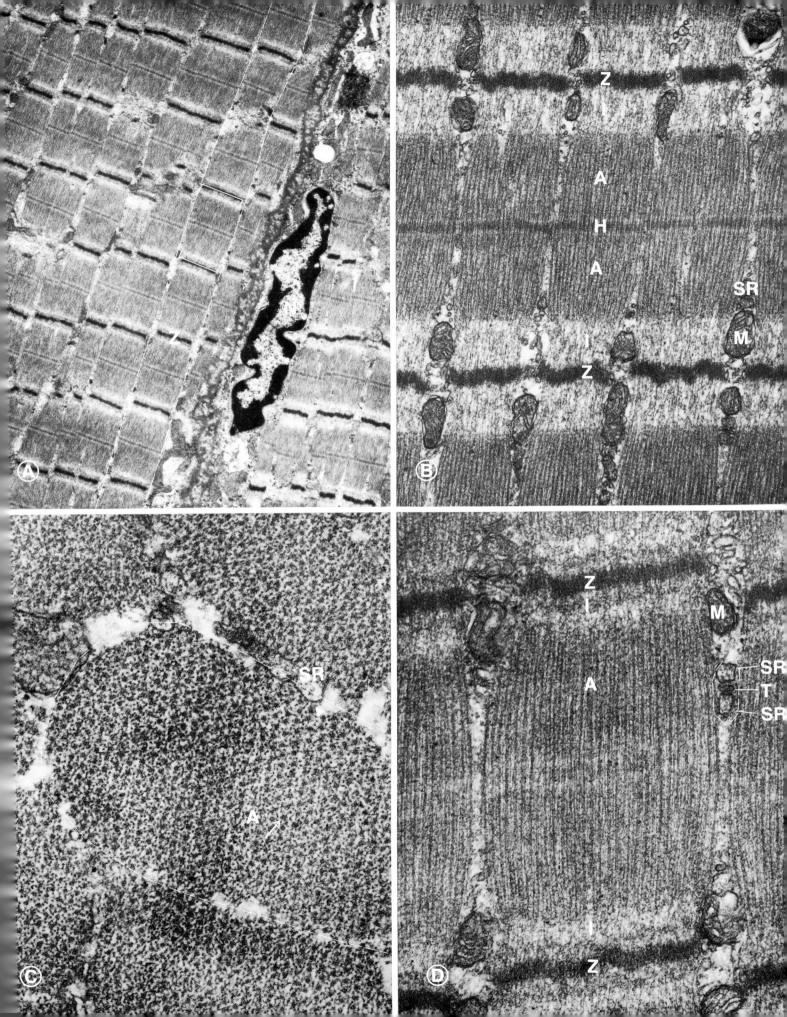

Plate 7–3

The Heart: Cardiac Muscle

The human heart is a powerful pump that propels blood to all parts of the body rapidly. During strenuous exercise, for example, the left ventricle of the heart is capable of pumping 12 gal/min into the aorta. This flow rate is greater than that of a garden hose turned on full. The tremendous pumping force of the heart is generated by a special kind of muscle called cardiac muscle. Cardiac muscle is similar to skeletal muscle in that it is striated, its fibers are organized into myofibrils, and the fundamental unit of contraction is the sarcomere. There are, however, many significant differences between cardiac and skeletal muscle, as seen in Figures A and B.

Figure A is a low-magnification electron micrograph of a cross section through the atrium of the heart of the squirrel monkey. The wall of the heart, like that of large blood vessels, consists of three distinct regions. The innermost region that lines the lumen (L) of the heart, the *endocardium* (EN), consists of a thin layer of endothelial cells and some loose connective tissue. Most of the mass of the heart is contained within the muscular *myocardium* (MYO). The outermost region of the wall of the heart is the *epicardium* (EPI), an envelope of dense connective tissue containing both collagenous and elastic fibers.

The contractile force of the myocardium is supplied by cardiac muscle fibers. Unlike the skeletal muscle fiber, which is a syncytium, each cardiac muscle fiber consists of a number of branched cardiac muscle cells aligned end to end. Consequently, each cardiac muscle cell—which measures around 100 μm in length and 15 μm in width—is much smaller than a typical skeletal muscle fiber. The size of a cardiac muscle cell is evident in Figure A, in which the lateral boundaries of a single cell are marked with a dotted line.

The details of cardiac muscle microanatomy are illustrated in Figure B, a higher magnification electron micrograph of the myocardium of the monkey heart. Here, as in Figure A, the lateral boundaries of a single cardiac muscle cell are indicated by a dotted line. Within this cell, several longitudinally oriented myofibrils (MF) are marked by brackets. As in skeletal muscle, each myofibril consists of a series of contractile units, or sarcomeres, aligned end to end. Numerous mitochondria (M) are present between adjacent myofibrils. These large, abundant mitochondria supply the ATP essential for muscle contraction, which, in cardiac muscle, must occur many times per minute for life to go on.

One of the most interesting features of cardiac muscle is the specialized junctions—the intercalated disks—by which cardiac muscle cells contact and adhere to one another. As mentioned previously cardiac muscle cells are branched. The branches of one cardiac muscle cell join the branches of another muscle cell in such a way that the cells are linked end to end. The intercalated disk (ID), a dense line, is evident where the branches meet, as illustrated in Figure B. It performs several important functions. First, it acts as an adhesive structure that holds together the tips of abutting branches of adjacent cardiac muscle cells, thus preventing them from being pulled apart when the muscle fiber contracts. Second, it provides for electrical continuity between adjacent cardiac muscle cells; that is, ionic currents may pass freely from one cell to another through specialized regions within the intercalated disk.

The intercalated disk is capable of performing several functions because it contains several different kinds of intercellular junctions. Intermediate junctions perform an adhesive function. Gap junctions allow certain ions to pass, providing electrical continuity between adjacent cells. Desmosomes act as "spot welds," also serving to hold the adjacent cells together. Taken together, the intercalated disks allow the individual cells within a cardiac muscle fiber to act together as if they were a syncytium.

Figure A. Electron micrograph of cross section through the atrium of the squirrel monkey heart. CT, connective tissue; EN, endocardium; EPI, epicardium; L, lumen of atrium; MYO, myocardium; dotted line, outline of individual cardiac muscle cell. 2,800 X

Figure B. Longitudinal section through portions of several cardiac muscle fibers. A, A-band; Co, collagen fibrils; I, I-band; ID, intercalated disk; M, mitochondria; MF, myofibril; Z, Z-line; dotted line, outline of individual cardiac muscle cell. 16,000 X

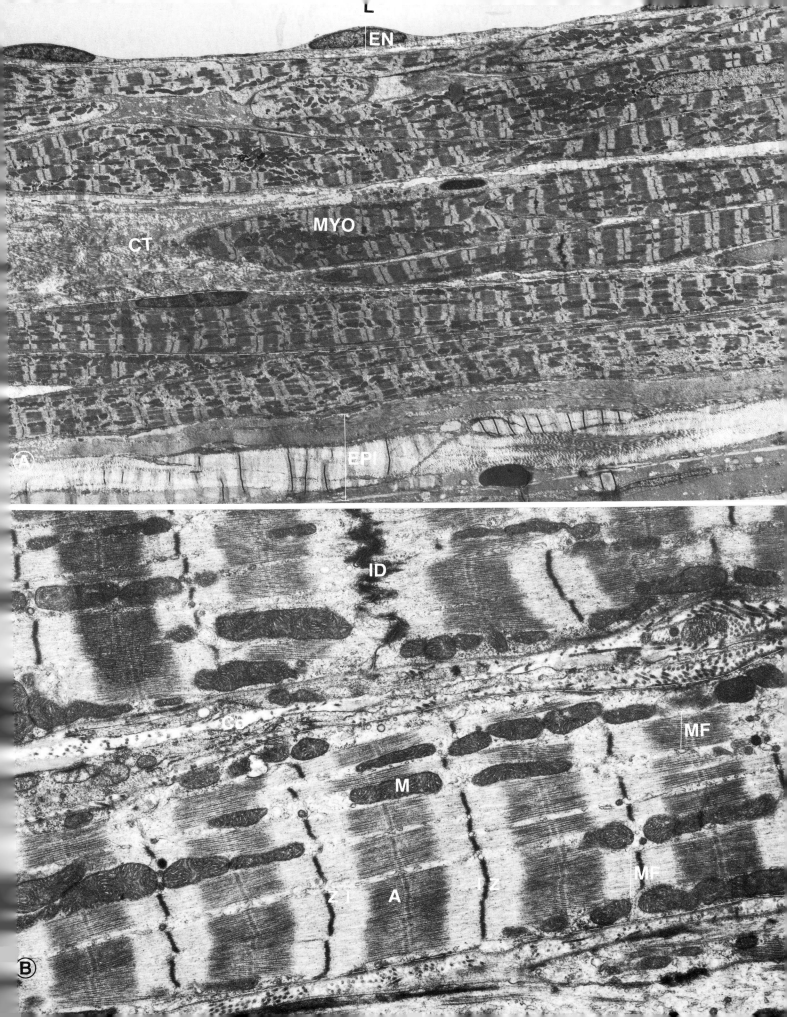

Plate 7–4

Smooth Muscle

Smooth muscle is quite different in structure and function from skeletal and cardiac muscle in several important respects. When viewed with the light or electron microscope, smooth muscle displays no striations. A given smooth muscle fiber is quite small (averaging some 5 to 10 μm in width and 20 to 200 μm in length), tends to contract rather slowly, and has only one centrally located nucleus. Instead of being associated with the voluntary movements of the outer body, as is skeletal muscle, or with the rhythmic contractions of the heart, as is cardiac muscle, smooth muscle tends to be associated with the involuntary movements of the viscera, respiratory system, and circulatory system.

In the alimentary canal, for example, smooth muscle is responsible for the *peristaltic* movements that propel food on its course as it undergoes the process of digestion. The position of smooth muscle within the wall of the intestine is illustrated by light microscopy in Figure A. Here, the smooth muscle fibers are organized into two distinct sheets running at right angles. The inner circular layer of smooth muscle is shown in cross section (XS); the outer longitudinal layer is shown in long section (LS). Since each smooth muscle fiber is fusiform, or spindle-shaped, it will look more or less circular when cut in cross section and long and thin when cut lengthwise. This difference is more clearly shown in Figure B, an electron micrograph of a serial section cut from the same specimen depicted in Figure A. Here, each smooth muscle fiber is surrounded by connective tissue (CT) that serves to bind the individual fibers into a functional sheet of smooth muscle tissue. In this field of view, small autonomic nerves (N) that innervate the smooth muscle are evident, as are blood capillaries (C) and lymph capillaries (LC).

Portions of several smooth muscle fibers are shown at higher magnification by electron microscopy in Figures C and D. Figure C, a longitudinal section, shows the centrally located nucleus (N) surrounded by cytoplasm that contains many fine filaments. These filaments, called myofilaments, resemble the thin actin filaments observed in skeletal and cardiac muscle. A glance at Figure C shows at once that smooth muscle is not organized neatly into sarcomeres. Although many studies have revealed the presence of both actin and myosin within smooth muscle, the precise relative arrangement of actin and myosin within the smooth muscle fiber awaits discovery.

Figure D is a cross section of a single smooth muscle fiber taken through the center of the cell at the level of the nucleus (N). The nucleus is folded upon itself, suggesting that the cell was fixed in the contracted state. The thin filaments, presumably made of actin, are evident everywhere. A few thick filaments, which may represent myosin, are detectable. At the periphery of the cell, a number of dense bodies (D) are intimately associated with the plasma membrane. Many workers in the field think that these dense bodies provide attachment sites for the myofilaments. During the process of smooth muscle contraction, the myofilaments pull against these dense bodies. Because the dense bodies are attached to the plasma membrane, the cell shortens. When the cell contracts, a number of pits, called *caveolae* (arrows), become evident at the cell surface. Outside of the plasma membrane, the smooth muscle fiber is covered by a glycoprotein coat similar to the basement membrane (*) that is closely associated with fine collagen fibrils (Co).

Figures A and B. Light and electron micrographs of smooth muscle in the wall of the small intestine of the macaque. C, capillary; CT, connective tissue; LC, lymphatic capillary (Figure B only); LS, smooth muscle in longitudinal section; N, nerve; XS, smooth muscle in cross section; Figure A, 710 X; Figure B, 1,300 X
Figure C. Longitudinal section through several smooth muscle fibers. N, nucleus. 16,000 X
Figure D. Cross section through one smooth muscle fiber. Co, collagen fibrils; D, dense body; N, nucleus; arrows, caveolae; *, basement membrane. 22,500 X

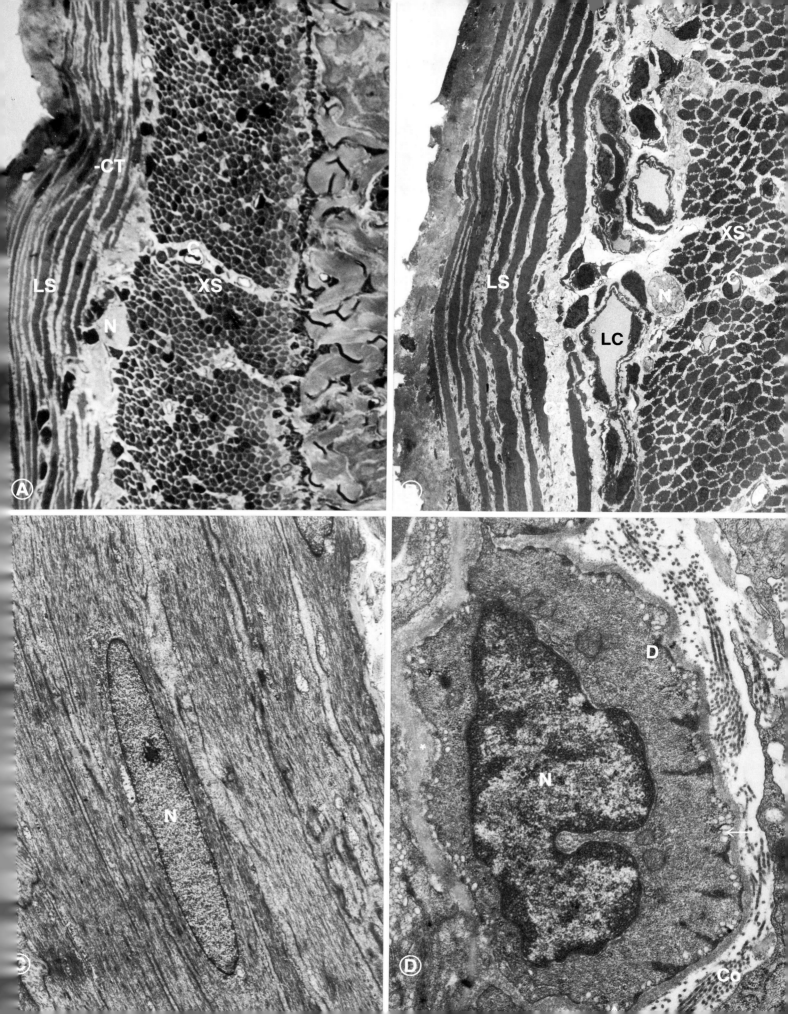

8

Nerves

Overview

The latest estimates place the number of nerve cells in the human nervous system at *100 billion.* (The number of nerve cells in the nervous system is similar to the number of stars in our galaxy). In addition, each nerve cell can receive input from 1000 other nerve cells and send information to up to 1000 nerve cells. The tremendous complexity of the nervous system raises a question that puzzles neurobiologists of a philosophical bent: can the brain ever understand itself?

We cannot now understand the nervous system; it is too complex, and we don't know enough about it to explain basic phenomena, such as what a thought is, or how memory works. Nevertheless, great strides have been made in our understanding of the nervous system within the past century. We do, for instance, know a great deal about the structure and function of individual nerve cells.

The nerve cell, or *neuron,* is the functional unit of the nervous system. Neurons are concerned with information transfer. There are three basic phases of information transfer in which neurons participate. First, they receive inputs from the environment, other neurons, or both. Second, they transmit information from one point in space to another. Third, they integrate and process information. Because neurons located in different places within the nervous system vary in structure, it is difficult to pinpoint a "typical" neuron. Nevertheless, some structural features that are common to

many neurons allow us to make some general statements about "the nerve cell." Figure 8-1 is a simplified drawing of a *motor neuron,* a nerve cell that causes a muscle to contract. The motor neuron has a large cell body, or *soma,* in which the nucleus resides. The cytoplasm around the nucleus is often called the *perikaryon.* The cell body gives rise to a very long and slender cylindric cytoplasmic extension, the *axon,* that goes from the cell body to the muscle fibers innervated by the motor neuron. The axon may branch along its length, and each branch may have many functional endings that connect with many muscle fibers.

The point at which the axon makes functional contact with the muscle fiber is called the *motor end plate,* or the *myoneural junction.* Information travels along the axon to the muscle fiber in the form of an action potential, a kind of electrical excitation that does not decrease in strength with distance. The action potential originates at the initial segment of the axon as a result of electrical excitation the motor neuron receives from other nerves. These signals are received by the *dendrites* and cell body of the motor neuron. The dendritic tree is a vast system of branched cytoplasmic extensions that bring information from other neurons into the motor neuron itself. The motor neuron, then, has dendrites that serve as the input stage, a cell body that is a receiving and integrating center, and an axon that carries information away from the cell body to the "target" cells of the

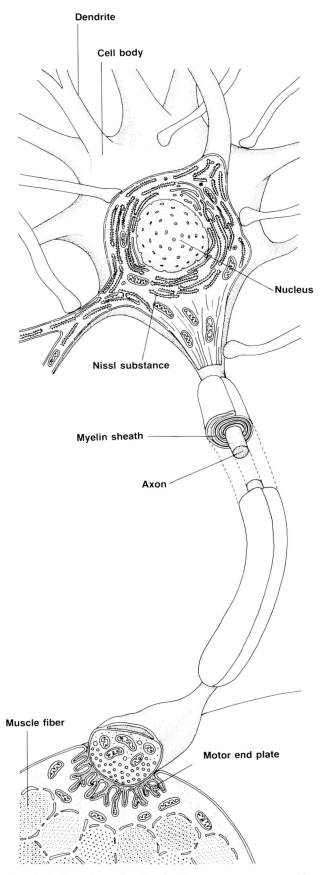

Dendrite

Cell body

Nucleus

Nissl substance

Myelin sheath

Axon

Muscle fiber

Motor end plate

motor neuron—the muscle fibers with which it makes functional connections.

The *nervous system* is a giant, integrated communications network. For simplicity, neurobiologists have subdivided the nervous system into several categories, which, being artificial, overlap biologically. The nervous system is commonly subdivided into three major categories: the *central nervous system,* the *peripheral nervous system,* and the *autonomic nervous system.* The central nervous system is that part of the nervous system consisting of the brain and spinal cord. The peripheral nervous system is that part of the nervous system consisting of the nerves *outside* the brain and spinal cord. The autonomic nervous system, which is subdivided into the *sympathetic* and *parasympathetic* nervous systems, is that part of the nervous system that participates in the regulation of the activity of smooth muscle, cardiac muscle, and glands. The overlap between the central, peripheral, and autonomic nervous systems underlies the operation of an integrated nervous system. Consider, for example, a motor neuron that innervates a runner's gastrocnemius (calf) muscle. The cell body of that neuron is in the spinal cord and hence is in the central nervous system. Its axon, which leaves the spinal cord and travels to the gastrocnemius in a large nerve trunk, is in the peripheral nervous system.

In addition to neurons, the nervous system contains supporting cells called *neuroglia,* also known as glia or glial cells. Just as there is a variety of nerve cells, so is there a variety of glial cells. One example of a glial cell is the *Schwann cell*—the cell that generates the *myelin sheath* that covers many large axons in the peripheral nervous system. Another example of a glial cell is the *oligodendrocyte* which generates the myelin sheath of some axons within the central nervous system. In general, nerve cells cannot exist without glia, and they die very quickly without their support. A related distinguishing feature of nerve cells in the human nervous system is that nerve cells are a static cell population. Unlike epithelial cells, they do not turn over during the life of the individual. Once the cell body of a neuron dies, it is lost for all time, and cannot be replaced by mitotic activity of other cells. (There is one known

FIG. 8–1. Drawing of a ''typical'' motor neuron, not drawn to scale, showing its major component parts.

exception to this rule; olfactory receptor neurons, described in Chapter 20, *do* turn over during life, and lost cells can be replaced by mitotic activity of basal cells). Consequently, neuronal degeneration can have disastrous effects. In the crippling disease poliomyelitis, for example, the polio virus takes residence in the cell bodies of motor neurons within the ventral horn of the spinal cord. If the viruses kill the cell body, the motor neuron dies, its axon degenerates, and the individual can no longer move the muscle fibers originally innervated by the destroyed neurons. The severity of the ensuing paralysis depends upon the number and location of the infected motor neurons.

Given the complexity of the nervous system, the objective of this chapter is to present the microanatomy of several prototypes of major classes of nerve cells in order to facilitate their recognition and understanding in histological material. The chapter starts with the motor neuron described above and moves on to describe myelinated nerve fibers, unmyelinated nerve fibers, the myelin sheath, the synapse by which nerve cells communicate with one another, and ganglion cells of the autonomic nervous system. Careful study of the light and electron micrographs should greatly facilitate your recognition and understanding of nerves encountered in sectioned material.

Plate 8–1

The Motor Neuron

Plate 8–1

The Motor Neuron

The motor neuron, such as the one depicted at right, is one of the largest kinds of nerve cell in the nervous system. Motor neurons are important to proper body function because they are responsible for exciting the skeletal muscles that power our voluntary movements. Each motor neuron houses its cell body within the spinal cord. From there, it sends a long axon out into the periphery; the axon terminates by making synaptic contact with one or more skeletal muscle fibers. Take, for example, one of the motor neurons that innervates the muscles that move one of your toes. Its cell body, which measures some 50 μm in diameter, is in your spinal cord; its axon, some 3 m long, travels out of the spinal cord, down your leg, and into your foot to its point of contact with the specific muscle fibers it innervates. Consequently, the cell body is charged with the manufacture and maintenance of a vast amount of axoplasm. It is not surprising, then, that the cell body of the motor neuron contains much of the biosynthetic material essential for large-scale macromolecular synthesis.

Figures A and B at right are a matched pair of light and electron micrographs of serial sections taken through the ventral horn of the spinal cord, a region inhabited by many motor neurons. In this field, the same motor neuron is seen by light and electron microscopy. The large cell body, or soma, contains a round, centrally located, euchromatic nucleus (N) with a conspicuous nucleolus. In the light micrograph, the cell body contains a large quantity of highly basophilic material known as *Nissl substance* (Ni). Also called Nissl bodies, the basophilic material consists of the cytoplasmic machinery responsible for protein systhesis: the rough endoplasmic reticulum and a large number of free ribosomes. When viewed by electron microscopy (Figure B), the granular nature of the Nissl substance is evident even at this relatively low magnification. The granular appearance of the Nissl substance is created by the large population of ribosomes, which look like small dark dots in thin sections. Some large, electron-dense inclusions represent *lipofuscin granules* (L), often called "wear and tear granules," which are darkly pigmented, membrane-limited bodies that are secondary lysosomes filled with indigestible material sequestered from the rest of the cytoplasm. Since neurons are not replaced by mitotic activity, the number of lipofuscin granules within motor neurons tends to increase with age.

Although the geometry of the motor neuron is not evident in sectioned material (see Figure 8-1 for an illustration of a motor neuron), some of its cytoplasmic extensions are evident in the photomicrographs at right. A large dendrite (D) reaches out from the right side of the cell body. At the left of the cell body, one of many smaller incoming dendrites (D) may be seen. Surrounding the motor neuron are a number of components of the spinal cord, such as capillaries (C) and myelinated nerve fibers (NF).

Figures A and B. Matched pair of light and electron micrographs of serial thick and thin sections taken through the anterior (ventral) horn of the spinal cord. C, capillary; D, dendrite of motor neuron; L, lipofuscin granules; N, nucleus; NF, cross section through myelinated nerve fiber; Ni, Nissl substance; S, soma (cell body) of motor neuron. 2000 X

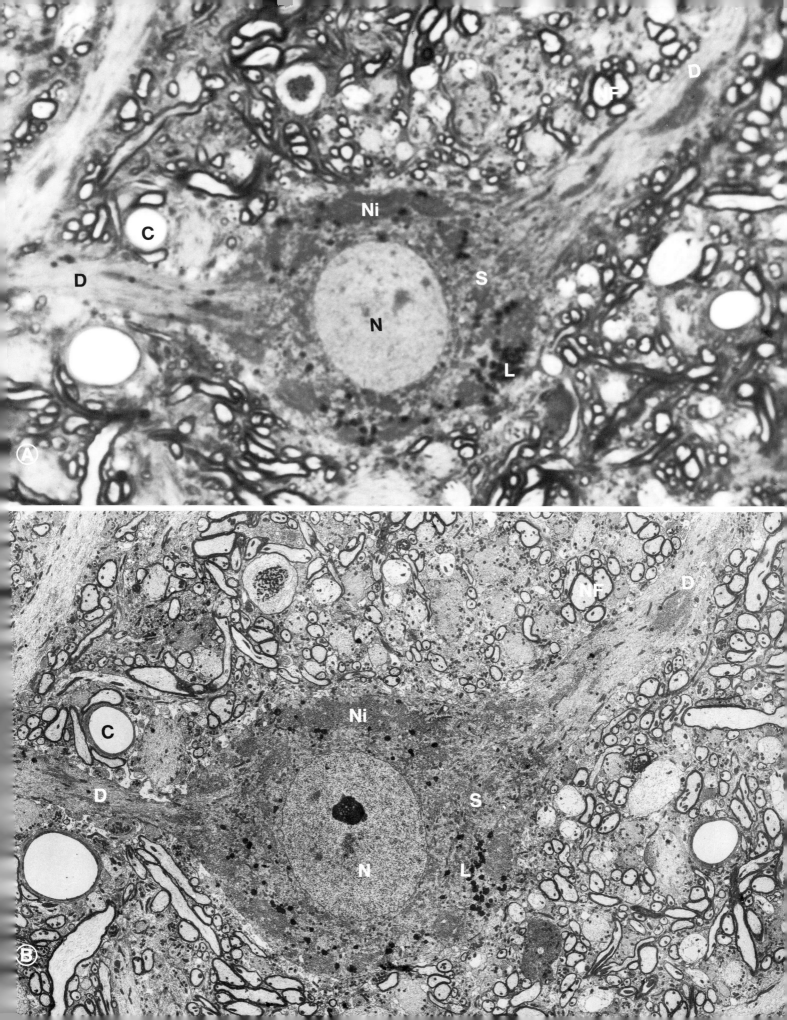

Plate 8–2

The Myelinated Nerve Fiber

As described in the previous plate, each motor neuron has an *axon* that extends from the nerve cell body to the axon's destination, a skeletal muscle fiber. Plate 8–2 is an electron micrograph of a longitudinal section taken through a group of large myelinated axons of motor neurons that course through a peripheral nerve. Because each axon is tubular, its profile, when cut in longitudinal section, resembles a soda straw split in half. In Plate 8–2, each axon (A) contains a core of pale axoplasm. The axoplasm contains many slender mitochondria (arrowhead) and is supported by cytoskeletal elements including microtubules and neurofilaments. The microtubules and neurofilaments, too small to be individually resolved at this magnification, appear as wispy strands. Each of these axons is covered by an electron-dense myelin sheath (M). The myelin sheath, composed of the compressed, spiral wrappings of the plasma membrane of a Schwann cell, acts as an electrical insulator. The nuclei (N) of several Schwann cells are evident near the top of the field of view. At the periphery of the myelin sheath, a thin layer of Schwann cell cytoplasm (∗) is visible.

At many points along the length of the myelin sheath are discontinuities in the myelin called **Schmidt-Lantermann clefts.** Their function is unknown. Other discontinuities in the myelin sheath, called the **nodes of Ranvier** (not shown here), are better understood. They represent gaps between the myelin sheaths laid down by Schwann cells that lie next to one another along the length of the axon. (If you were to firmly grasp a garden hose in both hands, the hose would represent the axon, each hand would represent a Schwann cell and the myelin sheath beneath it, and space between your hands spanned by the naked hose would represent a node of Ranvier.) The nodes of Ranvier, which may be spaced at 1-mm intervals from one another along a large axon, accelerate the rate at which the nerve impulse travels along the axon. Nerve impulses can travel rapidly. Large axons, such as those of motor neurons, can reach 30 μm in diameter and have a conduction velocity of 100 m/sec. In contrast, small axons, such as those of olfactory receptor neurons, may be as small as 0.1 μm in diameter and have a somewhat sluggish conduction velocity of 0.5 m/sec.

The relatively "empty" appearance of the axoplasm (A) is due largely to the absence of cytoplasmic organelles associated with protein synthesis. The axon has neither rough endoplasmic reticulum nor free ribosomes. Consequently, its protein must come from a distant source—the cell body. Protein synthesized in the Nissl substance within the nerve cell body travels down the axon by an active, energy-dependent process known as *axoplasmic transport.* Although rates of axoplasmic transport vary in different axons, and even within the same axon, a good average rate of transport observed in many axons is about 1 mm/day. The rate of regeneration of severed axons proceeds at the same rate—about 1 mm/day. Should the axon of a neuron be severed but its cell body and Schwann cell sheath remain intact, a new axon, derived from materials synthesized in the cell body, can grow down through the Schwann cell sheath and reestablish its original pattern of connection.

Electron micrograph of a longitudinal section through axons of motor neurons within a peripheral nerve. A, axon; CT, connective tissue of endoneurium; M, myelin sheath; N, nucleus of Schwann cell; ∗, cytoplasm of Schwann cell; arrow, Schmidt-Lantermann cleft; arrowhead, mitochondrion in axoplasm. 1,400 X

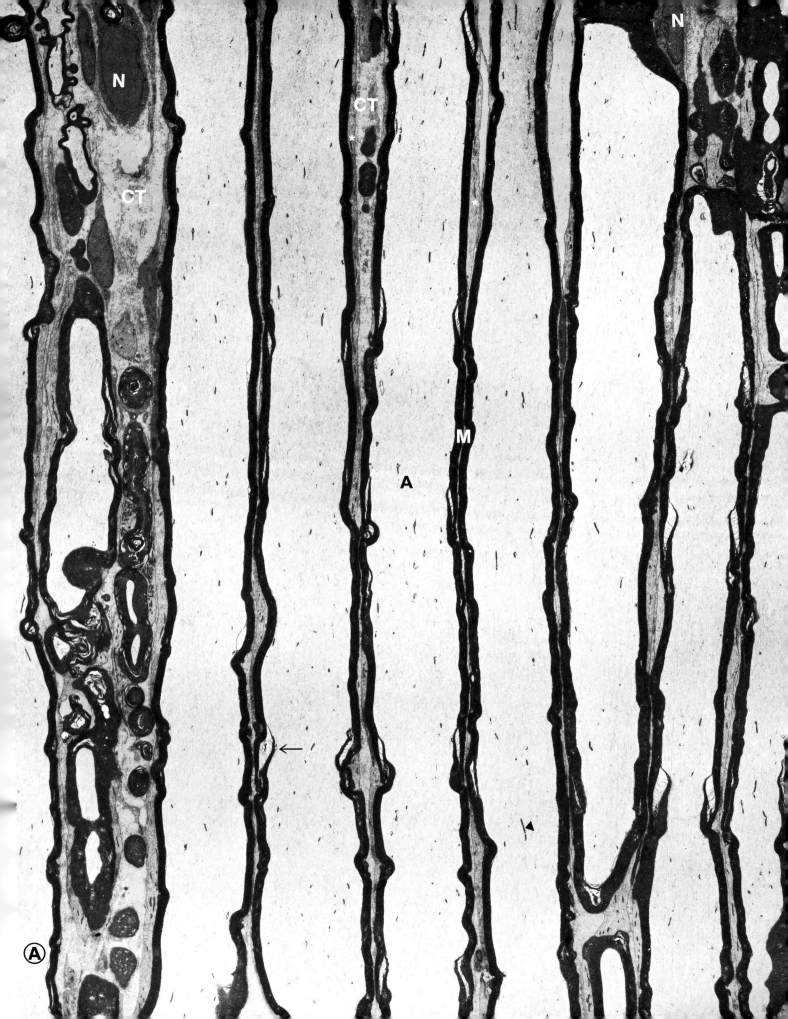

Plate 8–3

The Unmyelinated Nerve Fiber

As described in the overview to this chapter, the term "nerve fiber" commonly refers to a single axon and its sheath. Plate 8–2 showed the myelinated nerve fiber. Plate 8–3 shows the unmyelinated nerve fiber. An unmyelinated nerve fiber, as its name indicates, does not have a myelin sheath; its sheath, in the case of a peripheral nerve, consists of a Schwann cell and its basement membrane.

The plate at right is an electron micrograph of a cross section taken through a small peripheral nerve found in the spermatic cord of the squirrel monkey. Much can be learned from close study of this micrograph, since it contains a variety of permutations and combinations of axons and their sheaths. At lower left in the field, for example, a cross-sectional image of a small myelinated axon (M) is evident. Here, the Schwann cell responsible for the formation of the myelin sheath has been cut at the level of its nucleus (N'). Note that a single Schwann cell typically ensheathes a single axon in the peripheral nervous system. At the top of the field, an axon undergoing myelination is visible (AM). Here again, a single Schwann cell is associated with a single axon. The remainder of the field, however, is filled with unmyelinated axons. In some cases, a single unmyelinated axon is encased within the cytoplasm of a single Schwann cell (A). In other cases, many unmyelinated axons are surrounded by the cytoplasm of one Schwann cell. In the nerve bundle labeled A', for example, 15 unmyelinated axons are invested by one Schwann cell. A more striking example is evident at far left within the plate; a bundle of unmyelinated axons are arranged radially at the periphery of a small nerve bundle, in the center of which sits the large nucleus (N) of a Schwann cell.

All of the nerve fibers within this small peripheral nerve are surrounded by a delicate support system of loose connective tissue fibrils (CT) that comprise the *endoneurium.* The connective tissue of the endoneurium is elaborated by a small number of fibroblasts, one of which (F) is present in the center of the field of view. The perimeter of the peripheral nerve is, in this case, defined by a sheath called the *perineurium* (P), which consists of cells and connective tissue. Large peripheral nerves are surrounded by a thicker sheath called the *epineurium.* Small peripheral nerves such as the one shown here, however, do not have an epineurium and are protected by a perineurial sheath alone.

Electron micrograph of a cross section taken through a small peripheral nerve in the spermatic cord of the squirrel monkey. A, single unmyelinated axon in Schwann cell sheath; A', group of unmyelinated axons ensheathed by a single Schwann cell; AM, axon undergoing the process of myelination; CT, connective tissue fibrils of the endoneurium; F, fibroblast; M, myelinated axon; N, nucleus of Schwann cell that invests many unmyelinated axons; N', nucleus of Schwann cell that ensheathes one myelinated axon; P, perineurium. 17,600 X

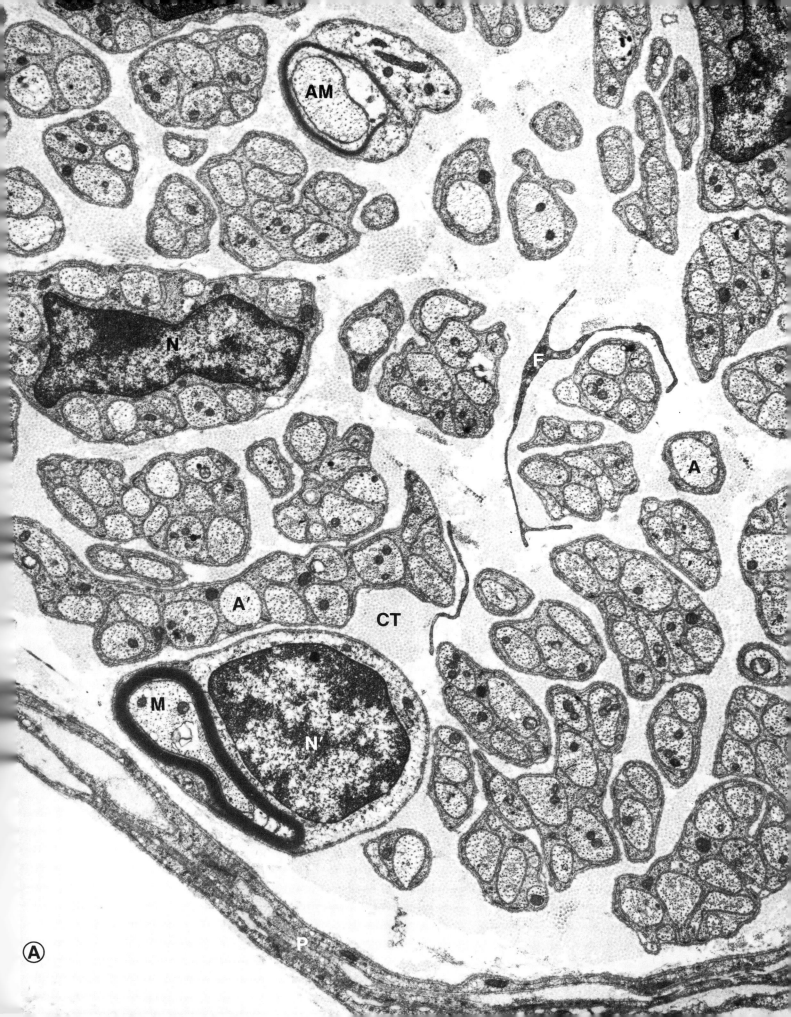

Plate 8–4

The Myelin Sheath And The Synapse

Two important components of the nervous system—the myelin sheath that surrounds many axons and the *synapse* that provides a mechanism for communication of excitation between neurons—are illustrated by electron microscopy in Figures A and B at right. Figure A is a cross section taken through a small myelinated axon found within the spinal cord. The axon itself (A) contains a mitochondrion (M), a few microtubules (Mt), and many neurofilaments (Nf). In addition to providing cytoskeletal support to the axon, the microtubules and neurofilaments are believed to participate in the process of axoplasmic transport described in Plate 8–2. The cell membrane of the axon (arrow) is surrounded by a myelin sheath (MS), which when examined closely has a laminated appearance. The layers of the myelin sheath consist of tight, spiral wrappings of the plasma membrane of the Schwann cell that surrounds the axon. During the process of myelination, the Schwann cell spins around the axon and wraps it with layers of its plasma membrane, much as a spider wraps up a fly in its web. With each successive revolution of the Schwann cell, the cytoplasm is squeezed out from between the neighboring layers of cell membrane. The result of these complex maneuvers, the myelin sheath, is an effective electrical insulator that isolates the activities of large axons.

Whereas the myelin sheath is an electrical insulator, the synapse is just the opposite: it is the site of the communication of excitation between nerve cells. Figure B is an electron micrograph of an unusual situation in which four axons (A1, A2, A3, and A4) are making synaptic contact with a single dendrite (D). In this image, part of the dendrite is sandwiched in between the adjacent axon terminals, forming a series of crests of dendritic cytoplasm (C). At the right side of the field, a single crest of dendritic cytoplasm makes synaptic contact with two separate axon terminals (A3, A4). Here, the fine structure of the synapse is apparent. At the point of synaptic contact between axon and dendrite, the space between adjacent cell membranes is expanded to form the *synaptic cleft.* A number of *synaptic vesicles* (SV), filled with *neurotransmitter* material, are clustered within the axon terminal near the synaptic cleft. When the axon is electrically stimulated—that is, when an action potential arrives at the axon terminal—some of the membrane-limited synaptic vesicles fuse with the axon cell membrane and liberate their contained neurotransmitter into the synaptic cleft. The liberated neurotransmitter alters the electrical properties of the postsynaptic dendrite cell membrane, thereby either exciting or inhibiting the dendrite. In this way, neurons can "speak" to one another via chemical synapses.

Not all synapses are chemical; some are electrical, centering their function around the *gap junction,* or *nexus.* The gap junction permits certain ions to flow between adjacent cells. Since currents in nerves are carried by ions in solution, ionic continuity between cells creates electrical continuity between cells. Although electrical synapses are common, they are outnumbered by chemical synapses.

Figure A. Electron micrograph of a cross section taken through a small myelinated axon in the spinal cord. A, axon; MS, myelin sheath; M, mitochondrion; Mt, microtubule; Nf, neurofilament; SV, synaptic vesicle in nearby nerve terminal; arrow, plasma membrane of axon; arrowhead, mesaxon (point at which cell membrane folds upon itself) of Schwann cell. 68,000 X

Figure B. Electron micrograph of a series of synapses in the brain. A1, A2, A3, and A4, separate synaptic endings, each from a different axon; C, crest of dendrite cytoplasm; D, dendrite; M, mitochondrion; Mt, microtubule; S, synapse; SC, synaptic cleft; SV, synaptic vesicle. (Micrograph of "crest" synapse courtesy of Dr. Tom Mehalick.) 57,500 X

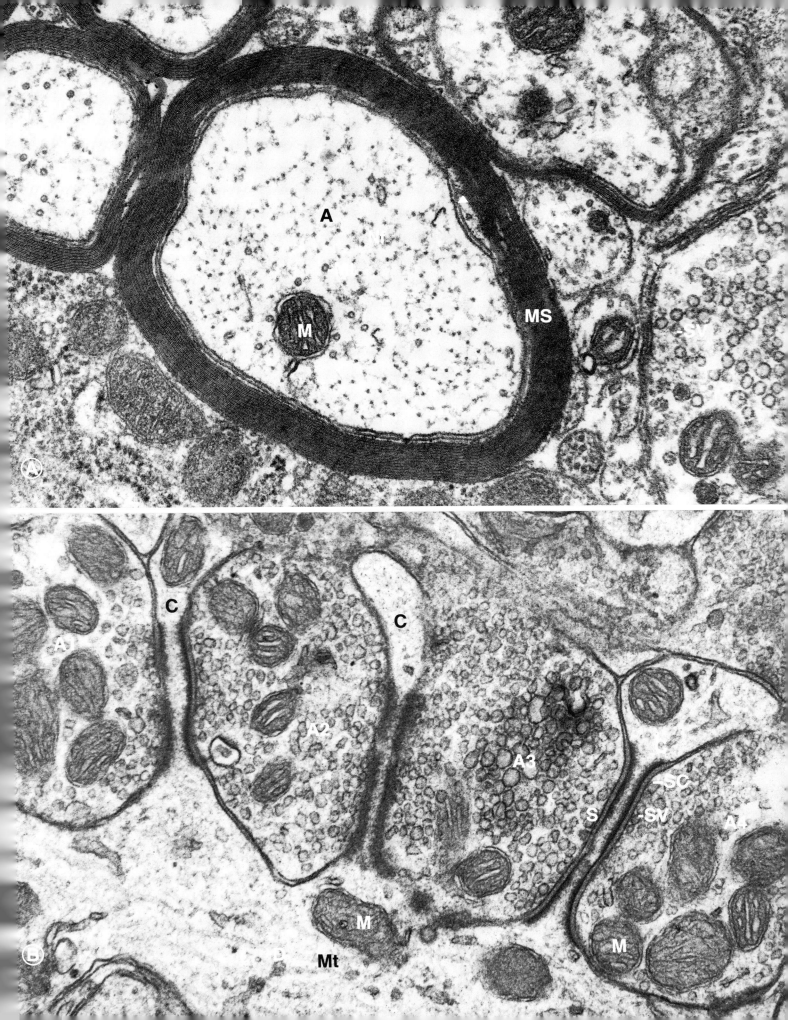

Plate 8–5

Ganglion Cells Of The Autonomic Nervous System

The autonomic nervous system consists of motor neurons that participate in the regulation of a variety of "involuntary" visceral activities. Whereas the motor neurons of the peripheral nervous system innervate skeletal muscle fibers that power voluntary movements, the motor neurons of the autonomic nervous system innervate smooth muscle fibers that power involuntary movements of such structures as the gut, blood vessels, and sweat glands. In addition, the myoepithelial cells associated with glands such as the salivary glands are regulated by motor neurons of the autonomic nervous system.

The autonomic nervous system is not a system unto itself; despite its name, it does not act autonomously. Instead, its functions and its neurons are closely tied to the central and peripheral nervous systems. Many of the cell bodies of autonomic neurons reside within the central nervous system. Whereas the motor neurons of the peripheral nervous system are arranged so that one motor neuron, with its cell body in the spinal cord, transmits activity to a particular muscle, the autonomic nervous system employs two motor neurons arranged in series. The first neuron, located in the brain or spinal cord, sends its axon out and makes contact with the second neuron in the series, which is usually located in a ganglion or plexus close to the structure whose activity it mediates. An example of the second neuron in the series, often called an autonomic *ganglion cell*, is illustrated at right.

Figure A is a light micrograph of a section taken through the submaxillary ganglion in the vicinity of the salivary glands. Here, the ganglion cells are seen to be large cells with round, pale nuclei (N). In autonomic ganglion cells, the prominent nucleolus (Nu) is often placed off center. The cytoplasm, or perikaryon, has an abundance of Nissl substance (NS) that makes the ganglion cells appear more dense than the nerve fibers (NF) that course past them. In the connective tissue (CT) surrounding the ganglion, a capillary (C) is evident, as are several mast cells (M).

The same ganglion cells are seen in greater detail in the electron micrograph in Figure B. This photomicrograph was taken of a serial thin section cut adjacent to the thick section depicted in Figure A. Here, the large, round nucleus (N) of the ganglion cells is mostly euchromatic; a thin ring of heterochromatin is closely applied to the inner margin of the nuclear envelope. In this image, the Nissl substance, which appeared as dense, amorphous material by light microscopy (Figure A), consists of cisternae of the rough endoplasmic reticulum (RER) interspersed with thousands of free ribosomes (R). The nerve fibers (NF) that run around the ganglion cells are small, unmyelinated fibers. Their small size becomes apparent when you notice that most of them are dwarfed by the nuclei of the Schwann cells (SN) that ensheath them. Small, unmyelinated nerve fibers are often difficult to identify by light microscopy. Comparison of light and electron micrographs of the same bundles of small nerves, such as those depicted in Figures A and B, can facilitate the recognition of small unmyelinated nerves in histological sections.

Figure A. Light micrograph of the submandibular ganglion of the rat. C, capillary; CT, connective tissue; M, mast cell; N, nucleus of autonomic ganglion cell motor neuron; NF, nerve fibers; NS, Nissl substance; Nu, eccentrically placed nucleolus in ganglion cell nucleus; SN, Schwann cell nucleus. 2,500 X

Figure B. Electron micrograph of serial thin section taken through the same ganglion cells shown in Figure A. CT, connective tissue; N, nucleus of autonomic ganglion cell; NF, nerve fibers; R, free ribosomes; RER, rough endoplasmic reticulum; SN, Schwann cell nucleus. 4,000 X

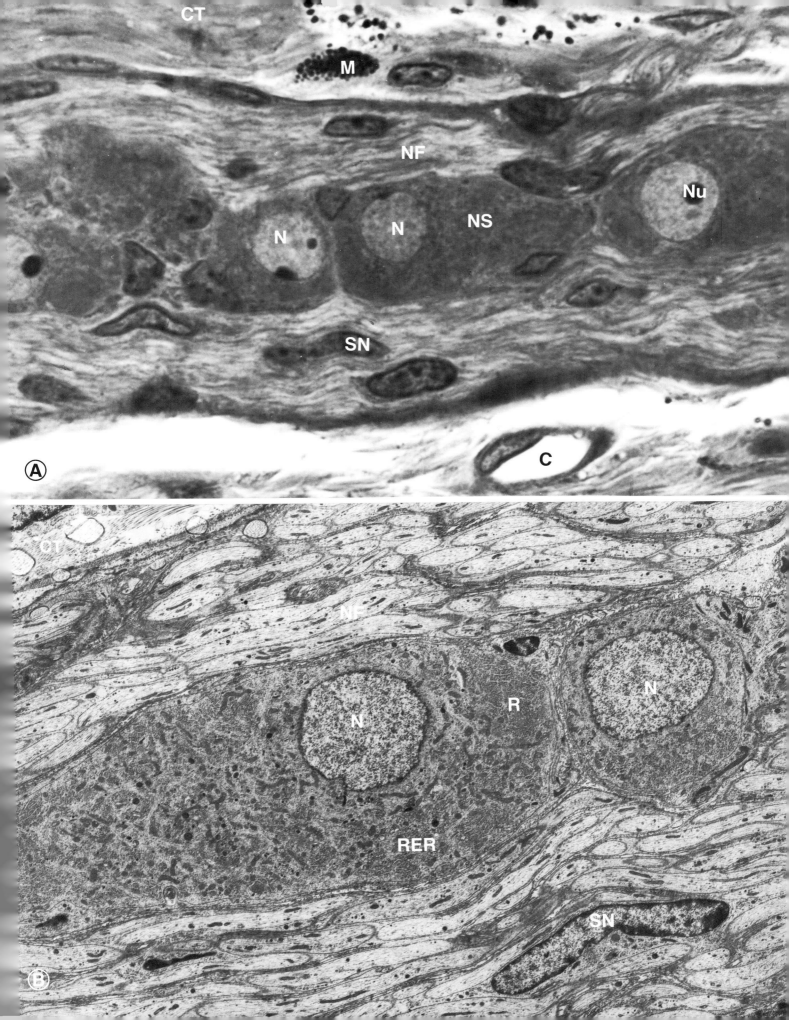

9

Skin

Overview

The skin, or integument, is a highly complex organ that performs many necessary functions. Skin is in a sense a container; it is the outer boundary of the physical being, the major material interface between a human being and the outside world.

Human beings are made mostly of water and, being warm-blooded creatures, must operate at a relatively constant body temperature. Because temperature and relative humidity of the atmosphere can vary greatly, human skin—which has an extremely large surface area—has many major tasks, including retaining water and regulating temperature. In addition, skin provides protection against the damaging effects of ultraviolet radiation from the sun, serves as a site of synthesis of vitamin D, and provides an exquisitely sensitive sensory surface that keeps an individual "in touch" with his or her immediate surroundings. All the while, the skin serves to protect delicate underlying soft tissues from physical damage imposed by contact with hard objects among which land-dwelling vertebrates such as man must move.

How can a single organ perform such a variety of important, life-sustaining functions? To answer this question, we must look to the carefully designed architecture of the skin and its many integumentary derivatives. The basic design of the skin centers around its subdivision into two major components: the superfi-

cially located *epidermis,* which is an epithelium, and the elaborate connective tissue layer beneath it called the *dermis,* or the *corium.* The structure of the epidermis and dermis varies considerably in different parts of the body. In areas of thick skin such as the soles of the feet, both epidermis and dermis are much thicker and tougher than they are in the thin skin that covers the eyelids.

The epidermis is a keratinized stratified squamous epithelium made up of four histologically distinct regions. At the surface, the *stratum corneum,* which is in direct contact with the environment, consists of flat, lifeless plates of *keratin.* These keratinized plates, called squames, are periodically lost from the surface and replaced by mitotic activity of cells in deeper layers. The keratin that fills the squames is a tough, durable, waterproof protein that is formed within cells of the *stratum granulosum,* the region just beneath the stratum corneum. Although the precise intracellular mechanisms of keratinization await discovery, two conspicuous classes of cytoplasmic inclusions—keratohyalin granules and *tonofilaments*—are evident in the cells of the stratum granulosum (called *keratinocytes*) that are undergoing keratinization. Beneath the stratum granulosum lies the *stratum spinosum,* also called the "spiny layer" or the "prickle cell layer." The large, polygonal cells of the stratum spinosum are attached to one another by desmosomes—cell junctions that form many tiny "spot welds" between the plasma membranes of adjacent cells. Beneath the stratum spinosum lies the deepest region of the epidermis, the *stratum germinativum.* The large cells of the stratum germinativum proliferate by mitosis at a relatively rapid rate and supply cells that serve to replace those lost at the surface of the skin. Daughter cells produced within the stratum germinativum move upward through the epidermis, undergo the process of keratinization, and take up residence in the stratum corneum as surface squames.

The epidermis, like all epithelia, is avascular. The dermis, on which it rests, is a highly vascular bed of connective tissue that is subdivided into several regions. The uppermost region, called the *papillary layer,* makes direct contact with the basement membrane that underlies the epidermis. Made of loose connective tissue, the papillary layer in thick skin is thrown into conspicuous folds called *dermal papillae* and is responsible for the ridges that make fingerprints. Beneath the thin papillary layer lies the *reticular layer* of the dermis, an extensive feltwork of collagen and elastic fibers classified as dense irregular connective tissue.

In addition to blood vessels and nerves, the dermis houses a number of important integumentary derivatives such as hair follicles, sebaceous glands, and sweat glands. These will be depicted and described in more detail in the remainder of this chapter. In addition, the skin is generously supplied with sensory receptors such as *pacinian corpuscles, Meissner's corpuscles,* and *Merkel's cells,* all of which serve important and specific mechanoreceptive functions.

Plate 9–1

Thick Skin: The Epidermis

Although often thought of as a simple sheet of tissue, the skin is truly an organ, one of the largest and most complex of the organs in the human body. The skin is a covering and as such performs many functions. Of all the skin covering the body, none is tougher or thicker than that covering the palms of the hands and the soles of the feet. The toughness and thickness of palmar and plantar skin makes its inclusion in a single thin section for electron-microscopic investigation difficult. Fortunately, the skin of the fingertip is much thinner and more delicate and yet retains all the histologic landmarks of thick skin.

Figures A and B at right are a matched pair of light and electron micrographs of serial cross sections taken through the skin of the fingertip of the squirrel monkey. Like all skin, it is made up of two major regions—the epidermis, a keratinized stratified squamous epithelium, and the dermis, a thick underlying layer of connective tissue. Here, the epidermis is so extensive and thick that it nearly fills the field. Only a small part of the dermis in the form of the edge of a dermal papilla (DP) is visible. (Dermal papillae are ridges that project into the epidermis, push it up, and are responsible for the complex patterns of whorls and lines in fingerprints).

Skin has many functions, one of which is protecting the underlying soft, wet tissues from abrasion and dehydration. The protective function of the skin resides in the physical properties of the flattened, horny cells, or squames, that cover its surface. The superficial layer of the epidermis, the stratum corneum (SC), consists of dead cells very much like flat scales that are filled with the fibrous protein keratin.

These cells are periodically shed from the surface of the skin. In some cases, they are rapidly worn away by physical contact with tennis rackets, lawn mowers, or, in the case of the squirrel monkey, branches. The tough, expendable surface cells would be of little use unless they were regularly replaced, and it comes as no surprise that they are, due to the special properties of the remainder of the epidermis upon which the stratum corneum sits.

Replacement of worn-out surface squames is ultimately a function of mitotic activity in the deepest layer of the epidermis, the stratum germinativum (SG). The stratum germinativum lies atop the dermis and consists of a single layer of large, polygonal cells. As mitotic activity occurs, daughter cells migrate upward into the next layer, the stratum spinosum (SS). The cells of the stratum spinosum have a spiny appearance because of the large number of small desmosomes that bind them together. As cells move upward through the stratum spinosum, they synthesize keratin. When their cytoplasm contains a noticeable number of dark, electron-dense keratohyalin granules, the cells form a layer known as the granular layer, or stratum granulosum (SGr). As the cells move upward through the stratum granulosum, their cytoplasmic organelles degenerate and the cells become packed with keratin, until, in the clear layer, or *stratum lucidum* (SL), they have no nuclei and are completely devoid of organelles. The keratinized cells then migrate (or rather are pushed) up into the horny layer, or stratum corneum, where they serve to protect the body until lost to the outside world.

Figures A and B. Matched pair of light and electron micrographs of serial thick and thin cross sections through the skin of the fingertip of the squirrel monkey. DP, dermal papilla; E, duct of eccrine sweat gland; SC, stratum corneum; SG, stratum germinativum; SGr, stratum granulosum; SL, stratum lucidum; SS, stratum spinosum; arrow, surface opening of eccrine sweat gland. 1,900 X

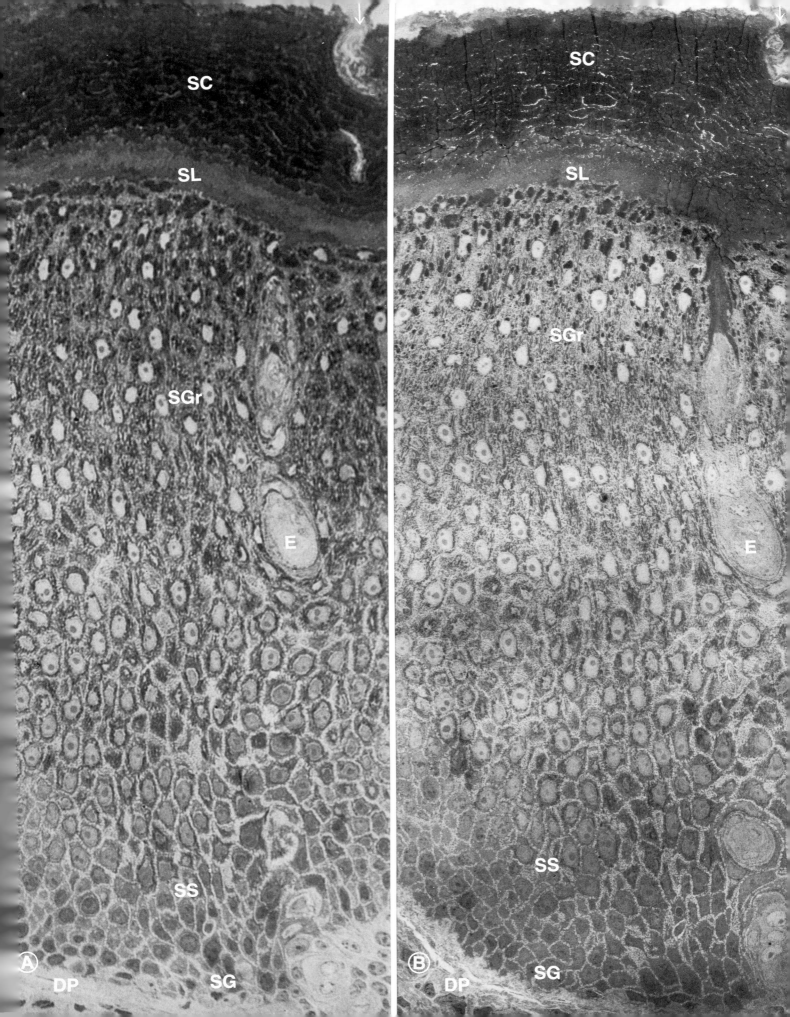

Plate 9–2

Thin Skin: The Scalp

Figures A and B, a matched pair of light and electron micrographs of serial cross sections taken through the monkey scalp, portray the microanatomy of thin skin. To observe the vast difference between thick and thin skin, compare the images at left to those of thick skin shown in Plate 9–1. What strikes the eye at once is how delicate the epidermis of thin skin appears when compared with that of thick skin. In the scalp at right, for example, the epidermis (E) measures 25 μm at its thickest point. The stratum corneum (SC), well over 1 mm thick in the sole of the foot, is only 2.5 μm deep in the scalp. In thin skin, the layers of the epidermis can be difficult to distinguish from one another. The stratum corneum, here composed of 10 to 12 layers of flattened, keratinized scales, is distinct and easy to recognize. The deeper layers, however, appear more homogeneous and tend to blend in with one another. The cells of the stratum granulosum (SGr), just beneath the stratum corneum, are long, thin cells with oval nuclei. Although their cytoplasm contains tonofilaments and keratohyalin granules, these are not as conspicuous as in thick skin. Beneath the stratum granulosum lies the stratum spinosum (SS), filled with large, polyhedral cells that contain round, centrally located nuclei. The many desmosomes (arrow) that serve to conjoin adjacent cells appear as dark dots under the light microscope (Figure A) and as electron-dense bars in the electron microscope (Figure B).

The basal cells—the cells of the stratum germinativum (SG)—are large, isodiametric cells that rest upon the finely fibrillar basement membrane (B). Their round, euchromatic nuclei possess prominent nucleoli; both of these features of nuclear structure indicate that basal cells are active in the transcrip-

tion of messenger RNA. The basal cells are mitotically active as well. Following cell division, some of the daughter cells remain in the stratum germinativum, where they continue to serve as stem cells. Others, however, migrate upward through the epidermis, become keratinized, and ultimately take station as squames in the stratum corneum. Surface squames are periodically shed from the skin. Consequently, the rate of turnover of epidermal cells is high and varies with location in the body. Whereas thin skin may experience complete renewal of its stratum corneum in a week or two, thick skin may require upward of 1 month to undergo complete cellular replacement. The mitotic potential of the basal cells is manifest not only in the generation of cells to replace those lost in the normal course of events, but also in the regeneration of cells lost by injury. The healing power of skin is truly remarkable.

The basal layer of the epidermis sits atop a thin basement membrane (B) that, in turn, rests upon the dermis (D). As described briefly in the overview, the dermis consists of two regions: the papillary layer, just beneath the epidermis, and the deeper reticular layer. In the figures at right, only part of the papillary layer is shown. In the scalp, the papillary layer is a 50 μm-thick region of loose connective tissue made up of a diffuse network of collagen fibrils (CF) that support small blood vessels, nerves, and various cells of the immune system. Here, a small bundle of unmyelinated nerves (N) is evident. Although small nerve bundles are initially quite difficult to recognize in the light microscope, you can learn to identify them by comparing their images as shown in light and electron micrographs of the same magnification.

Figures A and B. Matched pair of light and electron micrographs of serial thick and thin sections taken through the scalp of the squirrel monkey. B, basement membrane; CF, collagen fibrils; D, dermis; E, epidermis; F, fibroblast; N, small nerve bundle; SC, stratum corneum; SG, stratum germinativum; SGr, stratum granulosum; SS, stratum spinosum; arrow, desmosomes in stratum spinosum. Figure A, 3,000 X; Figure B, 3,400 X

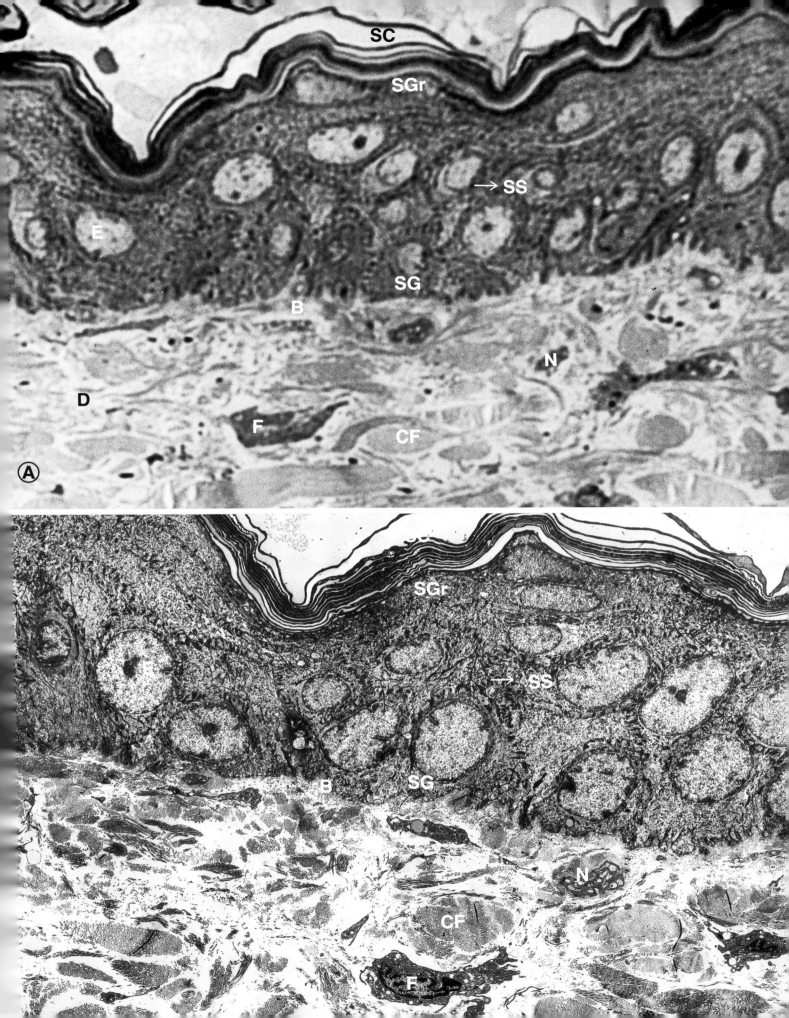

Plate 9–3

Skin: Epidermal Derivatives

Many of the important functions of skin are carried out not only by the dermis and epidermis, as described earlier in this chapter, but also by highly specific skin structures collectively known as *epidermal derivatives.* Epidermal derivatives include such structures as hairs, *sebaceous glands, apocrine sweat glands,* and *eccrine sweat glands.* The first three of these are captured in a single plane of section in the photomicrographs at right.

Figures A and B are a matched pair of light and electron micrographs of serial horizontal sections taken through the skin of the scalp of the squirrel monkey. Here, the knife has passed through the dermis and has caught a *hair follicle* (HF) in cross section. Closely associated with the hair follicle are a sebaceous gland (SG), the duct of an apocrine sweat gland (A), an arrector pili muscle (M), and a pigment cell, or melanocyte (MC). This cluster of structures is embedded in the feltwork of collagenous fibers (CF) and elastic fibers, which are woven together to form the connective tissue that gives strength and substance to the dermis. The sebaceous gland, apocrine gland, and arrector pili muscle are all located next to the hair follicle for one simple reason: their functions are closely related to the proper biologic functions of hair.

The hairs that cover your scalp and much of your body are derived from invaginations of the epidermis called hair follicles. As seen in the figures at right, the hair follicle is a multilayered tube of cuboidal cells that surrounds a central *hair shaft* (HS). During the growth of a hair, cells of the hair follicle become keratinized. As they differentiate, they are packed into the shaft of the hair in a very precise manner. Continuous addition of new cornified cells to the base of the hair shaft pushes the hair outward through the surface of the skin. Since hair, like the stratum corneum of the skin, consists of keratinized cells, it is essentially lifeless. To maintain its elasticity and water-repellant properties, it must be constantly coated with oily secretions. These are provided by the sebaceous glands. As shown at right, sebaceous glands consists of cells that fill themselves with lipid droplets. During secretion, whole cells filled with lipid are released by *holocrine secretion* from a short duct that opens at the base of the hair. During times of fright, excitement, or low temperature, hairs quite literally stand on end. Movement of hair is brought about by muscles associated with the base of the hair called arrector pili muscles. It is believed that movement of hair by the arrector pili muscles compresses the sebaceous gland, causing its oily secretion to be expressed onto the base of the hair at the surface of the skin.

Two major types of sweat glands—apocrine glands and eccrine glands—are present in skin. Eccrine glands, not depicted here, are responsible for the watery sweat used for temperature regulation. Apocrine glands are quite different. They secrete a highly proteinaceous material, chemically specific for each individual, that provides a chemical "fingerprint" that can readily be detected by the olfactory system. Apocrine glands release their secretion onto the skin surface at the base of the hair shaft. Consequently, the hair serves as a carrier for apocrine secretions, which are thought to contain, among other things, *pheromones.* (Pheromones are chemical attractants, mediated by olfaction, that affect members of the opposite sex). The duct of the apocrine gland at right consists of large, cuboidal cells, rich in lipid droplets, that have a brush border. The entire complex of epidermal derivatives depicted here is richly supplied by capillaries (C).

Figures A and B. Matched pair of light and electron micrographs of serial horizontal sections taken through the scalp of the squirrel monkey. A, duct of apocrine sweat gland; C, capillary; CF, collagenous fiber; HF, hair follicle; HS, hair shaft; M, arrector pili muscle; MC, melanocyte; SG, sebaceous gland. 1,000 X

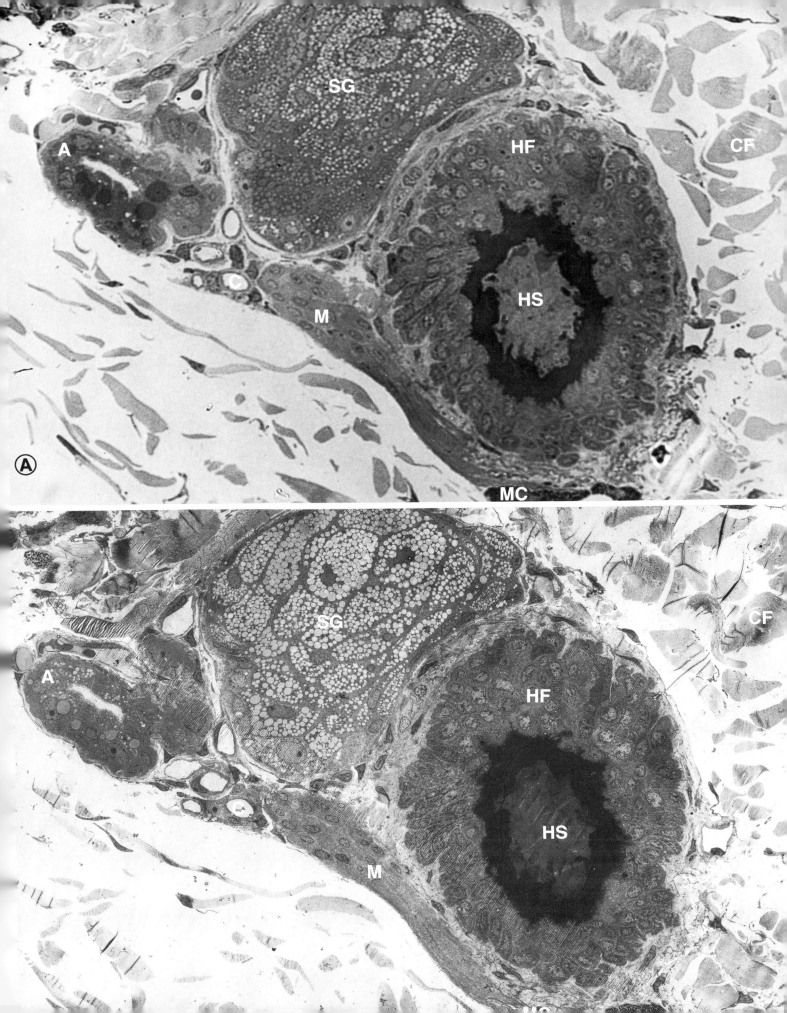

The Circulatory System 10

Overview

The human body is a well-constructed collection of trillions of cells. As indicated in Chapter 1, each of those cells needs essential raw materials such as food, water, and oxygen to survive. Because most of the body's cells are distant from food and air, these materials must be brought to them, and waste products generated by the cells must be carried away.

In keeping with our oceanic origins, human cells, like those of all Metazoa, are made mostly of water. Consequently, they are surrounded by extracellular tissue fluids that, in turn, are water based. As a result, the major task of the digestive and respiratory systems is to take in food and gases, respectively, and put them into solution or suspension in a watery medium. That aqueous medium, the blood, is enclosed within a hydraulic system of tubes and pumps designed to transport fluid to and from all the body's cells and tissues. This blood vascular system is subdivided into two major circuits: the pulmonary circulation, which takes blood to and from the lungs, and the systemic circulation, which carries blood to and from the rest of the body.

The circulatory system is a closed hydraulic system powered by a pump—the highly efficient heart—that weighs less than a pound. At rest, it pulses at around 70 beats per minute—a rate that results in approximately 40 million heartbeats each year. Exercise increases this number of dramatically: for example, during strenuous exercise, the pulse rate can rise to 180 heartbeats per minute, and the blood can flow out of the, aorta to the tissues at a volume in excess of 30 L (7.5 gallons) per minute. In a highly trained athlete, that number can reach 12 gallons per minute. Given a total blood volume of 6 L, the heart can cycle all of the blood through the body many times per minute. Consequently, blood coming out of the heart exits the ventricles at high pressure. This high pressue is handled by a series of thick-walled, resilient distribution tubes called *arteries.* The arteries lead to thin-walled exchange vessels called *capillaries,* in which the crucial exchange of materials between blood and tissue fluids occurs. As illustrated in Plate 10–4, the capillaries are surrounded by extremely thin walls that facilitate the passage of materials across them. The capillaries, in turn, lead to a series of relatively thin-walled collecting tubes called *veins,* which carry the blood back to the heart at moderately low pressure.

The microarchitecture of the heart—arteries, veins, and capillaries—is reflected in their functions. The close and strikingly obvious correlation between structure and function in the heart and vessels of the blood vascular system greatly simplifies understanding their histologic organization. The distribution vessels, the arteries, handle large volumes of blood at high pressure. Consequently, one would predict that the arteries closest to the heart would be big bored and thick walled, and those farthest from the heart, small bored and thin walled. This prediction holds true not only for arteries but also for veins: veins closest to capillaries are small and thin walled, and those near the heart, large and thick walled.

No discussion of the circulatory system would be complete without emphasizing that it is composed of the blood and lymph vascular systems. Unlike the blood vascular system, the lymphatic circulation has no heart of its own. Instead, lymph—a viscous, creamy fluid devoid of red blood cells—picks up materials from the tissue fluids via blind-ended, thin-walled lymph capillaries. These lymphatic capillaries flow into larger vessels that pass lymph through lymph nodes. Lymph, which is picked up from the tissue spaces, is delivered into the blood vascular system at the subclavian vein; close to the neck, a large lymphatic vessel enters the wall of the subclavian vein and empties its contents into the lumen of that blood vessel. As a result, the blood and lymph vascular systems, although made up of a separate system of tubes, eventually connect with one another.

Plate 10–1

The Aorta And Vena Cava

Many of the body's blood vessels have a common pattern of organization, exemplified by the body's largest artery and vein—the *aorta* and the *vena cava.* Figure A is a light micrograph of a cross section taken through the wall of the aorta of the squirrel monkey. Figure B is a light micrograph of a similar section through the vena cava of the same animal. Figure C is a low-magnification electron micrograph of the inner portion of the wall of the same vena cava shown in Figure B.

The aorta, like all large blood vessels, has a wall composed of three layers—the *tunica intima,* the *tunica media,* and the *tunica adventitia.* As shown in Figure A, the innermost layer, the tunica intima (TI), borders on the lumen of the vessel (L) and is lined by a single layer of flattened endothelial cells (arrow). The endothelial cells are supported by a thin bed of subendothelial connective tissue that, in turn, rests upon a thick sheet of elastic tissue called the internal elastic membrane (EM). The internal elastic membrane forms a boundary between the thin tunica intima and the middle layer, the thick tunica media (TM).

The aorta, the largest blood vessel in the human body, can deliver 12 gal of blood per minute to the general circulation under conditions of strenuous exercise. The aorta's ability to handle that large volume of blood, forcefully pumped in pulsatile bursts from the left ventricle of the heart, resides in the great strength and resilience of its tunica media. The strength of the tunica media comes from its collagen fibers; the resilience, from large sheets of elastic fibers. These elastic sheets (E), each flat and perforated by holes like a slice of Swiss cheese, appear as black, wavy lines when viewed in cross section in

Figure A. The elasticity of the aorta permits it to expand when it receives the large bolus of blood from the heart delivered by ventricular contraction (systole), and to recoil when the left ventricle relaxes (diastole). In addition to being quite elastic, the aorta is very muscular; Figure A reveals large numbers of smooth muscle fibers (S) in the tunica media. The aorta's collagen fibers give it great strength and set limits to its ability to stretch under pressure.

The tunica adventitia (TA) forms the outermost layer of the aorta. Only partially included in the field of view in Figure A, the adventitia is a loosely woven envelope made up of collagen fibers, a few elastic fibers, and some smooth muscle fibers. Small autonomic nerves and blood vessels that serve the aorta course through the adventitia.

The vena cava, shown in Figure B, returns circulating blood to the heart. Because blood pressure within the vena cava is much lower than in the aorta, the vena cava's wall is much thinner (compare Figures A and B, photographed at the same magnification). The tunica media of the vena cava contains far less elastic tissue than that of the aorta.

The wall of the vena cava is shown by electron microscopy in Figure C. Here, a few blood cells remain in the lumen (L), stuck to the endothelium that lines the vessel. The inner surface of the vena cava depicted here is thrown into folds. The tunica intima (TI) contains surface endothelial cells (arrow), subendothelial connective tissue (CT), and a few smooth muscle fibers (S). Beneath the wavy profile of the innermost elastic sheets lies the tunica media, which consists of connective tissue, numerous smooth muscle fibers (S), and a few strands of elastic tissue (E).

Figure A. Light micrograph of cross section through the aorta of the squirrel monkey. 330 X
Figure B. Light micrograph of cross section through the vena cava of the squirrel monkey. 330 X
Figure C. Electron micrograph through inner portion of the same vena cava shown in Figure B. 1,150 X
CT, subendothelial connective tissue; E, elastic sheets; EM, internal elastic membrane; L, lumen; S, smooth muscle; TA, tunica adventitia; TI, tunica intima; TM, tunica media; arrow, endothelium.

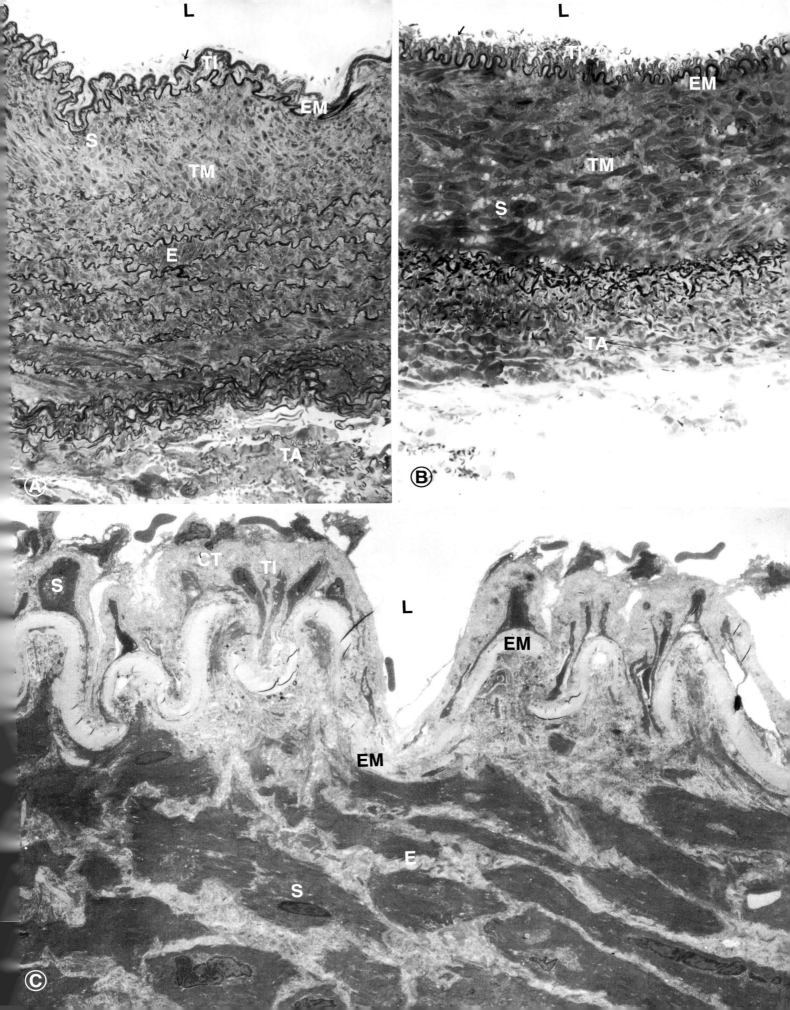

Plate 10–2

Medium-Sized Artery And Vein

One of the most common and frustrating obstacles faced by students of microanatomy is the differential identification of arteries and veins in sectioned material. Careful study of Figures A, B, and C at right should help solve that problem.

Figure A is a light micrograph of a cross section through a medium-sized artery (A) and vein (V) from the testis of the squirrel monkey. Because the tissue was fixed by intravascular perfusion, the vessels contain no blood and their walls are dilated—unlike the constricted walls of the aorta and vena cava shown in Plate 10–1. The artery has a much thicker wall in proportion to its lumen than does the neighboring vein. In addition, the profile of the artery is almost perfectly circular, whereas that of the vein is somewhat irregular. These characteristics, which provide key visual cues to the histologic identification of artery and vein, originate in the comparative ultrastructures of the vessels' walls. This difference is evident in Figures B and C, which are electron micrographs of the walls of the same artery and vein shown in Figure A.

In Figure B, the wall of the medium-sized artery is seen to consist of the three basic layers previously described in the aorta—the tunica intima (TI), the tunica media (TM), and the tunica adventitia (TA). Here, the tunica intima consists of a single layer of endothelial cells (E) and is therefore quite thin. A well-developed internal elastic membrane (EM) lies between the intima and media. The tunica media contains seven concentric layers of smooth muscle fibers (SM) whose fusiform nuclei are cut in longitudinal section. The smooth muscle fibers are spiralled in a tight helix; consequently, their contraction can dramatically reduce the caliber of the vessel, thereby restricting blood-flow through the artery itself. Hence, medium-sized arteries such as this one are commonly called *distributing arteries.* Their capacity to rapidly change in diameter—to open and close under control of autonomic nerves (N)—can distribute blood-flow differently to various organs in the body as needed.

Outside the muscular tunica media lies the tunica adventitia, a loosely woven meshwork of collagenous connective tissue (Co) secreted by a sparse population of fibroblasts (F). In this section, the profiles of several small, unmyelinated autonomic nerves are evident as they course through the loose connective tissue of the adventitia.

The ultrastructure of the wall of a medium-sized vein is illustrated in Figure C. As in the artery just described, the tunica intima (TI) consists of a single layer of endothelial cells (E). A thin internal elastic membrane (EM) is present, beneath which lies the tunica media (TM). In this vein, the tunica media is seen to consist of only two concentric layers of smooth muscle fibers (SM). As is evident in Figures A, B, and C, the thin, somewhat flaccid wall of the vein has a much less massive tunica media than does the artery. Because the tunica media and tunica adventitia of the artery and vein are similar, the different relative properties of the walls of the two kinds of vessels, which allow for their identification in sectioned material, originate in the ultrastructure of the tunica media.

Figure A. Light micrograph of a cross section through a medium-sized artery and vein from the testis of the squirrel monkey. A, artery; V, vein. 438 X

Figures B and C. Electron micrographs of cross sections taken through the walls of the same artery (Figure B) and vein (Figure C) shown in Figure A. Co, collagen fibrils; E, endothelial cell; EM, internal elastic membrane; F, fibroblast; N, nerve; SM, smooth muscle; TA, tunica adventitia; TI, tunica intima; TM, tunica media. Figure B, 3,300 X; Figure C, 8,900 X

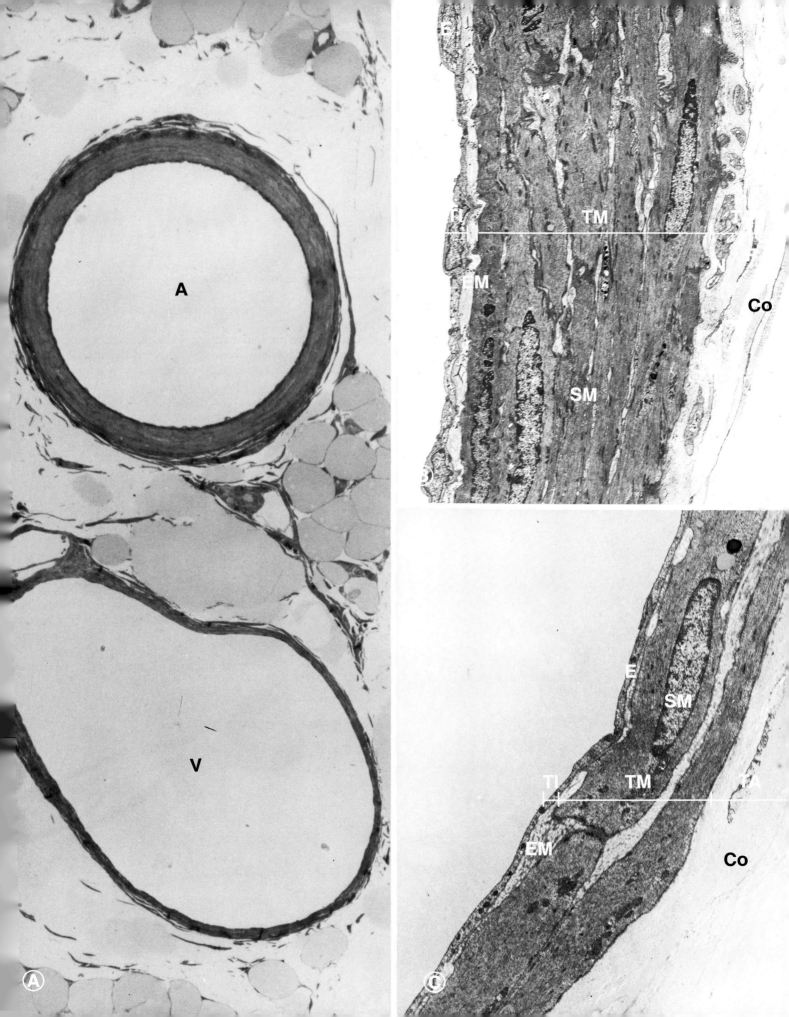

Plate 10–3

Arterioles, Capillaries, And Lymphatic Vessels

Whereas medium-sized arteries serve to distribute blood to organs, *arterioles* move blood within organs. Arterioles, having an outer diameter of 0.1 mm or less, are the smallest of all arteries. Because the limit of resolution of the human eye is about 0.2 mm, arterioles are too small to be seen with the naked eye. Like the medium-sized (distributing) arteries described in Plate 10–2, the walls of arterioles are capable of graded contraction during vasoconstriction, permitting them to direct bloodflow to different regions within the organ they serve.

Figure A is a low-power electron micrograph of a longitudinal section through a small arteriole within the colon. A chain of red blood cells (R) are lined up in single file within its lumen. The lumen is lined by a monolayer of endothelial cells (E). A thin sheet of elastic tissue, the internal elastic membrane (EM), separates the tunica intima (TI) from the tunica media (TM). In this arteriole, the tunica media consists of a single layer of smooth muscle fibers (SM) that are wrapped about the arteriole's long axis like the coils of a spring. Since the arteriole is embedded within an organ, no true tunica adventitia is present. Instead, a thin layer of collagenous connective tissue (Co) binds the vessel to surrounding tissues.

Arterioles eventually lead to capillaries, in which the major functions of the circulatory system are carried out—the vital exchange of nutrients, gases, and metabolites between blood and tissue. Figure B, an electron micrograph of a cross section through a continuous capillary, shows that the capillary is ideally suited for the diffusion of gases and exchange of materials across its wall. First, the ultra-thin walls favor gas diffusion. Second, hundreds of *micropinocytotic vesicles* (arrow), shown at high magnification in the inset, serve to shuttle nutrients and waste products back and forth between the circulating blood and the cells and tissue spaces next to the capillary. The wall of the capillary shown in Figure B consists of a single endothelial cell (E) rolled into a tube. The endothelial cell's nucleus (N) is evident, as is a tangentially sectioned red blood cell (R) in the lumen. The capillary is surrounded by a thin, delicate basal lamina (arrowhead).

When viewed with the light microscope, small blood vessels and small lymph vessels can easily be mistaken for one another. Under the electron microscope, however, their ultrastructural differences become readily apparent. Compare, for example, the images in Figures B and C. Figure B is the capillary we have just described; Figure C is a lymph capillary. Its wall is extremely thin, consisting of the attenuated cytoplasm of a single thin, flattened endothelial cell (E). The shape of the lymph capillary is irregular, in part because the lymphatic circulation has no heart. Instead, lymph is passively propelled through its vessels by the movement of neighboring muscles. Consequently, lymph circulates at very low pressure, and its flaccid, thin-walled vessels present irregular—and often collapsed—profiles in sectioned material. The lumen (L) is quite large compared to the thin wall; the wall is held in place by a delicate skein of collagen fibrils (Co). Red blood cells are never seen in healthy lymphatic vessels. Lymphocytes, however, are often evident, especially in inflamed or infected regions of the body.

Figure A. Electron micrograph of longitudinal section through an arteriole. Co, collagen fibrils; E, endothelial cell; EM, internal elastic membrane; R, red blood cell; SM, smooth muscle; TI, tunica intima; TM, tunica media. 9,140 X
Figure B. Electron micrograph of cross section through a continuous capillary. E, endothelial cell; N, nucleus of endothelial cell; R, red blood cell; arrows, micropinocytotic vesicles; arrowhead, basal lamina. Inset, same capillary wall at higher magnification. 15,000 X; inset, 35,500 X
Figure C. Electron micrograph of cross section through a lymphatic capillary. Co, collagen fibrils; E, endothelial cell; L, lumen. 5,100 X

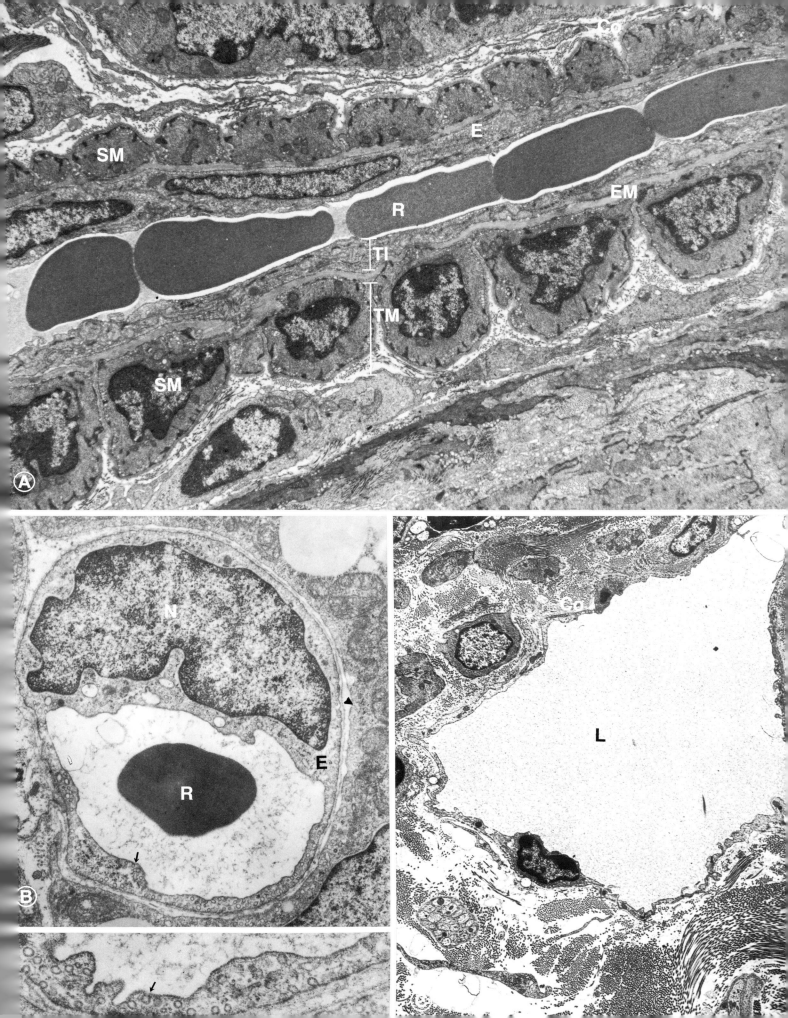

Plate 10–4

The Heart: The Wall Of The Atrium

The heart is a truly amazing organ. Although it beats cyclically and constantly throughout life, the heart is so quietly efficient that we often go about our business quite unaware of its vigorous activity. The human four-chambered heart consists of two *atria,* which receive venous blood, and two *ventricles,* which pump blood independently to the body and lungs. The microanatomy of the heart reflects its function; it is a highly muscular pump, held together by connective tissue, that receives blood from the venous circulation and pumps it into the arterial circulation at high pressure.

The microanatomy of the monkey heart is illustrated at right. Figures A and B are a matched pair of light and electron micrographs of serial sections taken through a thin portion of the atrium, chosen because other parts of the heart are far too thick and bulky to fit into the confines of a single thin section. In these illustrations, the lumen (L) of the heart is at the top of the photomicrograph; the outside of the heart, or epicardium (Ep), is at the bottom. The microanatomic organization of the heart parallels that of the larger blood vessels; it is built up of three major layers. On the inside of the heart, a thin inner lining called the endocardium (E) corresponds to the tunica intima of a blood vessel. A thick, muscular middle layer, the myocardium (M), corresponds to the tunica media of a blood vessel. The myocardium, a powerful mass of cardiac muscle, does the active pumping of blood. An outer layer of connective tissue, the epicardium (Ep), is homologous to the tunica adventitia of a blood vessel. The similarity in structure between heart and blood vessel is no accident; its origin is in vertebrate evolution, during which the heart is thought to have originated as a well-placed expansion of a muscular blood vessel.

Because Figures A and B are serial sections, much can be learned about the microanatomy of the heart by first finding specific structures as seen by light microscopy (Figure A) and then looking at precisely the same structures shown in greater detail by electron microscopy (Figure B). In these images, the endocardium (E) consists of a thin layer of endothelial cells underlain by a small amount of connective tissue. The myocardium, by contrast, is massive and consists of many cardiac muscle fibers running in a variety of different directions. Intercalated disks (arrowhead), characteristic of cardiac muscle, are visible even at this comparatively low magnification. A vein (V) is evident running through the myocardium, as are many small capillaries (C). The heart is well supplied with blood, and its high degree of vascularity is consistent with its continuous activity. At the point where the myocardium and the epicardium (Ep) meet, a bundle of small nerves (N) is evident. Difficult to identify by light microscopy (Figure A), their nature is obvious when viewed by electron microscopy (N, Figure B). Deeper in the epicardium (Ep) may be seen an arteriole (A), cut in longitudinal section. In Figure A, the elastic tissue of the internal elastic membrane (arrow) shows as a dark-staining line; that same structure, when viewed by electron microscopy in Figure B, appears as an electron-lucent, clear line (arrow).

Figures A and B. Matched pair of light and electron micrographs of serial thick and thin sections taken through the atrium of the heart of the squirrel monkey. A, arteriole; C, capillary; E, endocardium; Ep, epicardium; L, lumen of atrium; M, myocardium; N, nerve; V, vein; arrow, internal elastic membrane of arteriole; arrowhead, intercalated disk. 1,000 X

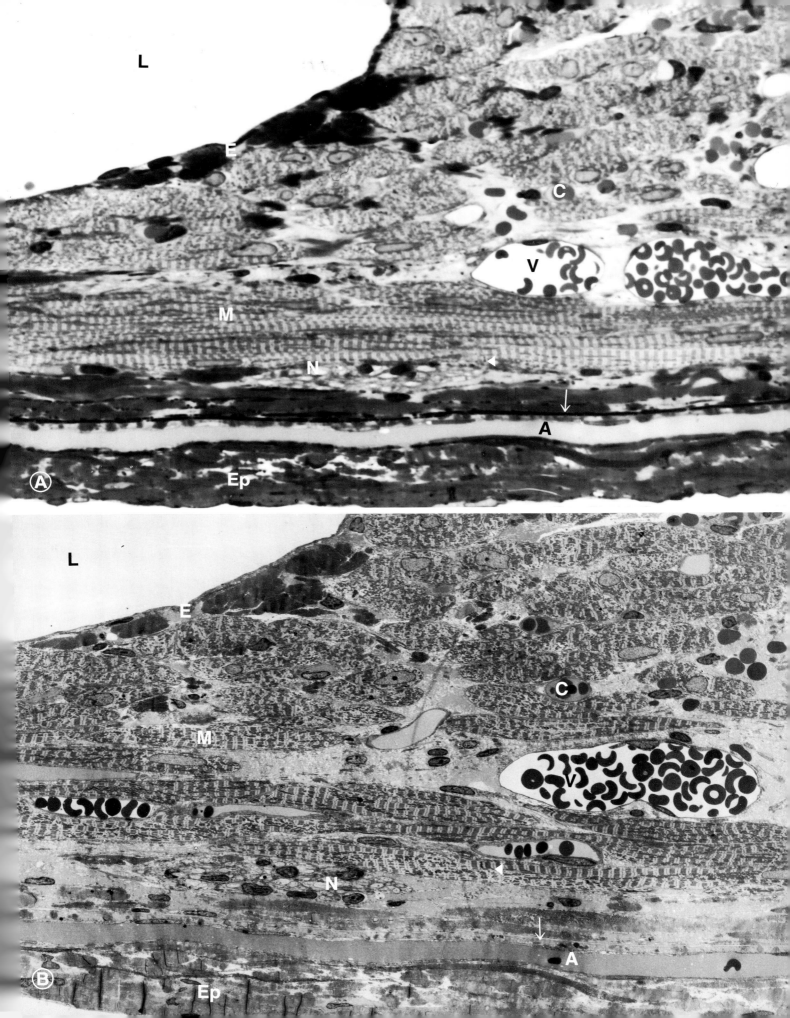

11

The Respiratory System

Overview

The primary function of the respiratory system is to provide oxygen to, and remove carbon dioxide from, the circulating blood. To accomplish this task, the respiratory system must take in oxygen from the atmosphere and deliver it directly to the red blood cells. The red blood cells, or erythrocytes, course through the general circulation and exchange oxygen for carbon dioxide with each of the body's many trillions of cells.

The microanatomic architecture of the respiratory system is highly complex. Despite its structural complexity, the respiratory system can be easily understood if you remember that it is constructed to perform one major function: to exchange gases between blood and air. Gas exchange between blood and air occurs across the thin walls of tiny hollow sacs called *alveoli*, which lie within the lung at the distal end of the respiratory tree. When inhaled air arrives at an alveolus, it can go no further; it remains there until it is moved out by exhalation to make room for fresh, oxygen-rich air taken in with the next breath.

Much of the respiratory system is designed to deliver air to the alveoli. The major parts of the respiratory system through which air passes are the *nasal cavity*, the *pharynx*, the *larynx*, the *trachea*, the *bronchi*, the *bronchioles*, the *terminal bronchioles*, the *respiratory bronchioles*, the *alveolar ducts*, the *alveolar sacs*, and finally the alveoli. All of the airways

from the nasal cavity through the terminal bronchioles are called *conductive airways*, since no gas exchange occurs across their walls. The respiratory bronchioles, alveolar ducts, alveolar sacs, and alveoli are called *respiratory airways*, since gas exchange does occur across their walls.

When one breathes in, air is drawn into the nasal cavity, in which a number of processes prepare the air for passage into the delicate alveoli. First, the air is warmed by blood that flows through a rich capillary bed that underlies the nasal mucosa. Next, the air is moistened by the blanket of watery mucus that lines the nasal epithelium. Secreted by both goblet cells and a well-developed system of submucosal glands, the mucus that covers the epithelial lining of the nasal cavity and other conductive airways also serves to purify the air by surface adsorption of potentially harmful substances including airborne particles such as asbestos and water-soluble gases such as sulfur dioxide. Toxic materials unsuitable for inhalation will in all likelihood be detected by a battery of exquisitely sensitive olfactory receptors located deep within the nasal cavity that will alert the individual to their presence.

Having passed through the nasal cavity, pharynx, and larynx, air enters the trachea, a short tube roughly the width of a garden hose with walls that are reinforced by cartilage. The trachea then bifurcates to form two smaller bronchi that enter the lungs. The bronchi branch repeatedly into smaller subunits—the bronchioles, terminal bronchioles, and respiratory bronchioles. The respiratory bronchioles give rise to alveolar ducts; these, in turn, lead to alveolar sacs, which are lined with alveoli.

The microanatomy of five of these airways— the trachea, bronchioles, terminal bronchioles, respiratory bronchioles, and alveoli—will be described in this chapter. The histologic organization of the nasal mucosa and the olfactory mucosa will be described in Chapter 20.

Plate 11–1

The Trachea

After inhaled air has passed through the nose, pharynx, and larynx, it enters the trachea. The trachea is a thick-walled tube, some 12 cm in length, that directs air down toward the pair of primary bronchi that enter the lung. The entire wall of the trachea of the mouse, which was selected because its small size permits inclusion in a single photographic field, is shown in cross section by the light microscope in Figure A. The trachea's inner surface, facing the lumen (L), is lined by a pseudostratified columnar epithelium that contains ciliated cells, goblet cells, and basal cells. Even at this relatively low magnification, motile cilia (arrow) are evident at the epithelial surface, as are mucus droplets (arrowhead) atop the goblet cells.

The tracheal epithelium (E) lies atop a highly elastic lamina propria (LP), which grades into the submucosa (S). The well-developed submucosa contains conspicuous rings of hyaline cartilage (C) that keep the trachea open when the neck is bent or turned. The cartilage is covered by a tough perichondrium (P), which, in the outer region of the wall, is covered by the adventitia (A), a sheath of loose connective tissue that envelops the outer surface of the trachea. This spatial arrangement of component tissues—epithelium, lamina propria, subcosa, and adventitia—is common to many of the body's interior tubular systems.

The epithelium, lamina propria, and part of the submucosa are shown in greater detail in Figure B and C, a matched pair of light and electron micrographs of serial cross sections through the trachea of the monkey. The pseudostratified columnar ciliated epithelium of the monkey trachea is much thicker than that of the mouse depicted in Figure A. The goblet cells (G), as the name suggests, have a goblet-shaped cytoplasm filled with mucus droplets that displace the nucleus and biosynthetic machinery toward the basal pole of the cell. The ciliated cells (Ci) appear much darker and have numerous motile cilia projecting from the cell surface. Taken together, these two cell types generate the mucociliary blanket that protects the inner tracheal surface. The goblet cells, along with large submucosal glands, produce and secrete the mucus; the cilia move mucus toward the mouth. In this way, foreign materials that enter the respiratory system are entrapped by the sticky mucus and are rapidly moved toward the throat to be swallowed or expectorated. At the bottom of the epithelium are the basal cells (B), stem cells that replace worn-out ciliated and goblet cells.

The epithelium rests upon a well-developed basement membrane (BM), readily visible by light and electron microscopy. The basement membrane, in turn, rests upon the lamina propria (LP), a network of loose connective tissue that, in the trachea, is rich in elastic fibers. Because the tracheal epithelium, like all epithelia, is avascular, it must receive nutrients and oxygen from the rich bed of capillaries (Ca) that flow through the lamina propria. Cells of the immune series, such as plasma cells (*), are common in the lamina propria, as are the flattened profiles of elastin-producing and collagen-producing fibroblasts (F).

Beneath the lamina propia lies the submucosa (S), which here contains hyaline cartilage (C). Deeper in the respiratory system, the cartilage becomes less and less prominent until it is absent from the bronchioles, as depicted in Plate 11–2.

Figure A. Light micrograph of cross section through mouse trachea. A, adventitia; C, cartilage; E, epithelium; L, lumen; LP, lamina propria; P, perichondrium; S, submucosa; arrow, motile cilia; arrowhead, mucus droplet. 610 X

Figures B and C. Matched pair of light and electron micrographs of serial sections through the trachea of the macaque. B, basal cell; BM, basement membrane; Ca, capillary; Ci, ciliated cell; C, cartilage; F, fibroblast; G, goblet cell; L, lumen; LP, lamina propria; S, submucosa; SG, submucosal gland; *, plasma cell. 740 X

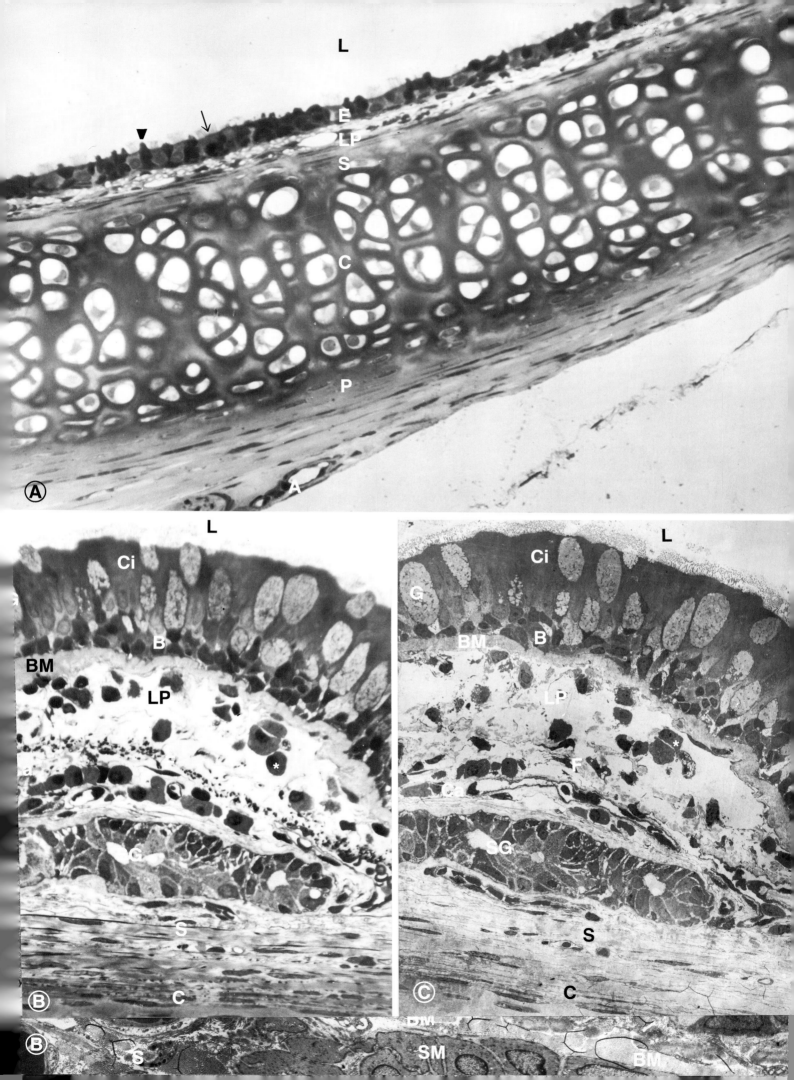

A

L

E
LP
S

C

P

A

B

L

Ci

B

BM

LP

*

SG

S

C

B

S

C

L

Ci

G

BM

B

LP

F

Ca

*

SG

S

C

BM

SM

BM

Plate 11-4

The Respiratory Bronchiole And Alveolus

The respiratory bronchiole, the first of the airways to participate in true gas exchange, is shown at low magnification by the electron microscope in Figure A. Its wall has a patchy appearance; the epithelium in different patches can vary from simple cuboidal to simple squamous. To see this, follow the respiratory bronchiole in Figure A from left to right. Initially, when the epithelium is cuboidal, Clara cells (C) are evident and the submucosa contains smooth muscle cells (S). Suddenly, the wall becomes extremely thin (arrow); simple squamous epithelium takes over, and the respiratory bronchiole's wall is thin enough to permit gas exchange. Then it thickens again. And so it goes along its length—alternating patches of thick (albeit not very thick) and thin epithelium form the wall of this first of the respiratory airways.

Respiratory bronchioles communicate with alveolar ducts, alveolar sacs, and alveoli (A). The delicate, lacelike structure of the alveolar portion of the lung is readily apparent in Figure A. The structure of the alveoli serves the primary functions of the respiratory system well. The microanatomy of the alveolus is simple to understand if you remember that air is in the alveolar spaces and blood is in the capillaries. The interalveolar septum is the ultra-thin "wall" of tissue that separates air from blood. Consequently, the interalveolar septum consists of two walls of simple squamous epithelium placed back to back: the epithelium of the alveolus and that of the capillary. The interalveolar septum can be so thin (0.1 μm) that it can be beneath the limit of resolution of the light microscope.

The fine structure of two alveoli and their associated capillaries is shown at intermediate magnification by electron microscopy in Figure B. This monkey's lung was fixed by immersion, and so its capillaries contain blood cells. (Organs fixed by in-travascular perfusion often have empty capillaries). Red blood cells (R), shaped like biconcave disks, are here cut in a variety of planes of section and display a variety of images. A lymphocyte (Ly) is present at upper right, as is part of a platelet. As mentioned above, the interalveolar septum that separates the alveolar air space from the capillary lumen can be extremely thin. The ultra-thin interalveolar septum is something of a bioarchitectural miracle, inasmuch as it consists of four elements sandwiched together: the cytoplasm of the thin type I alveolar cell; its basement membrane; the basement membrane of the capillary endothelial cell; and the cytoplasm of the capillary endothelial cell. In other places, usually near epithelial cell nuclei, the wall thickens and contains connective tissue rich in elastic fibers that facilitate elastic recoil of the lung during the breathing cycle.

Several other types of cells are associated with the alveolus. One, not shown here, has several names; it is called the *greater alveolar cell*, the *septal cell*, or the *pneumocyte type II*. Unlike the thin alveolar epithelial cells, the greater alveolar cell is bulky. Its cytoplasm contains large inclusions called lamellar bodies that are thought to contain surfactant. When released from the cell, surfactant spreads, reducing surface tension across the alveolus—surface tension that would otherwise collapse the ultra-thin alveolar walls when pressure drops at exhalation. Another type of cell quite commonly encountered in association with the alveolus is the *pulmonary alveolar macrophage*, or "dust cell." A single pulmonary alveolar macrophage (M) is evident in Figure B. These large cells glide along the interior of the alveolar walls, sweeping them clean by phagocytosis of foreign matter.

Figure A. Low-power electron micrograph of a monkey respiratory bronchiole. A, alveolus; C, Clara cell; Ca, capillary; L, lumen of respiratory bronchiole; S, smooth muscle; arrow, simple squamous epithelium. 645 X

Figure B. Portions of two alveoli and associated capillaries from the lung of the macaque. A, alveolus; Ca, capillary; Ly, lymphocyte; M, pulmonary alveolar macrophage; P, platelet; R, red blood cell. 3,800 X

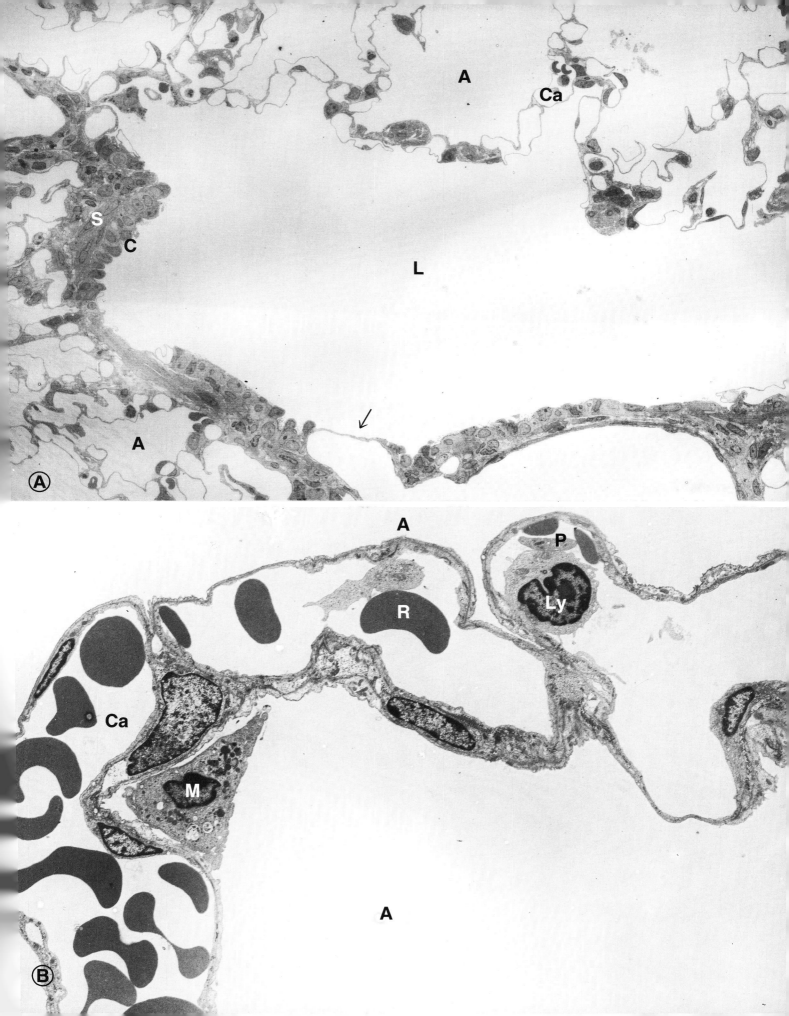

12

The Oral Cavity

Overview

Our bodies are made of matter. Consequently, the molecular building blocks for cells, tissues, and organs must be gathered from our surroundings. The portal of entry for the matter of which we are made is the subject of this chapter: the oral cavity.

Approximately 500 g (about 1 lb) of solid food and 2.5 L (about 6 lb) of water enter the oral cavity of the average person each day. (These figures are doubtless quite conservative for the average North American and vary considerably among nations, communities, and individuals.) By the time a person reaches age 25 he has taken 54,750 lbs (27.38 tons) of material into the oral cavity. At age 50, 109,500 lbs (54.75 tons) of food and drink have entered and passed through the oral cavity. By age 75, 164,250 lbs (82.125 tons) of material have been taken into the oral cavity, chewed, tasted, swallowed, and passed into the alimentary canal for further digestion and absorption.

The oral cavity performs its tasks efficiently, and usually quite pleasantly. This chapter will deal with three of the most important structures within the oral cavity: the *teeth,* the *tongue,* and the *salivary glands.*

When food is first taken into the mouth, it is reduced to small pieces suitable for swallowing by the cutting and grinding action of the teeth. Each of the 32 teeth is a highly complex organ.

The basic structure of the human tooth is illustrated in Figure 12-1. The exposed part of the tooth, called the *crown,* is covered by a cap of *enamel,* the hardest substance in the human body, which during tooth formation is laid down upon a core of *dentin.* Dentin, a hard, bony substance that constitutes the bulk of the tooth, surrounds a soft central cavity filled with *pulp.* Below the gumline lies the *root* of the tooth, covered by a modified bone called *cementum.* The cementum, in turn, is tightly attached to a ligament of dense connective tissue called the *periodontal ligament.* As is evident in Figure 12-1, the periodontal ligament anchors the tooth to the bony socket in which it sits.

The food that is chewed by the teeth is partially dissolved and put into suspension by the saliva, a complex liquid secreted by the salivary glands. The salivary glands secrete mucus, salts, water, and a digestive enzyme called *ptyalin,* an amylase that splits complex sugars such as starch and glycogen into simple sugars such as maltose and glucose. The dissolving action of saliva serves to intensify the taste of food in the mouth; this effect in turn promotes the secretion of digestive juices in the alimentary canal that receives swallowed food. The mucus secreted by the salivary glands lubricates the oral cavity and pharynx, facilitating swallowing.

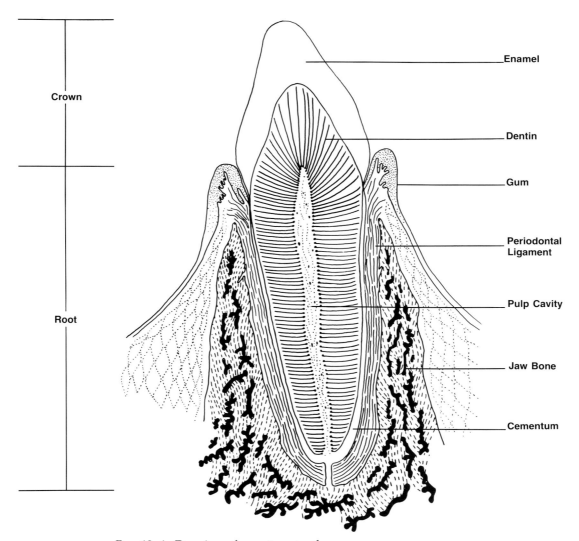

Crown

Root

Enamel

Dentin

Gum

Periodontal
Ligament

Pulp Cavity

Jaw Bone

Cementum

FIG. 12–1. Drawing of a mature tooth.

The salivary glands are compound tubuloacinar glands; they have a number of secretory units called *acini* that communicate with the oral cavity through a complex series of ducts. As shown in Figure 12-2, some acini contain *serous cells*, others contain *mucous cells*, and still others contain both serous and mucous cells. Each acinus empties its contents into a small duct called an *intercalated duct;* each intercalated duct, in turn, empties its contents into a larger *secretory duct.* The secretory ducts, also called *striated ducts,* modify the salt and water content of the saliva as demanded by conditions within the oral cavity.

While food is being chewed by the teeth and moistened, lubricated, and partially dissolved by the saliva, it is constantly being moved about by the tongue. The microanatomy of the teeth, tongue, and salivary glands will be illustrated and discussed in the following pages of this chapter.

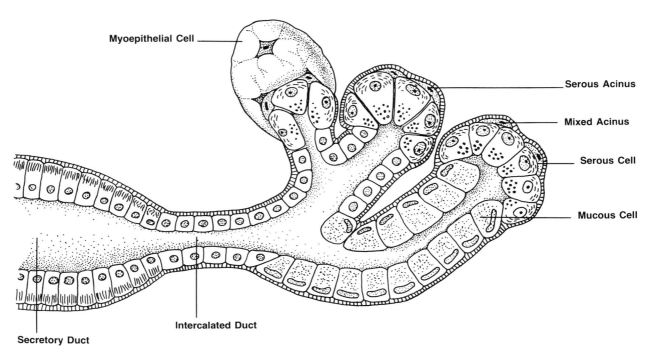

Fig. 12–2. Diagrammatic representation of a salivary gland showing several different kinds of acini.

Plate 12–1

The Developing Tooth

Plate 12–1

The Developing Tooth

Adult humans have 32 teeth, or 16 per jaw. We have incisors for cutting, canines for holding and tearing, and molars for grinding food. As omnivores—generalized eaters—we are endowed with the dental equipment necessary to perform a variety of tasks ranging from the grinding of carrots to the tearing of meat. Although canines and molars have different appearances, their general architectural plan is the same (see Figure 12-1). Plate 12–1 shows the structure of a developing tooth that has not yet erupted through the gumline.

Figure A is a light micrograph of a tooth at a relatively early stage of development. The future crown of the tooth points upward, the root points downward, and the jawbone (J), or the *alveolar bone* that will form the socket, is seen to the left. In the middle of the tooth sits the prominent pulp cavity (PC) that, at this stage of development, is filled with undifferentiated connective tissue cells called mesenchyme (M). The perimeter of the pulp cavity is lined with highly specialized cells called *odontoblasts* (O). Odontoblasts secrete dentin (D) which will eventually make up the bulk of the mature tooth. In the micrograph at right, the dentin is darkly stained. Just beneath the dentin and immediately above the layer of odontoblasts is a clear area made up of material called *predentin* (P). Just as bone's osteoblasts secrete osteoid, which later becomes mature, mineralized bone matrix, so do the tooth's odontoblasts secrete predentin, material that later becomes mature, mineralized dentin.

In the mature tooth, the outer surface is made of enamel. In the micrograph at right, specialized cells called *ameloblasts* (A) are shown in the act of secreting enamel (E). Normally, enamel lies right on top of dentin. Because of its hardness, however, enamel

often is distorted, displaced, or in some cases dissolved during the rather harsh decalcification procedures used to prepare teeth for microscopy. Here, the enamel has become separated from the underlying dentin by an artifactual space (S) that does not exist in life.

The relationship between dentin and enamel in the process of tooth development is dynamic. Early in the life of the tooth, when it is but a tooth germ, the odontoblasts at the perimeter of the pulp cavity are covered by a monolayer of ameloblasts. When the odontoblasts start to secrete dentin, they deposit it on their outer surface. Consequently, the newly formed dentin is laid down directly between the layer of odontoblasts and the layer of ameloblasts. When the ameloblasts are confronted by dentin, they are stimulated to secrete enamel, which they deposit on top of the layer of dentin. As a result, the inner core of dentin is covered by an outer coat of enamel, a pattern that is evident in the mature tooth.

Outside of the ameloblasts lies another epithelium, the outer enamel epithelium (OE), which at the base of the developing tooth is separated from the ameloblasts by a jelly-like mass of loose connective tissue called the *stellate reticulum* (SR). As the tooth matures and erupts through the surface of the gum, several events occur. The ameloblasts, being exposed, are rapidly worn away; consequently, enamel lost through decay or accident does not regenerate. The stellate reticulum is transformed from loose connective tissue into the periodontal ligament, which serves to keep the mature tooth firmly planted in its socket by binding the cementum at the root of the tooth to the bone of its socket.

Light micrograph of a developing tooth. A, ameloblasts; C, capillary; CT, connective tissue; D, dentin; E, enamel; J, jawbone (alveolar bone); M, mesenchyme that fills pulp cavity; O, odontoblasts; OE, outer enamel epithelium; P, predentin; PC, pulp cavity; S, artifactual space; SR, stellate reticulum. 210 X

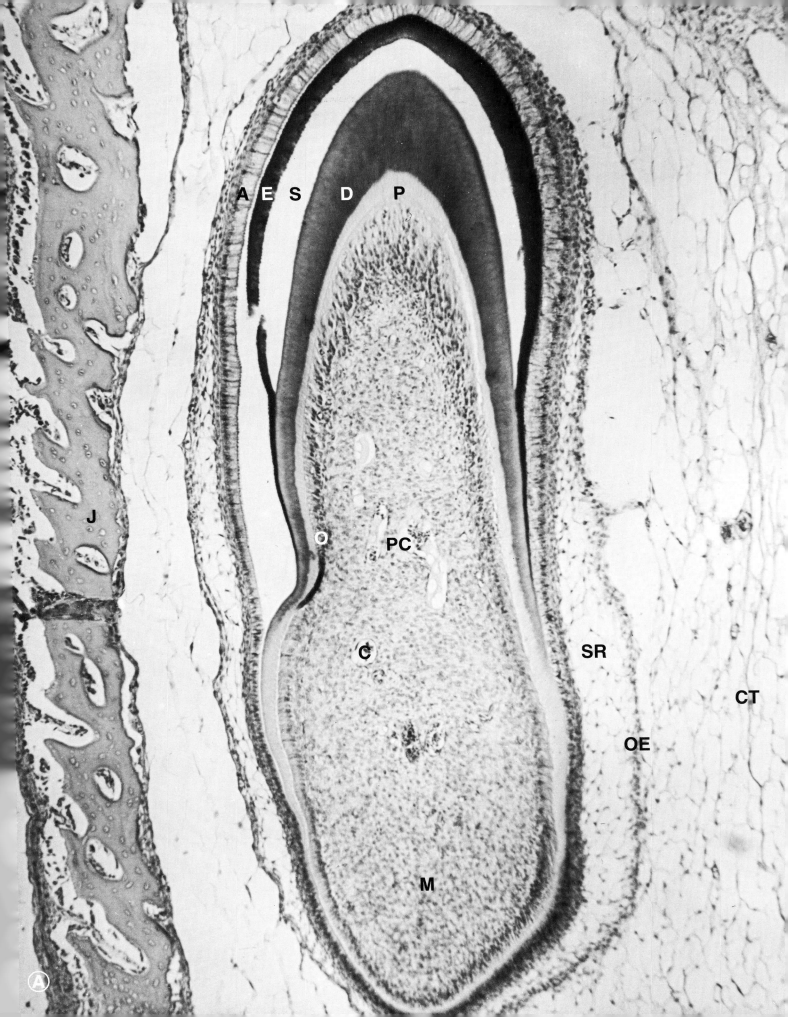

Plate 12–2

The Tongue, Part I

In order for the teeth to function properly, food must be placed between them so they can chop and grind it into small pieces suitable for swallowing. This placement is accomplished largely by the tongue, a sensitive, highly innervated, well-coordinated mass of muscle that sits in the middle of the mouth. In addition to moving food about in the mouth, the tongue performs sensory and secretory functions: it is equipped with chemosensitive taste buds that test food quality, mechanoreceptors that monitor texture, and salivary glands that lubricate its epithelial surface. In humans, the tongue is capable of extremely fine movements that permit speech.

Figure A is a light micrograph of a vertical section taken through the posterior portion of the tongue of the squirrel monkey. Here, the surface of the tongue is covered by a stratified squamous epithelium (EP). The superficial cells, although filled with keratin, still contain remnants of nuclei. Consequently, the epithelium is classified as nonkeratinized (some texts refer to it as parakeratinized). The epithelium is supported by an extensive lamina propria (LP). The lamina propria binds the epithelium to the underlying muscle mass (not evident in Figure A) that comprises the bulk of the tongue. The lamina propria is highly vascular, containing both blood capillaries (C) and lymphatic capillaries (L). The tongue is extensively innervated, and nerves (N) are clearly visible in the lamina propria. In the deeper layers of the lamina propria, salivary glands called *lingual glands* (LG) are evident. The secretory portions of the glands, filled with dark secretory vesicles, empty into ducts (D) that carry the saliva to the surface of the tongue.

Figure B is an electron micrograph of a serial section taken through the stratified squamous epithelium depicted in Figure A. The surface of the epithelium bears a series of ridges (arrow) that represent the bases of conical projections called *filiform papillae.* The filiform papillae, which do not contain taste buds, give a rough texture to the surface of the tongue that provides traction against material to be moved in the mouth. The filiform papillae are supported by projections of the lamina propria called *secondary papillae* (SP).

Figure C is an electron micrograph of a serial section taken through a deeper portion of the lamina propria shown in Figure A. Here, a relatively large nerve (N) and an accompanying small branch (N′) are viewed in cross section. Both myelinated and unmyelinated axons are present in these mixed nerves, and a capillary (C) runs through the center of the larger branch. The nerve is surrounded by secretory acini of lingual glands (LG). Several fat cells (A), or *adipocytes,* are present. Some of these structures are difficult to interpret by light microscopy alone. Fortunately, they are very easy to identify by electron microscopy. Try to find many of the structures shown in the light micrograph in Figure A in the electron micrographs in Figures B and C; this exercise will help you to develop the ability to instantly recognize the components of the tongue when you examine them in the light microscope.

Figure A. Light micrograph of vertical section through the tongue of the squirrel monkey. A, fat cell (adipocyte); C, capillary; D, duct of lingual gland; EP, epithelium; L, lymphatic capillary; LG, lingual gland; LP, lamina propria; N, nerve; SP, secondary papilla of lamina propria; arrow, base of filiform papilla. 340 X

Figure B. Matched electron micrograph of serial section through epithelium shown in Figure A. C, capillary; EP, epithelium; L, lymphatic capillary; LP, lamina propria; SP, secondary papilla of lamina propria; arrow, base of filiform papilla. 400 X

Figure C. Matched electron micrograph of serial section through lamina propria shown in Figure A. A, fat cell (adipocyte); C, capillary; LG, lingual gland; M, striated muscle fiber; N, nerve; N′, small branch of nerve. 775 X

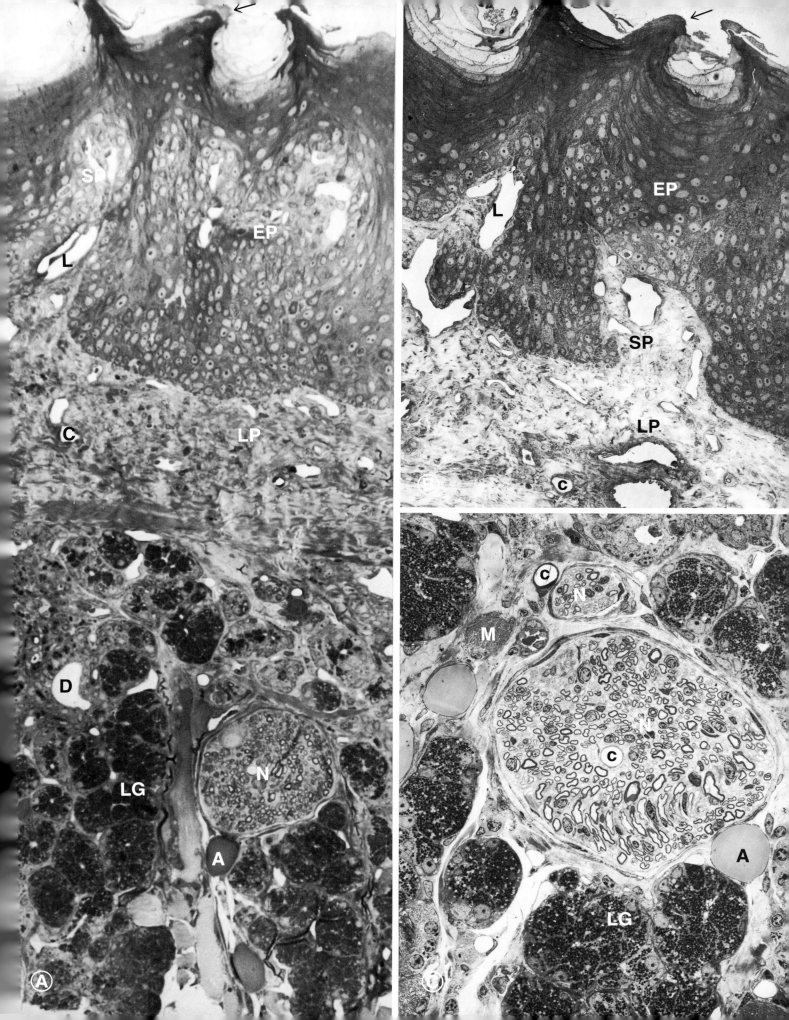

Plate 12–3

The Tongue, Part II

The human tongue has on its surface three types of projections, or papillae: filiform papillae, *fungiform papillae,* and *circumvallate papillae.* Of these, only the fungiform and circumvallate papillae are equipped with the chemoreceptive structures known as taste buds.

The base of the tongue contains a number of large, wartlike projections, the circumvallate papillae. Arranged in the shape of a V, these papillae, some 12 in number, provide a structural dividing line between the anterior and the posterior regions of the tongue. Each circumvallate papilla is a cylindric projection that is surrounded by a valley called the *circular furrow.* The lateral side of each papilla facing the furrow contains a large number of taste buds. These structures are evident in the micrographs at right.

Figures A and B are a matched pair of light and electron micrographs of serial sections taken through one side of a circumvallate papilla on the tongue of the squirrel monkey. Here, the upper surface of the papilla facing the oral cavity (OC) is at the top of the micrograph (Figure A); the circular furrow (F) that surrounds the papilla extends downward. The circumvallate papilla, like the rest of the tongue, is lined by a nonkeratinized stratified squamous epithelium (EP). The epithelium lies atop a lamina propria (LP) that sends a number of small projections, the secondary papillae (SP), up into the epithelium. The vast majority of the taste buds (T) of a circumvallate papilla are found on the lateral margins that line the circular furrow. The circular furrow provides a space in which saliva, bearing tastant molecules, can flow. Lingual glands, such as those described in Plate 12–2, open into the circular furrow at the base of the circumvallate papilla.

Each taste bud is a small, teardrop-shaped cluster of pale-staining cells that opens to the surface by means of a *taste pore* (arrow). An individual taste bud (T) is shown at higher magnification in the electron micrograph in Figure C. This taste bud is the same one indicated by the arrow in Figure B. (Its orientation, however, appears different, since the photograph has been rotated 90° so that the taste pore faces upward). The taste pore (arrow) is evident, as are the large, clear cells of the taste bud itself. Most of the cells in the taste bud are long, thin cells with round, basally located nuclei. The apical ends of the cells have microvilli that extend into a region called the taste pit that lies just beneath the taste pore. It is here that tastant molecules are thought to interact with taste cells in the process of chemoreception. The cells within the taste bud will be described in more detail in Chapter 20.

Figures A and B. Matched set of light and electron micrographs of serial vertical sections taken through a circumvallate papilla on the tongue of the squirrel monkey. EP, epithelium; F, circular furrow surrounding circumvallate papilla; LP, lamina propria; OC, oral cavity (Figure A only); SP, secondary papilla of lamina propria; T, taste bud, arrow, taste pore. Figure A, 280 X; Figure B, 500 X

Figure C. Electron micrograph of taste bud indicated by arrow in Figure B. EP, epithelium; F, circular furrow surrounding circumvallate papilla; T, taste bud; arrow, taste pore. 3,600 X

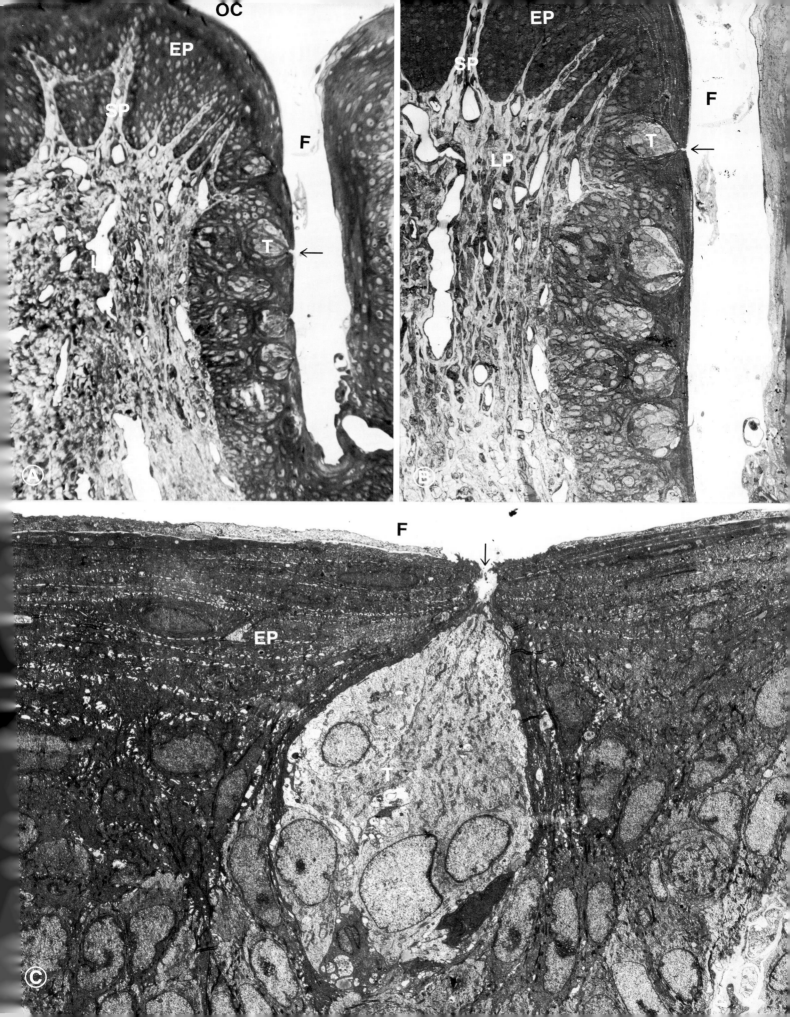

Plate 12–4

The Salivary Gland

When food enters the mouth, digestion begins. Digestion, the breakdown of large food particles into smaller ones, is facilitated in the oral cavity by the secretions of many different salivary glands. Taken together, the secretions are called saliva. Although saliva is often thought to be a simple substance, it is really quite complex, containing such chemical constituents as digestive enzymes (amylase), proteins, carbohydrates, mucoproteins, salts, and ions. Although there are thousands of ingredients in saliva, convention divides salivary secretions into two major categories: serous and mucous. Serous secretions, secreted by serous cells within salivary glands, are watery and nonviscous and tend to be proteinaceous. Mucous secretions, secreted by mucous cells within salivary glands, tend to be mucoid, viscous, and rich in polysaccharides and mucoproteins.

Secretory cells within salivary glands are grouped into acini. Each acinus contains serous cells, mucous cells, or both serous and mucous cells. All of these types of secretory acini are illustrated in Figures A and B at right, a matched pair of light and electron micrographs of serial sections taken through a salivary gland of the squirrel monkey. Serous and mucous acini look quite different from one another. Serous acini (S), for example, consist of dense, darkly stained, radially arranged pyramidal cells. Their large round nuclei are located at the base of the cell; the apical pole of the cell is packed with electron-dense secretory vesicles. Mucous acini, on the other hand, consist of pale, light-staining cells. The apical pole of the cell is filled with clear mucigen droplets; the cytoplasm and nucleus are compressed against the bottom of the cell. Other acini, called mixed acini (MS), contain both mucous and serous cells.

Whether mucous, serous, or mixed, all secretory acini within the salivary gland pour their secretions into a system of ducts, illustrated in Figure 12-2. The ducts range from very small to quite large. The smallest ducts are right at the neck of the acinus itself; the largest duct opens into the oral cavity. The smallest duct, the duct into which each acinus directly empties its contents, is the intercalated duct. As seen in Figures A and B at right, the intercalated duct (I) is a tiny tube lined by a simple cuboidal epithelium. Its diameter is smaller than that of a typical secretory acinus. (Were an acinus a grape, the intercalated duct would be its stem). The intercalated ducts, in turn, pour their contents into larger ducts, secretory ducts. A small secretory duct (SD), caught near its point of confluence with an intercalated duct, is evident in the micrographs at left. The structure of secretory ducts will be illustrated in more detail in Plate 12–5.

Within a salivary gland, the secretory acini are grouped together into distinct **lobules.** The individual lobules are separated from one another by strong connective tissue septa. Within a given lobule, the secretory acini and ducts are held together by a network of loose connective tissue that contains nerves, blood vessels, and many elements of the immune system. A careful look at the electron micrograph in Figure B will reveal small nerve branches (N), capillaries (C), and antibody-secreting plasma cells (*). These structures are also present in the light micrograph in Figure A.

Figures A and B. Matched pair of light and electron micrographs of serial thick and thin sections taken from a salivary gland of the squirrel monkey. A, fat cell (adipocyte); C, capillary; I, intercalated duct; M, mucous acinus; MS, acinus with both mucous and serous cells; N, nerve; S, serous acinus; SD, secretory duct; *, plasma cell. Figure A, 580 X; Figure B, 740 X

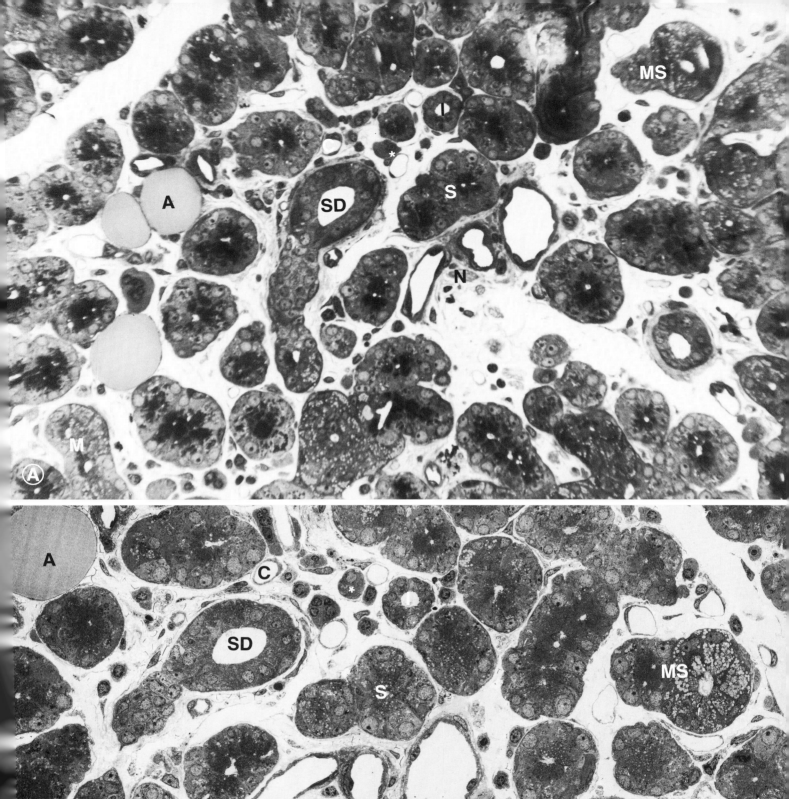
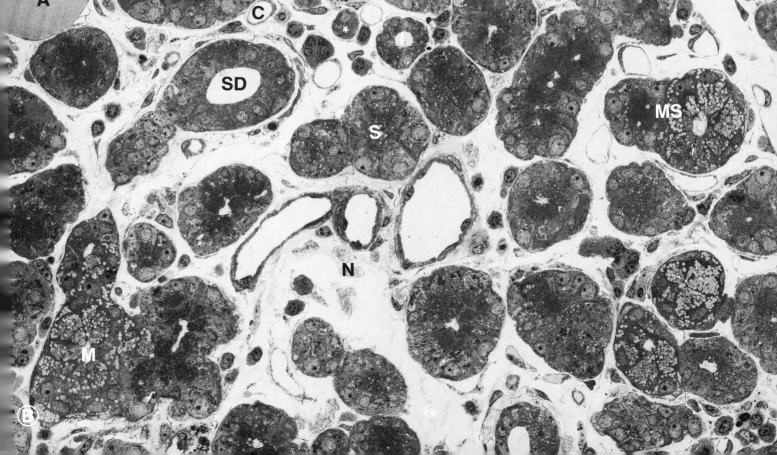

Plate 12–5

The Salivary Gland; Acini And Ducts

The three largest salivary glands in the oral cavity are the *parotid gland,* located in front of the ear; the *submandibular* (or *submaxillary) gland,* beneath the jaw; and the *sublingual gland,* under the tongue. The parotid is mostly serous; the submandibular gland is mixed, though it is more serous than mucous; and the sublingual gland, also a mixed gland, is far more mucous than serous.

The sublingual gland of the squirrel monkey is illustrated in the electron micrographs at right. Figure A depicts a number of typical secretory acini made of mucous cells. Each grape-shaped acinus appears round in cross section and consists of many mucous cells arranged around a small central lumen (L). On the very outside of each acinus sit one or two highly specialized contractile myoepithelial cells (arrow), frequently called *basket cells.* Each myoepithelial cell, shaped rather like an octopus, has its tentacle-like cellular extensions wrapped around the outside of the acinus. Under appropriate conditions of neuronal stimulation, the myoepithelial cells contract, expressing the salivary secretions into the small intercalated duct (I) that leads from each acinus. The myoepithelial cells, which are quite similar to smooth muscle cells, are spread so thinly that they are hard to see in low-magnification photomicrographs. In Figure A, they look like thin black lines and are most obvious around the perimeter of the intercalated duct (arrows, I).

The intercalated ducts lead to secretory ducts (SD), shown in Figure B. The histologic hallmark of the secretory duct is its very high density of mitochondria (Mi), which are for the most part aligned parallel to the long axis of the columnar cells that make up the duct's wall. When viewed at high magnification with the light microscope, these parallel, vertically oriented mitochondria appear as stripes, or striations. For this reason, secretory ducts are often called *striated ducts.* The mitochondria are intimately associated with the extensive basal infoldings of the plasma membrane of the cells of the secretory duct. Most cells with this configuration are active ion pumps—cells that pump ions against a concentration gradient, a process known as *active transport.* The cells of the secretory duct modify the saliva considerably, adding ions and water to the material produced by the acini. The water and ions are obtained largely from the blood circulating through the capillaries (C) that travel along the length of the duct.

In the image in Figure B, several unusual-looking secretory acini lie next to the secretory duct. These mixed acini contain both mucous (M) and serous (S) cells. The mucous cells are clustered about the center of the acinus. The serous cells are arranged in a crescent around the mucous cells and are frequently called *serous demilunes* because of their half-moon shape. The serous cells look quite different from the purely serous acini, such as the acinus depicted in Figure C. Here, each of the serous cells is shaped like a pyramid. Its broad base contains the nucleus (Nu), many stacked cisternae of the rough endoplasmic reticulum (RER), and a well-developed Golgi complex (G). The secretory vesicles (V) produced by the biosynthetic apparatus are clustered together in the narrow apical pole of the cell, ready to be released into the tiny lumen (L). Small capillaries (C) and nerves (N) pass close by. When viewed with the electron microscope, the secretory cells of serous acini clearly contain all the organelles necessary to produce large quantities of protein for export. They look quite similar to the secretory cells of the exocrine pancreas.

Figure A. Electron micrograph of mucous acini of the sublingual gland of the squirrel monkey. C, capillary; I, intercalated duct; L, lumen of acinus; arrows, myoepithelial cell. 1,850 X

Figure B. Mixed acini of same sublingual gland shown in Figure A. C, capillary; M, mucous cells; Mi, mitochondria; S, serous demilune; SD, secretory duct. 1,000 X

Figure C. Electron micrograph of serous acinus from squirrel monkey sublingual gland. C, capillary; G, Golgi complex; L, lumen; N, nerve; Nu, nucleus; RER, rough endoplasmic reticulum; V, secretory vesicles. 5,200 X

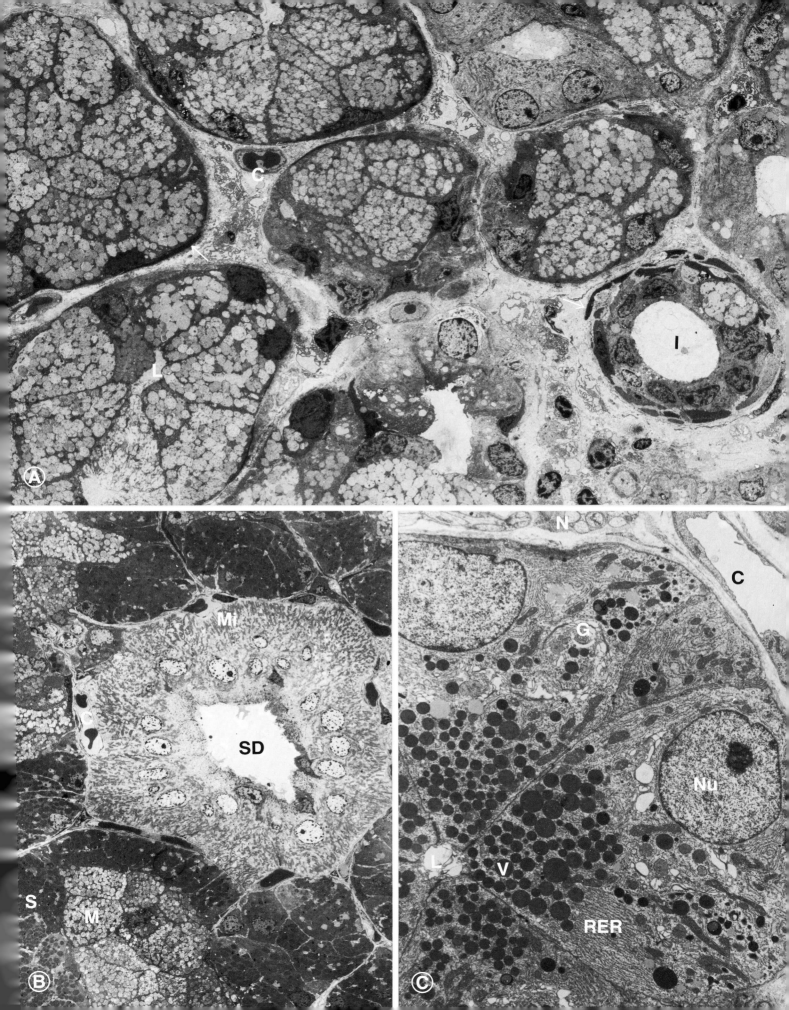

13

The Alimentary Canal

Overview

The microanatomy of the alimentary canal is easy to comprehend if you remember that in all superb designs—be they architectural, automotive, or biologic—*form follows function.* The species homo sapiens is organized as a two-hole open tube. Food makes a linear journey from one end of the tube to the other, with each segment of the alimentary canal performing a slightly different function. This process is reflected in (or, more correctly, permitted by) a series of successive microanatomic changes evident in samples taken at strategic points along the canal's length.

In this chapter, we shall follow the path of swallowed food as it enters the esophagus; is propelled into the stomach, wherein it is churned, acid-hydrolyzed, and stored; passes through the pyloric sphincter into some 30 ft of small intestine, wherein it is enzymatically digested and absorbed; and finally enters the colon, where water is resorbed, leaving concentrated waste ready for expulsion.

The primary function of the digestive system is, of course, to remove needed nutrients from food, get them into the general circulation, and leave waste materials behind. To do this, the alimentary canal must secrete chemicals that aid food breakdown, absorb and transport nutrient molecules to blood and lymph, and propel food along its length. Given these three processes, understanding the nature of the basic histologic plan of the alimentary canal is simple. Figure 13-1, a cross section through the wall of the small intestine, shows the elements of the basic histologic plan of the alimentary canal.

A surface epithelium of short-lived cells comes into contact with the food and, where appropriate, secretes chemicals and absorbs nutrients. Directly beneath the epithelium lies a thin layer of loose connective tissue, the lamina propria. The lamina propria contains cells of the immune series that fight unwanted, possibly infective foreign materials, and contains blood and lymph capillaries that not only take up digested nutrients, but also oxygenate and feed the epithelium.

The *muscularis mucosae,* difficult to identify in Figure 13-1, is usually a diffuse, ill-defined, gossamer-like skein of smooth muscle cells that imparts fine movements to the mucosa. Intestinal villi, for example, can shorten and wave about. Their movements result, in large part, from the efforts of the muscularis mucosae. Taken together, the epithelium, lamina propria, and muscularis mucosae form the *mucosa.*

Figure 13-1A. Light micrograph of a cross section through the jejunum of the squirrel monkey showing the basic histologic plan of the alimentary canal. 760 X

Figure 13-1B. Tracing of Figure 13-1A drawn to clarify the major components of the wall of the alimentary canal.

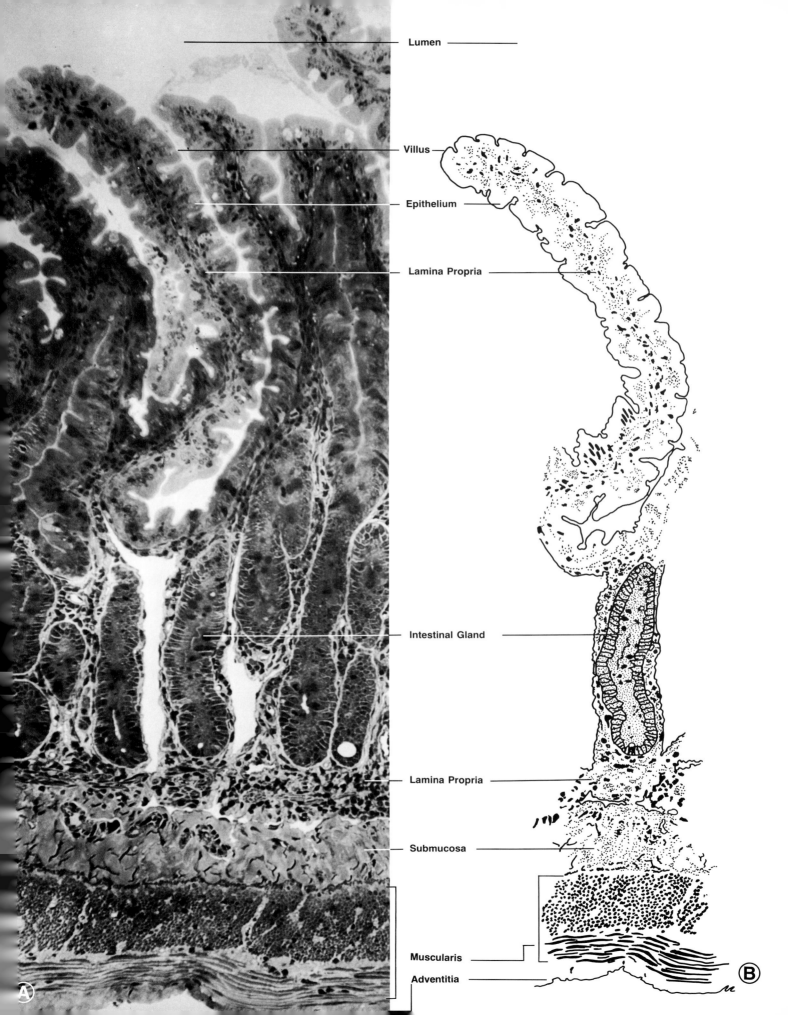

Lumen

Villus

Epithelium

Lamina Propria

Intestinal Gland

Lamina Propria

Submucosa

Muscularis

Adventitia

A

B

The *submucosa* is a bigger, tougher version of the lamina propria. A thick layer of dense connective tissue, the submucosa serves several functions. It binds the mucosa to a large muscle group, the *muscularis externa*; it contains a large population of immune cells, especially lymphocytes, that fight infection; it contains larger blood and lymph vessels whose finer branches enter the lamina propria; and, in the esophagus and duodenum, it can house submucosal glands.

The muscularis externa is a powerful group of smooth muscles set in bidirectional orienta- tions. The inner circular layer constricts the lumen; the outer longitudinal layer shortens the tube. Together, as in a worm, they cause peristaltic movements that not only propel food, but also provide the motive force for venous return of blood from the gut.

The entire gut is wrapped in a collagenous bag, the *adventitia,* which is a vascular, innervated extension of the mesenteries. The duodenum, applied against the wall of the body cavity, is covered by the *serosa,* an extension of the parietal peritoneum.

Plate 13–1

The Esophagus

Plate 13–1

The Esophagus

After food is swallowed, it enters the *esophagus*, the first part of the alimentary canal. The esophagus is a short tube, some 10 inches long, that leads from the mouth to the stomach. Because the function of the esophagus—to deliver food from mouth to stomach—is relatively simple, its microanatomic architecture is relatively simple as well.

As in all segments of the alimentary canal, the wall of the esophagus is histologically subdivisible into four major regions: the mucosa, the submucosa, the muscularis externa, and the adventitia. The mucosa (MUC) and submucosa (SUB) are illustrated at right. Figures A and B are matched light and electron micrographs of serial sections taken through the esophagus of a mouse, selected because its small size permits inclusion of most of the esophageal wall in a single cross section. The lumen (L) is at the top of the micrographs; the wall of the esophagus itself fills the rest of the field. The mucosa is made up of the epithelium (EP), the lamina propria (LP), and the muscularis mucosae. The mucosa lies atop the submucosa, which, in turn, is surrounded by the muscularis externa. The muscularis externa is wrapped in the baglike adventitia; neither the muscularis externa nor the adventitia are evident in the figures at right.

The esophagus is lined by a stratified squamous epithelium. In humans this epithelium is nonkeratinized, whereas in rodents it is lightly keratinized. Because the epithelium serves to protect the esophagus from abrasion by the fast-moving swallowed bolus of food, the degree of keratinization of the epithelium is largely a reflection of the amount of roughage in the animal's diet. As is the case in all stratified squamous epithelia, the flat surface cells, or squames, are periodically shed from the free surface and are replaced by the cells produced by the mitotic activity of the basal cell layer. In the figures at right, a single mitotic cell (arrow), caught in metaphase, has been cut in a pair of adjacent serial sections and photographed by light and electron microscopy.

The epithelium rests on a highly cellular lamina propria made of loose connective tissue. Beneath the lamina propria is the muscularis mucosae, which is conspicuous in the human esophagus. In the mouse esophagus shown at right, however, the muscularis mucosae is not a distinct layer. Instead, it consists of scattered smooth muscle fibers, too small to be readily detected at this comparatively low magnification.

The entire mucosa is supported by a strong submucosa, a bed of dense connective tissue that contains collagen fibers, elastic fibers, fat cells (A), and various vessels such as lymph capillaries (LC), blood capillaries (C), and postcapillary venules (V). The muscularis externa surrounding the submucosa propels food down the esophagus by peristaltic contractions. Several striated muscle fibers of the muscularis externa (M) are evident in the lower left corner of Figure B. In the upper esophagus, the muscularis externa is made of striated muscle; in the lower esophagus, as in the remainder of the alimentary canal, it consists of smooth muscle.

Figures A and B. Matched pair of light and electron micrographs of serial cross sections taken through the mouse esophagus. A, fat cell (adipocyte); C, capillary; EP, epithelium; L, lumen; LC, lymph capillary; LP, lamina propria; M, striated muscle fibers of muscularis externa (Figure B only); MUC, mucosa; SUB, submucosa; V, venule; arrow, cell in mitosis. 850 X

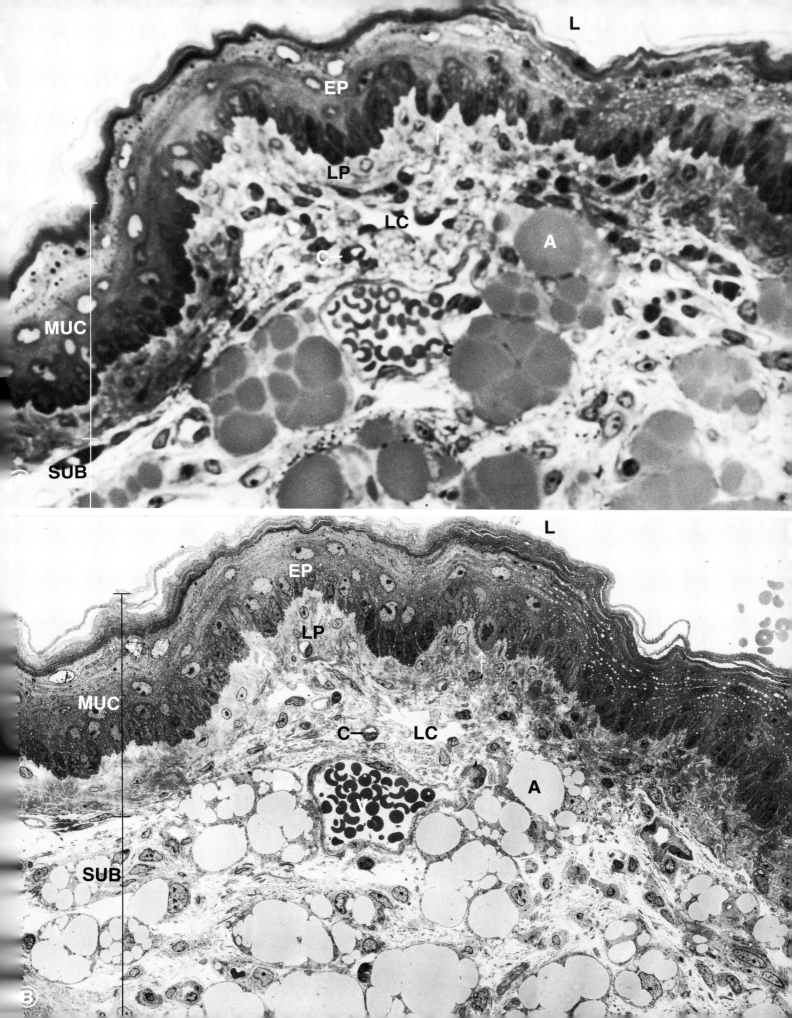

Plate 13–2

The Stomach

After a swallowed mouthful of food has passed through the esophagus, it arrives in the stomach. The stomach wall, illustrated in the matched pair of light and electron micrographs at right, is markedly different in function—and hence structure—from the esophagus. Whereas the esophagus is a relatively simple conduit for food, the stomach is a highly complex, muscular holding tank that doubles as a blender. Its mucosa houses glands that secrete enzymes and acids that accelerate the digestive process begun in the oral cavity. Although most absorption of digested food occurs further down in the alimentary canal in the intestines, some substances—water and alcohol, to name but two—are absorbed through the stomach wall and taken up into the general circulation.

The many functions performed by the stomach are reflected in its structural complexity. Initially, the microanatomy of the stomach wall can be difficult to comprehend. For example, histologic images often give the misleading impression that the surface of the stomach is thrown into small folds that resemble intestinal villi. In reality, the surface of the stomach is flat and perforated by conical invaginations called *gastric pits.* The gastric pits, in turn, are channels that lead to the *gastric glands.* The secretory products of the gastric glands, collectively called *gastric juice,* contain proteolytic enzymes and acids and are quite corrosive. Consequently, the lining of the gastric pits and the surface of the stomach consist of special protective cells called *surface mucous cells.*

Figures A and B at right are matched light and electron micrographs of serial sections taken through the stomach wall of the mouse, here selected because its small size permits inclusion of an entire cross section on an EM specimen support screen. The lumen (L) is at the top of the field of view. The inner surface of the stomach, lined by surface mucous cells (S), makes contact with the lumen and its contents. In Figure B, the mucus droplets that fill the apical pole of the cells are evident. Because the gastric pits (G) and the gastric glands tend to follow tortuous courses, some imagination is needed to see that the pits are continuous tunnels and the glands are simple tubes with cellular linings. The stomach, like the remainder of the alimentary canal, is lined by a simple columnar epithelium. The way in which this epithelium is bent, folded, and, in the case of the gastric glands, rolled into a tube can give the misleading impression that the epithelium lining the wall of the stomach is stratified.

The openings of several gastric pits (arrow) are evident in Figures A and B. Beneath the pits lie the gastric glands, whose lumens (*) open into the base of the pits. Close inspection of Figure B shows the profiles of several gastric gland lumens. Gastric glands are simple tubular glands whose walls are made up of several kinds of cells including *mucous neck cells, chief cells,* and *parietal cells.* The chief cells (C), whose cytoplasm is filled with secretory granules, make and release proenzymes such as pepsinogen. The parietal cells (P), also called *oxyntic cells,* secrete hydrochloric acid in surprisingly concentrated form. The tubular gastric glands are supported by the lamina propria which in the stomach is not the discrete layer it was in the esophagus. Beneath the gastric glands lies a well-developed muscularis mucosae (MM), under which lies the dense connective tissue of the submucosa (SUB). The submucosa, in turn, is surrounded by the contractile muscularis externa (ME), which, in the stomach, usually consists of three concentric layers: a circular, an oblique, and a longitudinal layer. The entire stomach is covered by the connective tissues of the adventitia (A).

Figures A and B. Matched pair of light and electron micrographs of serial sections through the stomach. A, adventitia; C, chief cell; G, lumen of gastric pit; L, lumen of stomach; ME, muscularis externa; MM, muscularis mucosae; P, parietal cell; S, surface mucous cell; SUB, submucosa; arrow, opening of gastric pit; *, lumen of gastric gland. 1,100 X

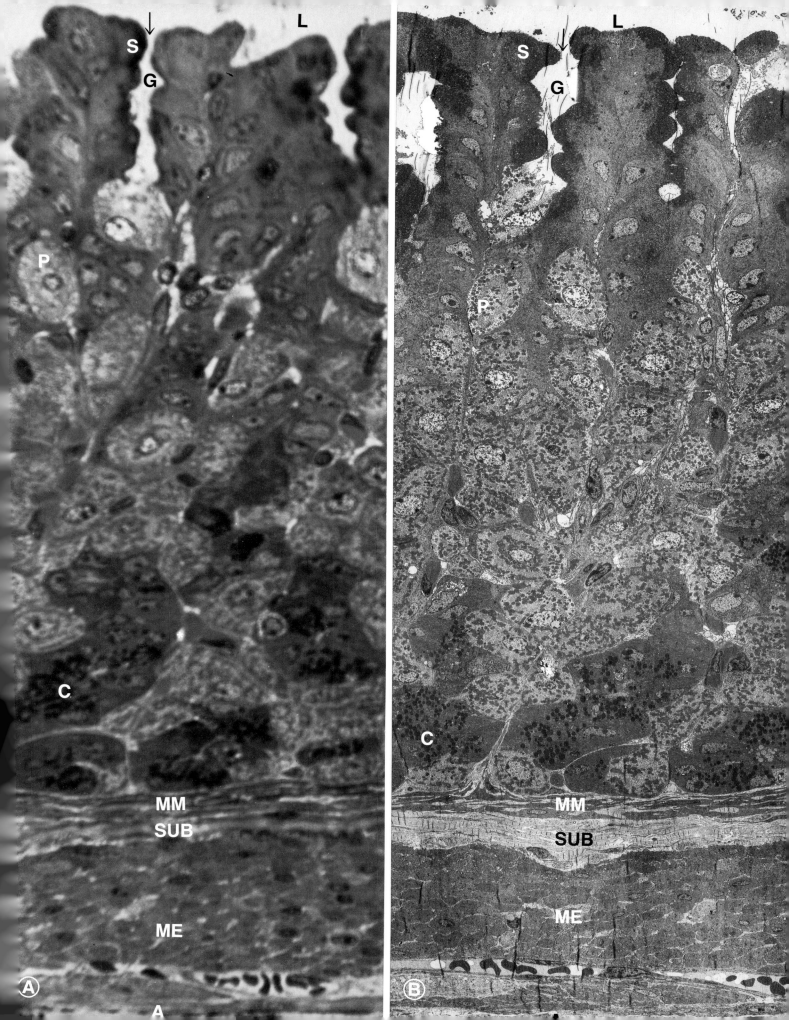

Plate 13–3

The Gastric Glands

Although most digestion of food occurs in the intestines, some preliminary processing occurs in the stomach. Here, the gastric juice secreted by gastric glands is mixed with the semisolid food received from the esophagus. Aided by the churning movements of the stomach's strong muscles, gastric juice converts material received from the esophagus into a pulpy mass of liquid called *chyme* that is suitable for delivery into the small intestine.

Gastric juice consists largely of secretions from two types of cells: chief cells (also called principal cells and zymogenic cells) and parietal cells. Both cell types inhabit gastric glands. Figure A, a low-magnification electron micrograph, shows the chief and parietal cells in position within a gastric gland; Figures B and C depict individual chief and parietal cells in greater detail.

Chief cells manufacture and secrete the proenzyme pepsinogen. Pepsinogen, which is made of protein, is released into the lumen of the stomach, where, at acid pH, it is converted to form *pepsin*, a proteolytic enzyme that cleaves peptide bonds. Because the chief cell is primarily a protein factory, its ultrastructure reflects the microanatomic features associated with the production of protein for export—a cytoplasm rich in rough endoplasmic reticulum and secretory granules. In Figures A and B, the basal pole of each chief cell (Ch) is loaded with densely packed cisternae of the rough endoplasmic reticulum (RER); the apical pole is packed with secretory granules (S). At lower left in Figure A, a group of chief cells is clustered about the tiny lumen (*) of a gastric gland.

Parietal cells are remarkably different in structure and function from chief cells. Parietal cells are not protein factories: instead, they secrete hydrochloric acid at astonishingly high (0.2-M) concentrations. Electron micrographs of parietal cells (Figures A and C) show an electron-lucent cytoplasm containing many mitochondria (M, Figure C). These mitochondria are essential for hydrochloric acid secretion. They provide energy in the form of ATP for the generation of hydrogen ion from carbon dioxide and water, a reaction mediated by the enzyme carbonic anhydrase. Hydrogen ions are pumped out across the parietal cell's surface into the lumen of the gastric gland. To facilitate this process, the surface area of the plasma membrane of each parietal cell is greatly expanded and is extensively invaginated to form a secretory canaliculus (Ca, Figure C).

Another class of cell, the *enterochromaffin cell,* (also called the argentaffin or argyrophil cell), is also present in the gastric glands (see Figures A and B). Enterochromaffin cells (E), which require special stains for viewing with the light microscope, are endocrine cells, secreting several biologically active substances including the hormone *gastrin*. Gastrin is extremely important to proper stomach function; it promotes pepsinogen secretion by chief cells, promotes acid secretion by parietal cells, and facilitates movements of the stomach wall. Taken together, the secretory products of the three types of cells in the gastric glands—chief cells, parietal cells, and enterochromaffin cells—all serve to prepare ingested food for entry into the next segment of the alimentary canal, the duodenum of the small intestine.

Figure A. Electron micrograph of gastric glands within the mouse stomach. C, capillary, Ch, chief cell; E, enterochromaffin cell; LP, lamina propria; MM, muscularis mucosae; P, parietal cell; RER, rough ER; S, secretory granules; *, lumen of gastric gland. 3,500 X

Figure B. Chief cell within gastric gland. Ch, chief cell; E, enterochromaffin cell; RER, rough ER; S, secretory granules. 5,600 X

Figure C. Parietal cell within gastric gland. Ca, secretory canaliculus; M, mitochondrion; P, parietal cell. 7,800 X

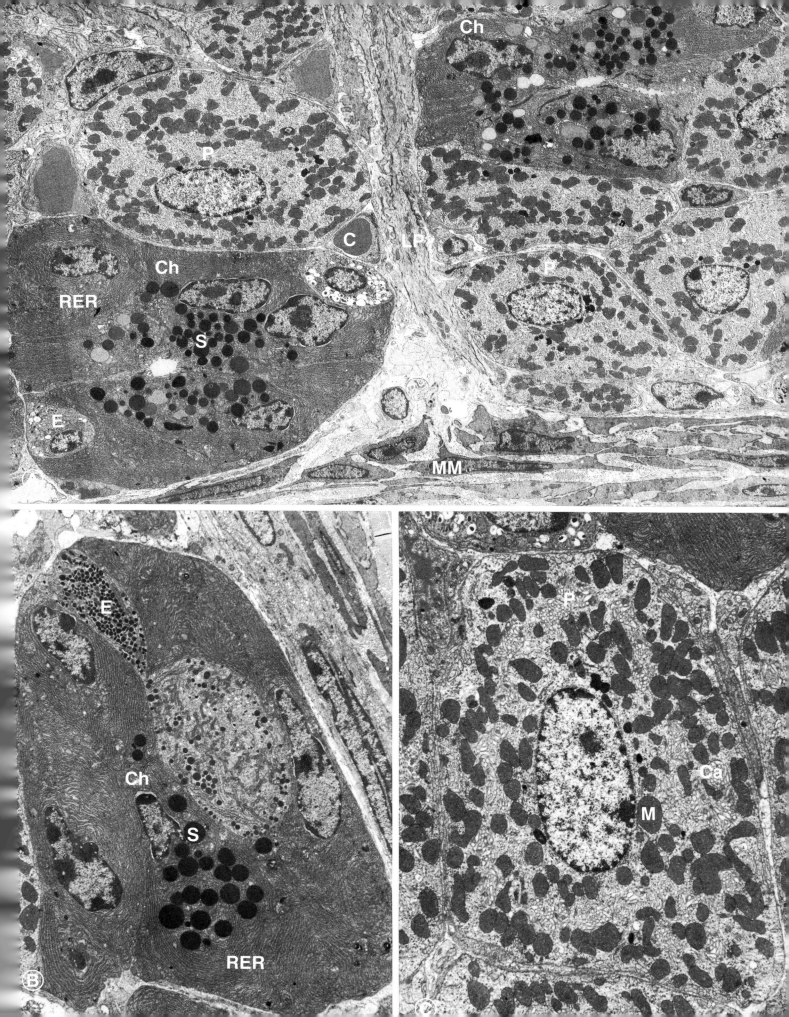

Plate 13–4

The Duodenum

Once the stomach has converted swallowed food into the pulpy mass called chyme, the pyloric sphincter—the muscular gateway into the intestine—opens. Chyme then passes from the stomach into the duodenum, the first segment of the small intestine. Here, digestion and absorption begin in earnest. In man, the entire intestinal tract measures some 30 ft in length. Most of this long tube is small intestine, which is anatomically divided into three segments, the duodenum, the jejunum, and the ileum. The wall structures of these three segments share the common plan presented in the overview. Despite their common pattern of organization, however, the duodenum, jejunum, and ileum do have distinct histologic features that render them identifiable in sectioned material.

Of the three segments of the small intestine, the duodenum is the shortest. Measuring a mere 10 in. in length, the duodenum is highly efficient in the digestion and absorption of food. It receives digestive enzymes from the pancreas and bile from the liver, which accelerate the digestion of materials in the intestinal lumen. The microanatomic organization of the duodenum reveals a number of structural specializations designed to increase its surface area, a feature crucial to an organ engaged in absorption.

First, the wall of the duodenum is thrown into large folds, the *plicae circulares,* which are visible to the naked eye. Second, the mucosa of the duodenum is organized into a series of small projections, shaped like cactus leaves, called villi, evident with the aid of the light microscope. Third, the surface of the epithelial cells atop the villi is highly modified to form microvilli—tiny fingerlike projections of the plasma membrane, visible at the level of the electron microscope. These three orders of folding—the plicae circulares, the villi, and the microvilli—provide three stages of surface area amplification not only for the duodenum, but for the jejunum and ileum as well.

Figures A and B are a matched pair of light and electron micrographs of serial sections taken through several villi (V) and part of the submucosa (SUB) of the duodenum. In these illustrations, the villi point to the right; the submucosa is at the left. Each villus is surrounded on all sides by the lumen (Lu) of the duodenum, normally filled with chyme received from the stomach. The villus is lined by a simple columnar epithelium (E) that may appear stratified when cut in oblique section. The free surface of the epithelium, as mentioned above, is covered by a prominent brush border made up of thousands of tiny microvilli. The epithelium is supported by a connective tissue core, the lamina propria (LP), which contains prominent lymph capillaries called *lacteals*. A single lacteal (L), cut along its length, is evident in the light (Figure A) and electron (Figure B) micrographs at right. Lacteals, with their thin walls and large-caliber lumens, often look like artifactual spaces under the light microscope. Because of their inherent low pressure they often collapse during tissue preparation and hence are hard to see. Lacteals are most conspicuous when filled with material recently absorbed by the villus.

At the base of the villi lie the intestinal glands—simple coiled tubular glands often called the *crypts of Lieberkuhn.* The intestinal glands contain mitotically active stem cells that replace intestinal epithelial cells constantly shed from the tip of the villus. Autoradiographic studies indicate that the life span of a typical intestinal epithelial cell is only 3 to 4 days.

Beneath the villi and intestinal glands sits the submucosa which in the duodenum contains conspicuous secretory glands called *Brunner's glands* (BG). These will be illustrated at higher magnification on the following plate.

Figures A and B. Matched pair of light and electron micrographs of serial sections taken through the mouse duodenum. BG, Brunner's glands; E, epithelium; IG, intestinal glands; L, lacteal; Lu, lumen of duodenum; LP, lamina propria; SUB, submucosa; V, villus; *, brush border. Figure A, 550 X; Figure B, 675 X

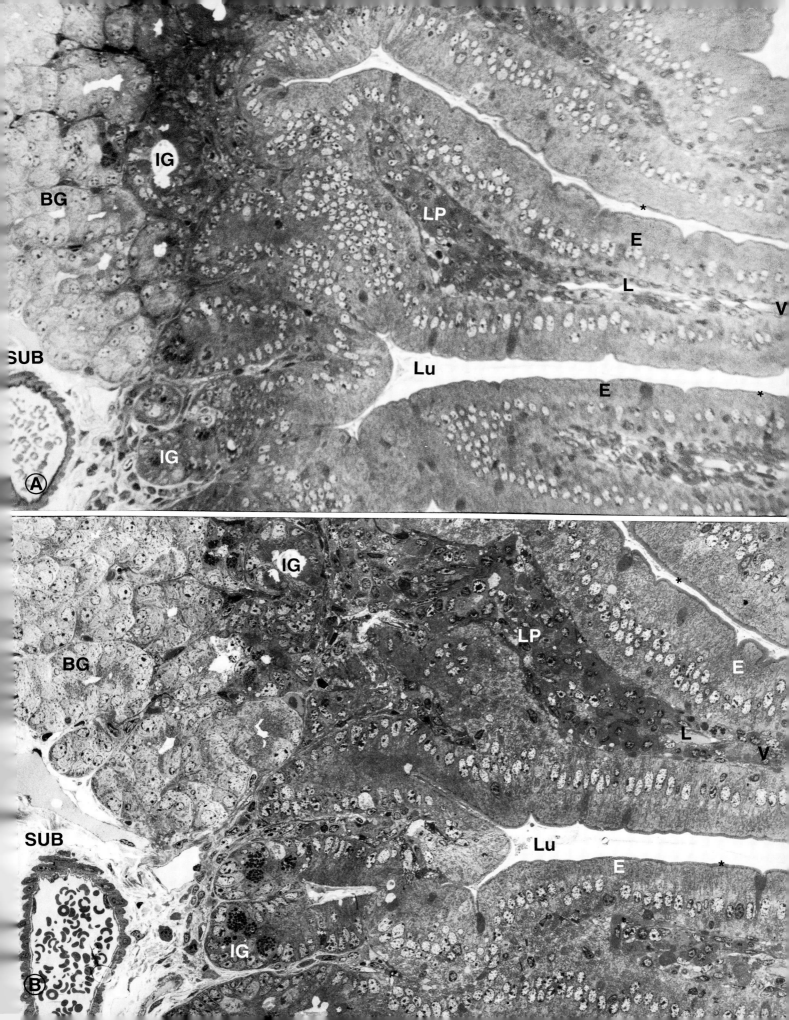

Plate 13–5

The Duodenum: Villus And Submucosa

Figure A is an electron micrograph of a longitudinal section through a single villus of the duodenum. In this image, two morphologically distinct types of cells inhabit the simple columnar epithelium—columnar absorptive cells (C) and goblet cells (G).

Within the intestinal lumen (Lu), complex foodstuffs undergo extracellular digestion; that is, they are broken down into simpler components by digestive enzymes from the pancreas and by bile from the liver. The end products pass from the lumen into the columnar absorptive cells, wherein further processing is carried out by the cytoplasmic machinery of the cells themselves. The nutrient materials are then transported from the columnar absorptive cells into the lamina propria (LP) that comprises the core of the villus. The lamina propria is richly supplied with lymphatic capillaries (lacteals, L) and blood capillaries (*) that deliver the absorbed nutrients to the general circulation. The circulation, in turn, distributes nutrients to all of the body's cells.

Within the lamina propria, tiny bundles of autonomic nerves (N) innervate the smooth muscle fibers of the muscularis mucosae that move the villi. In addition, many cells of the immune system reside in the loose connective tissue of the lamina propria. Several antibody-secreting plasma cells (P) are present in Figure A. Since the intestinal epithelium is in direct contact with the "outside world," it is a prime portal for entry of pathogenic microorganisms and antigens. Consequently, the establishment of an immunologic first line of defense within the lamina propria does much to combat infection and disease that could otherwise run rampant throughout the tissues of the intestine or, worse yet, invade the general circulation.

Part of the submucosa of the duodenum is illustrated in Figure B. Here, the base of the intestinal epithelium—composed of the intestinal glands—is at left; the submucosa is at right. The submucosa is a thick layer of dense connective tissue that contains collagen fibrils (Co), elastic fibers, cells of the immune series, lymph capillaries (L), blood capillaries (*), larger blood vessels such as arterioles (A), and nerves (N). In addition, the submucosa of the duodenum contains Brunner's glands (BG), which provide a convenient histologic marker for the duodenum, for they are not present in any other segment of the small intestine. Brunner's glands perform several crucial functions. They secrete bicarbonate ions, which buffer the acidic chyme received from the stomach. In addition, they secrete mucus that lubricates the epithelial surface over which the lumenal contents pass.

Figure A. Electron micrograph of longitudinal section through a villus of the duodenum. C, columnar absorptive cell; G, goblet cell; L, lymph capillary (lacteal); LP, lamina propria; Lu, lumen of duodenum; N, nerve bundle; P, plasma cell; *, blood capillary; arrow, brush border; dotted line, boundary between epithelium and lamina propria. 1,100 X

Figure B. Electron micrograph of upper part of the submucosa of the duodenum. A, arteriole; BG, Brunner's glands; Co, collagen fibrils; IG, intestinal glands (crypts of Lieberkuhn) at the base of the epithelium; L, lymph capillary; LP, lamina propria; N, nerve; *, blood capillary; dotted line, boundary between lamina propria and submucosa. 1,300 X

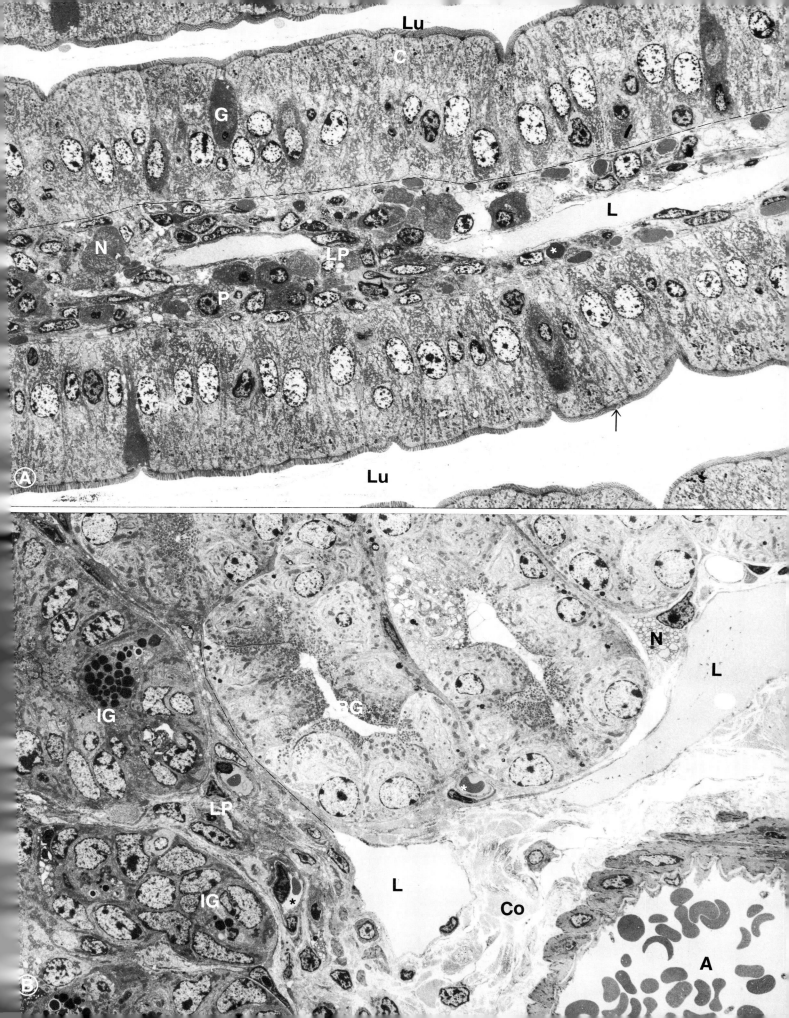

Plate 13–6

The Jejunum

Having run its course through the duodenum, the partially digested chyme enters the next segment of the small intestine—the *jejunum*. Some 8 ft long, the jejunum interconnects the duodenum with the ileum. Figures A and B at right are low-power electron micrographs of thin sections taken through the jejunum of the squirrel monkey. Figure A shows parts of several villi (V) projecting into the lumen; Figure B illustrates the lower aspect of the intestinal wall including the intestinal glands (IG), the lamina propria (LP), the submucosa (SUB), and part of the muscularis externa (ME).

The villus depicted in the center of Figure A has a convoluted profile, indicating that the villus was partially contracted at the time of fixation. Villi are motile; they pump up and down at a rate of 6 cycles/min, thereby maximizing surface exposure to gut contents and forcing nutrient-laden blood and lymph through capillaries and lacteals toward the larger plexus of vessels deep within the submucosa. Like the duodenum, the jejunum is lined with a simple columnar epithelium containing columnar absorptive cells (C) and goblet cells (G). The free surface is lined by a brush border (BB)—rows of tightly packed microvilli that provide a thirtyfold increase in epithelial surface area. The simple columnar epithelium covering the villus is in direct contact with the gut contents. The core of the villus is composed of the lamina propria (LP) and some smooth muscle fibers (*) sent in from the muscularis mucosae. In Figure A, part of the interface between epithelium and lamina propria has been marked with a dotted line. Within the core, the smooth muscle fibers are evident as dark, wavy, thin cells. The lymph capillaries, or lacteals, appear as thin-walled vessels that follow a tortuous course; they are easily distinguished from capillaries, because capillaries contain red blood cells and lymphatic vessels do not.

The lower portion of the wall of the monkey jejunum is illustrated in Figure B. Here we see the basal regions of the intestinal glands (IG) as they descend into the depths of the extensive lamina propria (LP). Within the lamina propria, one can see profiles of lacteals (La), capillaries (C), and numerous cells of the immune series. Fibroblasts abound amidst the network of connective tissue, as do scattered smooth muscle cells (*) of the muscularis mucosae. It is important to remember that often the muscularis mucosae is present not as a discrete layer of tissue, but rather as a series of smooth muscle fibers scattered throughout the lamina propria.

Beneath the highly cellular lamina propria lies the submucosa (SUB). Figure B clearly illustrates the dramatic difference between the appearance of the lamina propria and the submucosa; whereas the lamina propria consists of loose connective tissue, the submucosa is made up of dense connective tissue. The heavy sheets of collagen that make up the bulk of the submucosa are penetrated by lymph vessels (La), small arterioles (A), capillaries, and tiny nerve bundles. The submucosa acts, in a way, like a tubular tendon; it provides a substrate against which the large muscles of the muscularis externa (ME) can contract. The rhythmic contractions of the muscularis externa power the peristaltic waves that propel food distally down the length of the intestinal tract.

Figure A. Longitudinal section through the tip of a villus in the jejunum of the squirrel monkey. BB, brush border; C, columnar absorptive cell; G, goblet cell; L, lumen of intestine; LP, lamina propria; V, villus; *, smooth muscle fiber; dotted line, interface between epithelium and lamina propria. 1,300 X
Figure B. Electron micrograph of the lower aspect of the wall of the same jejunum. A, arteriole; C, capillary; IG, intestinal gland; La, lymph vessel (lacteal); LP, lamina propria; ME, muscularis externa; SUB, submucosa; *, smooth muscle fibers. 800 X

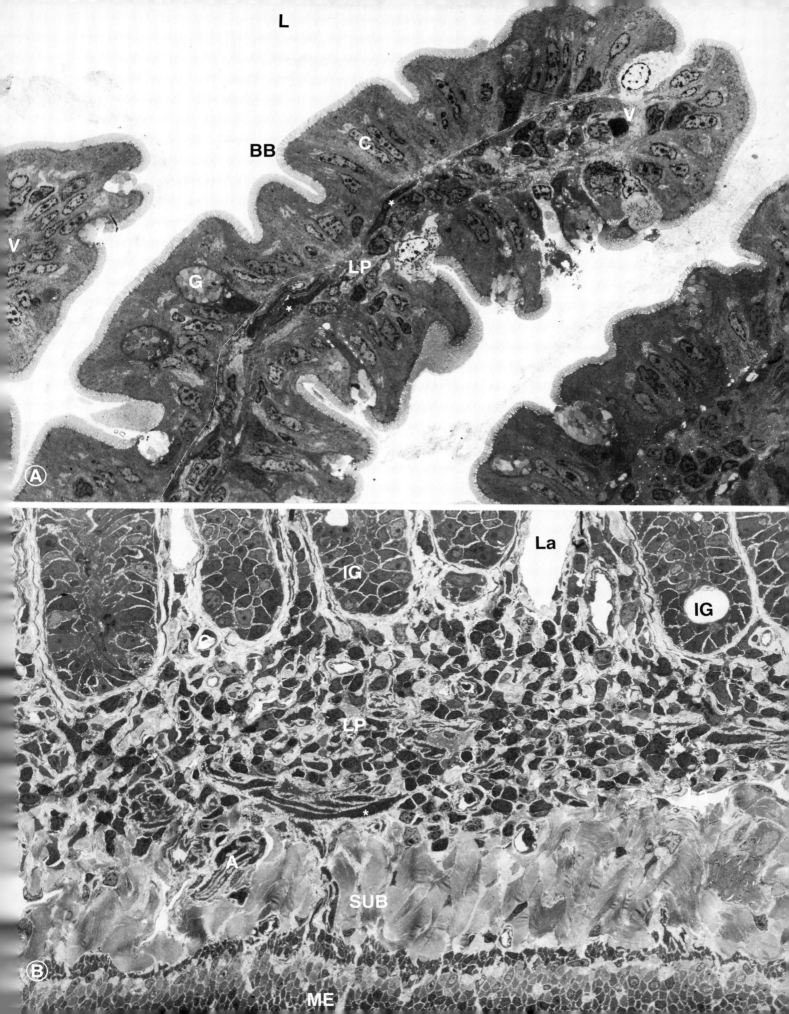

Plate 13–7

The Jejunum:
Intestinal Glands And Outer Wall

Figures A and B at right are a matched pair of light and electron micrographs of serial sections taken through the lower region of the wall of the monkey jejunum. The intestinal glands (IG) are near the top of the field; the lamina propria (LP) and submucosa (SUB) are in the middle; and the muscularis externa (ME) and adventitia (A) lie at the bottom of the field.

One of the features of intestinal microanatomy most difficult to visualize is the upward projection of the villi from the intestinal surface in contrast to the downward projection of the intestinal glands beneath the intestinal surface. Figures A and B illustrate the portion of the intestinal glands that lies beneath the intestinal surface; the intestinal surface is not evident in the image. (To locate the relative positions of villi and intestinal glands, see Figure 13-1.)

The simple columnar epithelium that lines each villus continues down through the intestinal surface as part of the epithelium that lines the intestinal glands. Each villus contains a central lacteal, or lymph capillary, that carries absorbed fats and other nutrients downward toward a plexus of lymph vessels deep in the submucosa. Each of these central lacteals continues downward from the villus, passes through the intestinal surface, and squeezes between adjacent intestinal glands en route to the submucosa. Several of these central lacteals (La) are clearly evident in Figures A and B. When seen with the light microscope, as in Figure A, these vessels can easily be mistaken for empty spaces in the tissue. The electron micrograph in Figure B reveals that they are not empty spaces at all, but rather represent the distended lumens of lymph vessels lined by a very thin endothelium. This delicate endothelium is underlain by long, thin smooth muscle fibers (*), derived from the muscularis mucosae, whose contractions help to compress the lymphatic vessel and pump the chyle absorbed from the intestinal lumen downward along the length of the lacteal.

This pumping motion imparted by the smooth muscles that lie along the length of the lacteal not only moves the chyle through the lacteal, but also compresses the adjacent intestinal glands. This action serves to move the secretions of the blind-ended tubular intestinal glands upward into the lumen of the jejunum.

The lacteals course through the highly cellular lamina propria that lies atop the submucosa. In the figures at right, the submucosa appears as a distinct layer of dense irregular connective tissue. Many arterioles (Ar) that penetrate the submucosa give rise to capillary (C) networks that supply the intestinal glands and villi with blood. In addition, the submucosa contains a fine network of autonomic nerves (collectively referred to as *Meissner's plexus*) that innervate the smooth muscles that move the intestinal mucosa.

A much larger group of autonomic nerves called *Auerbach's plexus* (AP) innervates the powerful smooth muscles of the muscularis externa. In the jejunum, the smooth muscle fibers of the muscularis externa are organized into two layers: the inner circular layer (IC) and the outer longitudinal layer (OL). The tissue at right has been cut in longitudinal section. Consequently, the smooth muscle fibers of the inner circular layer are shown in cross section; the fibers of the outer longitudinal layer are cut along their length. At the boundary between the inner circular and outer longitudinal layers, the nerve cells of Auerbach's plexus—autonomic neurons that assist in regulation of the peristaltic movements of the jejunum generated by the muscularis externa—are apparent.

At the bottom of the figure, the adventitia is evident. The adventitia, an envelope of loose connective tissue, wraps around the outside of the intestine and joins with itself to form the sheet of mesentery that suspends the small intestine from the dorsal body wall.

Figures A and B. Matched pair of light and electron micrographs of serial longitudinal sections taken through the lower half of the wall of the monkey jejunum. A, adventitia; AP, Auerbach's plexus; Ar, arteriole; C, capillary; IC, inner circular layer of muscularis externa; IG, intestinal glands; La, lacteal; LP, lamina propria; ME, muscularis externa; OL, outer longitudinal layer of muscularis externa; SUB, submucosa; *, smooth muscle in wall of lacteal. 770 X

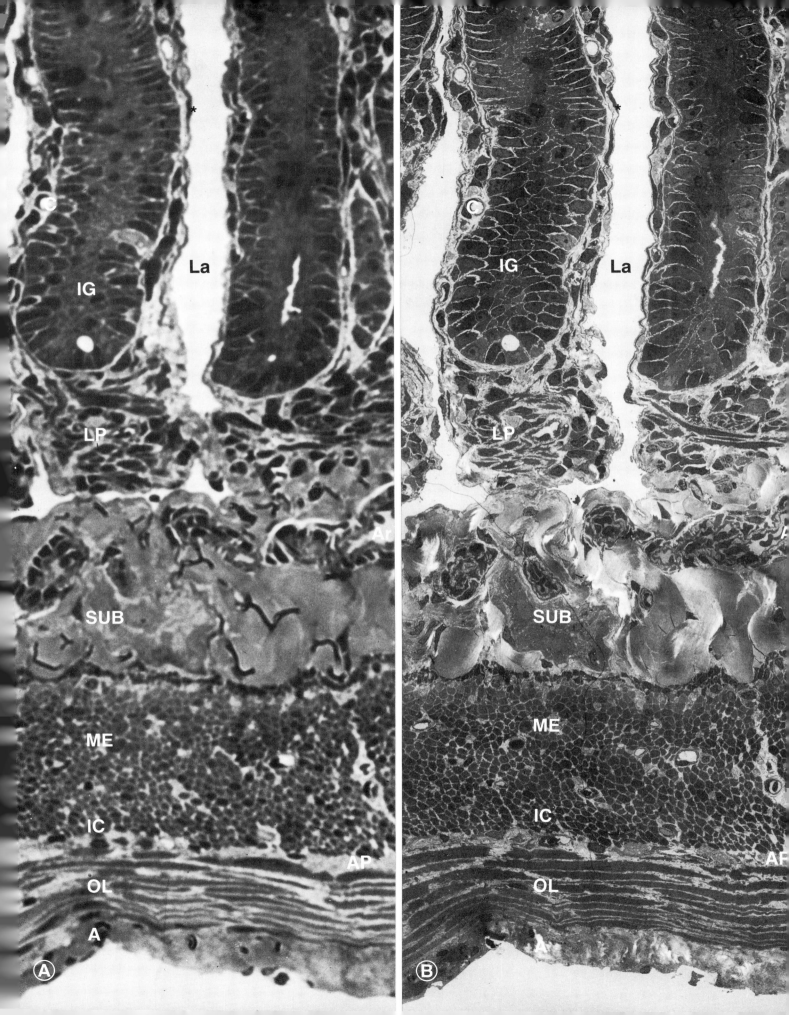

Plate 13–8

The Ileum

Figures A and B at right are low-power electron micrographs of the ileum, the most distal portion of the small intestine. The ileum, like the duodenum and jejunum, has villi that project into its lumen. The villi are lined by a simple columnar epithelium through which digested nutrients are absorbed.

Part of the epithelium lining a villus of the ileum is shown in Figure A. Here, two morphologically distinct types of cells, columnar absorptive cells (C) and goblet cells (G), lie side by side. The epithelial cells rest on a highly cellular lamina propria (LP); the brush border (BB) at their free surface is in direct contact with the lumen (L), which here appears as a narrow cleft between two closely spaced neighboring villi. The ileum has a much higher epithelial population of mucus-secreting goblet cells than the duodenum has, reflecting a histologic trend within the small intestine—i.e., the population density of goblet cells increases distally along the intestinal tract, because as food travels down the intestinal tract, more and more nutrients are absorbed, and the mass of material left behind in the gut lumen becomes more compact and requires more mucus to lubricate its passage. This histologic trend facilitates the identification of different regions of the small intestine.

The lower region of the wall of the ileum is illustrated in Figure B. Here, the basal portions of the intestinal glands (IG), the laminal propria (LP) that surrounds them, the submucosa (SUB), and the muscularis externa (ME) are evident. The submucosa of the ileum depicted in Figure B is different from that of the jejunum, illustrated in Plate 13–7. This difference is due not to specific differences in the construction of the jejunum and ileum, but rather to the different size of the animal of origin. The jejunum was obtained from a monkey, and the ileum, from the mouse. The smaller the animal, the more delicate the construction of its intestinal wall.

In figure B, a number of cells at the base of the intestinal glands have a distinct microscopic appearance. These cells are the *Paneth cells* (P)—cells that contain many large, electron-dense granules. It is thought that these dense granules contain lysozyme, an enzyme that breaks down bacterial cell walls. Paneth cells are believed to destroy certain intestinal bacteria by phagocytosis. Although Paneth cells can be found in all regions of the small intestine, they are normally most numerous in the ileum.

In addition to Paneth cells, the intestinal glands of the ileum contain intestinal epithelial cells, goblet cells (G), and dividing cells (M). The intestinal epithelial cells secrete an alkaline fluid that passes from the glands into the gut lumen. The dividing cells provide replacements for all classes of epithelial cells that are periodically shed from the tip of the villus. Autoradiographic experiments have shown that mitotic activity within the intestinal epithelium is restricted to stem cells that reside within the intestinal glands. Daughter cells migrate upward and differentiate into columnar epithelial cells or goblet cells. From birth to death, intestinal epithelial cells live some 3 to 4 days; consequently, the turnover of intestinal epithelial cells is high. It is no wonder that antimitotic drugs, such as those often administered in the course of cancer chemotherapy, have profound side effects on the digestive system.

Figure A. Electron micrograph of the simple columnar epithelium lining a villus of the mouse ileum. C, columnar absorptive cell; BB, brush border; G, goblet cell; LP, lamina propria; L, lumen of ileum. 3,800 X

Figure B. Electron micrograph of the same ileum showing the area beneath the intestinal surface. A, arteriole; G, goblet cells; IC, inner circular layer of muscularis externa; IG, intestinal glands; L, lumen of intestinal gland; LP, lamina propria; M, dividing cell; ME, muscularis externa; OL, outer longitudinal layer; P, Paneth cells; SUB, submucosa. 1,300 X

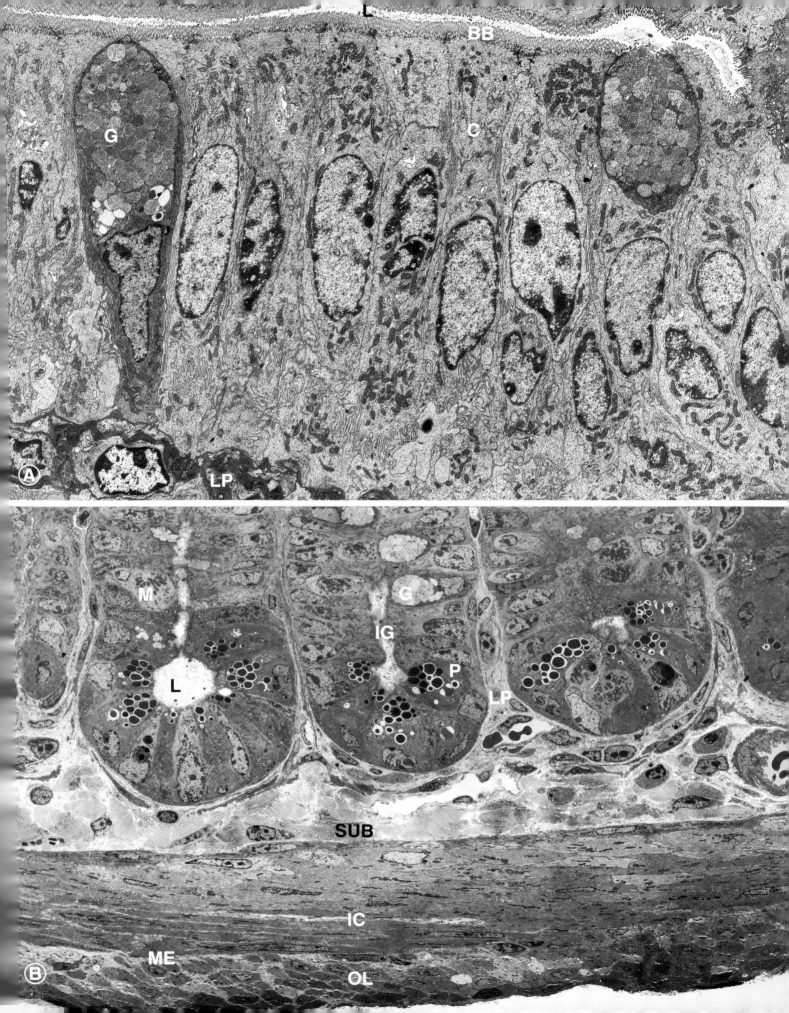

Plate 13–9

The Colon, Part I

During the process of digestion and absorption, the ingested material finally reaches the colon of the large intestine. The microanatomy of the colon is clearly illustrated at right by a matched pair of light and electron micrographs. Figure A is a light micrograph, and Figure B, an electron micrograph, of serial cross sections taken through the entire wall of the colon of the mouse.

The large intestine looks very different from the small intestine. First, it has no villi at all. The surface of the colon is quite flat and is perforated by holes that represent the openings (arrow) of intestinal glands (IG). The colon is primarily concerned with water resorption, a straightforward process that does not require the elaborate motile, absorptive, and conductive machinery of the villus. Second, the bulk of the mucosa of the colon is taken up by the intestinal glands. These are simple straight tubular glands that have a blind end near the submucosa (SUB) and an opening (arrow) at the intestinal surface. The lumen of the glands (Lu) can be followed for some distance within a single section because of the straight tubular nature of the colon's intestinal glands. Each intestinal gland is surrounded by a network of loose connective tissue, the lamina propria (LP), that contains collagen fibers, elastic fibers, smooth muscle fibers, and cells of the immune series such as antibody-producing plasma cells (*).

The mucosa of the colon is richly supplied with blood, evident in the micrographs at right. Here, an arteriole (A) passing between the lamina propria and the submucosa has been cut in longitudinal section. Although the arteriole is initially a bit difficult to identify in the light micrograph (Figure A), the electron microscope at the corresponding area in Figure B clearly resolves the cross-sectional images of the smooth muscle fibers wound spirally around the arteriole's contractile wall. Just above the arteriole lies a cross-sectional image of a thin-walled vein (V) filled with red blood cells.

Beneath the highly cellular lamina propria lies the dense connective tissue of the submucosa. Details of the construction of the submucosa are difficult to see at this relatively low magnification. At the junction between the lamina propria and the submucosa, however, some dark, thin lines that represent smooth muscle fibers of the muscularis mucosae are evident (arrowhead). Although these fibers can be seen with the light microscope (Figure A), they are more clearly illustrated by electron microscopy (Figure B). Repeated comparison of light and electron micrographs of serial sections through the same structures facilitates identification of the somewhat blurry images inherent in light micrographs of cells and tissues.

Beneath the submucosa lies the muscularis externa (ME), two sets of smooth muscle arranged in inner circular and outer longitudinal layers. Between the two layers is Auerbach's plexus (AP), a diffuse ganglion of autonomic nerves that assists in the regulation of the peristaltic movements of the intestine generated by the muscularis externa.

Figures A and B. Matched pair of light and electron micrographs of serial cross sections through the entire wall of the mouse colon. A, arteriole; AP, Auerbach's plexus; C, columnar absorptive cell; G, goblet cell; IG, intestinal gland; L, lumen of colon; Lu, lumen of intestinal gland; LP, lamina propria; ME, muscularis externa; S, artifactual space between submucosa and muscularis externa; SUB, submucosa; V, vein; *, plasma cell; arrow, opening of intestinal gland; arrowheads, smooth muscle fibers of muscularis mucosae. 550 X

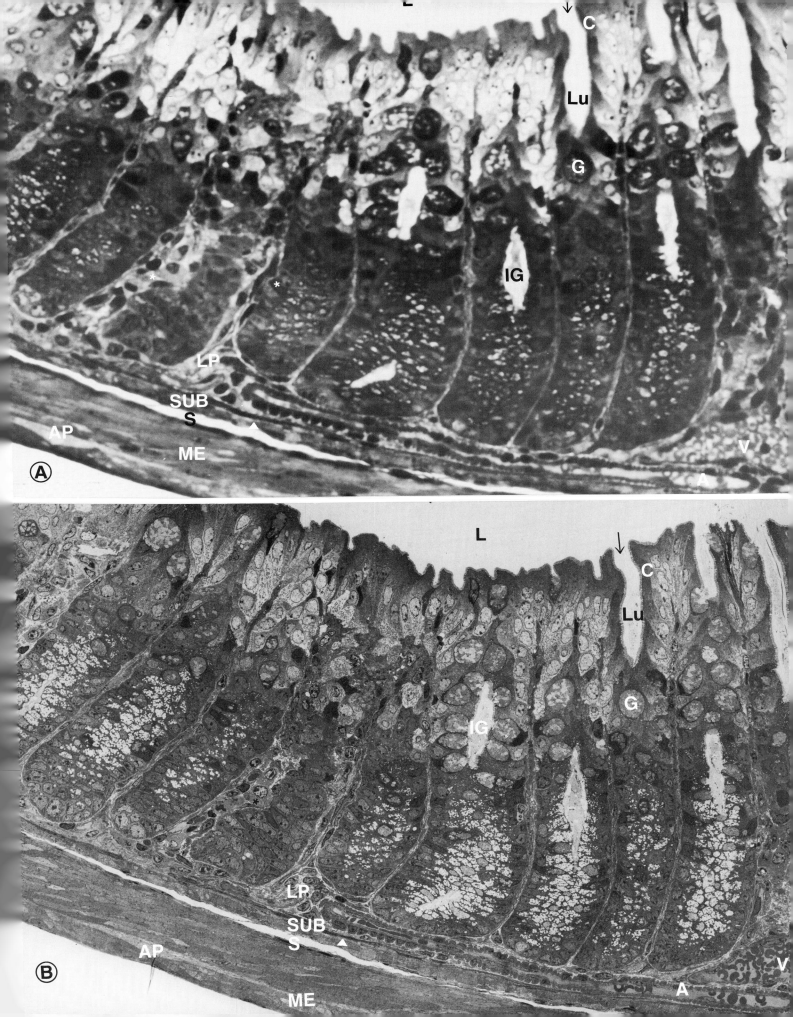

Plate 13–10

The Colon, Part II

Figure A at right is an electron micrograph of the free surface of the colon. Here, the simple columnar epithelium that lines the colon's surface comes into direct contact with the contents of the lumen (L) of the large intestine. The lumen of the colon is continuous with the lumen (Lu) of each intestinal gland, here seen as an invagination of the epithelial surface. The surface of the colon is flat and lacks villi; the clefts evident in the tissue in Figure A are invaginations of the surface, rather than spaces between adjacent projections.

As in the small intestine, the epithelium that lines the colon is composed of columnar absorptive cells (C) and goblet cells (G). The free surface of the colon's epithelium is a brush border (BB) made up of thousands of closely packed microvilli that greatly increase the surface area available for absorption. The apical surface of the goblet cell, too, bears a few short microvilli; these disappear when mucus is discharged onto the intestinal surface.

Goblet cells in several functional stages are evident in Figure A. Young goblet cells have a substantial amount of secretory cytoplasm dedicated to the elaboration of the many mucigen droplets that eventually come to fill the apical pole of the cell. At maturity, the secretory cytoplasm condenses and becomes dark-staining in the electron microscope. In the final stage of its life cycle, the goblet cell releases its complement of mucigen droplets. Once outside of the cell, the mucigen droplets coalesce to form mucus that coats the surface of the intestinal epithelium. A mature goblet cell (GD), caught in the act of releasing its mucus into the lumen (Lu) of an intestinal gland, is evident at the right side of Figure A. Nearby, several dying cells (D) may represent empty goblet cells that have spent themselves.

The basal portion of several intestinal glands (IG) of the colon is illustrated in Figure B. Many goblet cells (G), quite different in appearance from those at the free surface of the epithelium, line the lumen (Lu) of each gland. Few columnar absorptive cells are evident, and Paneth cells are quite rare in the colon's intestinal glands in healthy animals. A delicate lamina propria (LP) lies above a longitudinally sectioned arteriole (A)—the same arteriole photographed at lower magnification in Plate 13–9. Note the cross-sectional images of the many smooth muscle cells (SM) that are in the wall of the arteriole.

Beneath the lamina propria and the arteriole shown in Figure B, the images of smooth muscle of the muscularis mucosae (MM) are visible. The muscularis mucosae runs along the top of the submucosa (SUB). A small space (S), an artifact of tissue preparation, facilitates identification of the boundary between the submucosa and the muscularis externa (ME). Beneath the muscularis externa lies the serosa, a thin layer of connective tissue and mesothelial cells that line the outer surface of the large intestine.

Figure A. Electron micrograph of the surface of the colon. BB, brush border; C, columnar absorptive cell; D, dying cell; G, goblet cell; GD, goblet cell discharging mucus; L, lumen of colon; Lu, lumen of intestinal gland. 1,800 X

Figure B. Electron micrograph of the outer region of the wall of the mouse colon. A, arteriole; G, goblet cell; IG, intestinal gland; Lu, lumen of intestinal gland; LP, lamina propria; ME, muscularis externa; MM, muscularis mucosae; S, artifactual space between submucosa and muscularis externa; SM, smooth muscle in arteriole wall; SUB, submucosa. 1,900 X

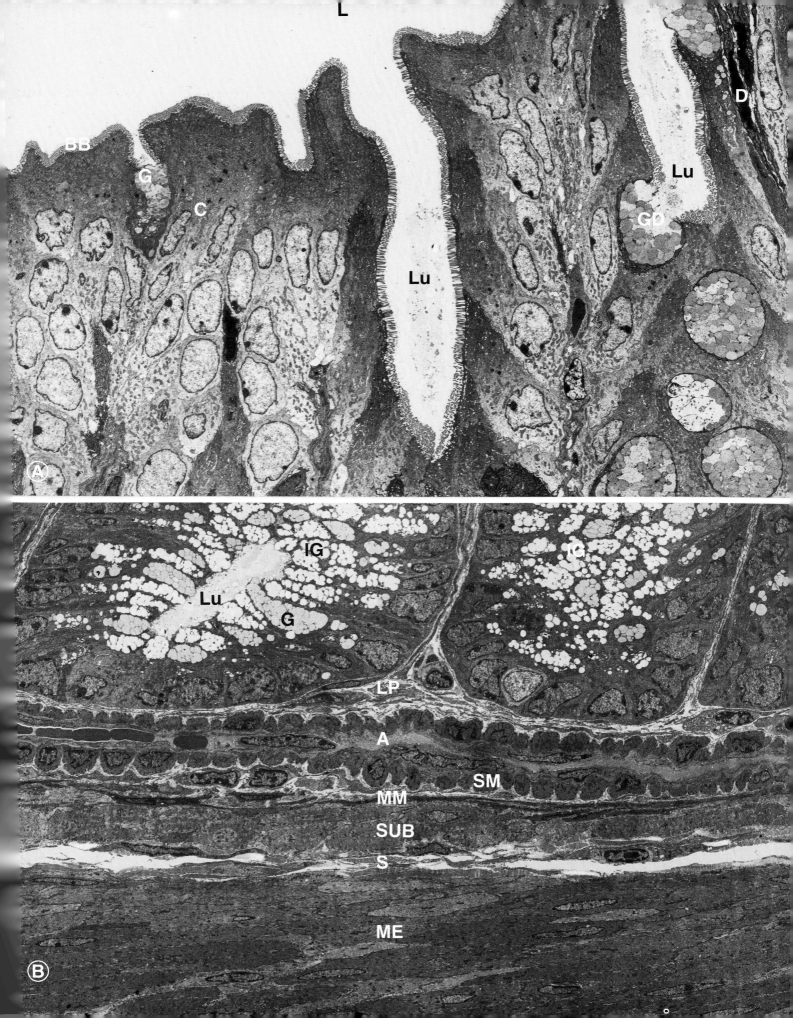

14

Pancreas, Liver, And Gallbladder

Overview

We now turn to three organs—actually, huge glands—that are intimately associated with the proper functioning of the digestive tract: the *pancreas, liver,* and *gallbladder.*

The pancreas, located near the duodenum, does double duty as an endocrine and an exocrine organ. The endocrine portion, called the *islets of Langerhans,* contains cells that secrete the hormones *insulin* and *glucagon.* The exocrine pancreas, described in this chapter, is a complex gland that contains many secretory units called acini arranged around a system of ducts. The ducts eventually combine to form the large *pancreatic duct* that carries *pancreatic juice,* a mixture of sodium bicarbonate and digestive enzymes, to the lumen of the duodenum of the small intestine. The microscopic anatomy of the pancreas is straightforward and needs little elaboration in this overview. (Chapter 1 provides a description of the functional unit of the exocrine pancreas, the pancreatic acinar cell.)

The gallbladder, a saclike structure appended to the liver, concentrates and stores bile for use by the small intestine in fat digestion. The microanatomy of the gallbladder, like that of the pancreas, is straightforward (see Plate 14–3).

The microscopic anatomy of the liver, however, unlike that of the pancreas and gallblad-

der, is difficult to understand. To do so requires an understanding of the *liver lobule,* a collection of efficiently placed vessels and cells that allows the liver to function as an extremely effective filter for the blood.

Thinking of the liver as a massive cross-flow filter helps in understanding its organization. The blood that leaves the digestive tract contains newly acquired macromolecules of all kinds. Were this blood to pass on to the rest of the body as is, individuals would become quite ill in short order, as there are many noxious substances that need to be treated before coming into contact with cells and tissues. The liver, then, is a sort of treatment plant placed in the path of the circulatory system between the gut and the rest of the body. The liver receives blood from the *portal vein,* a large vessel that drains the alimentary canal. The blood is guided through the liver by a series of very leaky capillaries called *sinusoids,* which are, in turn, in intimate contact with the cells of the liver itself, the *hepatocytes.* It is the hepatocytes that contain the elaborate enzymatic machinery that detoxifies noxious substances, packages glucose into glycogen, breaks down hemoglobin from dead red blood cells, and makes bile.

The liver has another, completely different blood supply—oxygenated blood, fresh from

164

the heart and lungs, that carries essential nutrients and gases to the hepatocytes. This blood comes into the liver via the **hepatic artery.** After the portal vein and the hepatic artery enter the liver, they branch many times to form smaller and smaller vessels that supply the lobules of the liver. At this level the microanatomy of the liver becomes complex and difficult to understand.

The lobule is best illustrated diagrammatically. Figure 14-1 shows one segment of a lobule that contains all of its major elements. Three of these elements—the portal vein, the hepatic artery, and the **bile duct**—are grouped together to form a **portal triad.** An ideal liver lobule, seldom seen in any given histologic section, consists of a group of portal triads arranged in circular fashion around a single central vein. Blood enters the lobule peripherally at the portal triad, flows centrally through the leaky sinusoids between rows of hepatocytes, and is collected by the central vein. The central vein, which carries blood away from the lobule, connects with larger vessels that carry blood out of the liver and back into the general circu-

lation. Materials are exchanged quite freely between the blood in the sinusoids and the hepatocytes. In addition, many macrophages, called **Kupffer cells** in the liver, are present near the walls of the sinusoids, where they police the area for unwanted particulate matter (including dead red blood cells).

Each lobule, then, positions hepatocytes and incoming blood in an ideal spatial array so that the hepatocytes can "treat" the blood before it is returned to the general circulation. Bile, made by hepatocytes from the breakdown of hemoglobin and other materials, flows from the hepatocytes into tiny channels between them called bile canaliculi. These bile canaliculi are not distinct vessels with walls of their own, but are channels that are lined by the cell membranes of adjacent hepatocytes. The bile canaliculi carry the bile outward from the hepatocytes to the portal triad, where the canaliculi join a branch of the bile duct. The bile duct carries bile to the gallbladder, where it is stored and eventually released into the lumen of the small intestine.

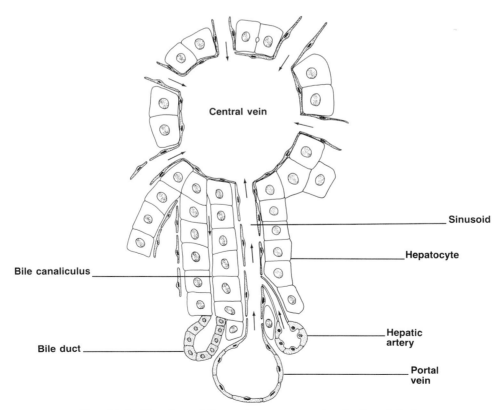

FIG. 14–1. Drawing of the major components of a liver lobule.

Plate 14–1

The Pancreas

The pancreas, a 9-in.-long digestive gland, is located next to the duodenum. Actually two glands in one, the pancreas has an endocrine portion that secretes hormones (insulin and glucagon) and an exocrine portion that secretes digestive enzymes. This plate will describe the exocrine pancreas.

The exocrine pancreas secretes copious amounts (1200 ml/day) of a watery substance called pancreatic juice, which is a mixture of sodium bicarbonate and digestive enzymes that travels through a system of pancreatic ducts and is released directly into the lumen of the duodenum. The sodium bicarbonate buffers the acidic chyme that enters the duodenum from the stomach; the digestive enzymes—trypsin, amylase, and lipase—break down the proteins, starches, and fats delivered to the duodenum from the stomach.

Figures A and B at right are a matched pair of light and electron micrographs of serial sections taken through the exocrine pancreas of the squirrel monkey. The histologic organization of the pancreas—especially the interrelationship of the secretory acini to the ducts—is difficult to visualize by light microscopy alone. Repeated comparison of the light and electron images at right will simplify that task considerably.

The pancreas contains thousands of acini. Each acinus is a near-spherical secretory unit—a ball of pyramid-shaped secretory cells (also called acinar cells) dedicated to the elaboration and release of digestive enzymes. The nucleus (N) of the acinar cell is located at the base of the cell. The secretory products are tightly packaged into dark-staining zymogen granules (Z) located at the apical pole of the cell. The zymogen granules are produced by an extremely well developed system of rough endoplasmic reticulum (RER) that fills the broad base of the acinar cell. Under the light microscope (Figure A), the nuclei and zymogen granules are clearly visible; the endoplasmic reticulum, however, is recogniza-

ble only because of its intensely basophilic–staining characteristics, which are not readily apparent in a black-and-white photograph.

In the electron micrograph, however, all of the components that are difficult to resolve by light microscopy are evident (Figure B). The rough endoplasmic reticulum (RER) appears as a series of closely apposed parallel cisternae. Interspersed among the cisternae of the rough endoplasmic reticulum are many mitochondria that supply ATP to fuel the energy-consuming process of protein synthesis. The digestive enzymes elaborated by the pancreatic acinar cell, like all enzymes, are made of protein. The pancreatic acinar cell, then, may be thought of as a protein factory—a cell that manufactures protein for export. The protein molecules are assembled from their constituent amino acids upon messenger RNA attached to the ribosomes; the assembled protein molecules are collected within the cisternae of the rough ER, ready for their transfer to the Golgi apparatus and subsequent packaging into membrane-limited zymogen granules.

Other cells found within the secretory acini of the exocrine pancreas are *centroacinar cells.* They are easy to identify in electron micrographs but can be difficult to spot in the light microscope. The same centroacinar cell has been identified (*) in Figures A and B at right. Close inspection of the centroacinar cell shown in Figure B will reveal that it is identical to the epithelial cells (E) that line the pancreatic duct (D). The cells appear similar because the centroacinar cells are really duct cells that interconnect each secretory acinus with a duct. Quite frequently, the plane of section will include part of an acinus and its duct. The cells of each acinus are arranged radially around a tiny lumen (L)—often not evident by light microscopy but readily visible by electron microscopy (Figure B). Because the lumen is coextensive with a duct, the centroacinar cells, as their name suggests, will appear in the center of each acinus.

Figures A and B. Matched pair of light and electron micrographs of serial thick and thin sections through the pancreas of the monkey. A, pancreatic acinar cell; C, capillary; D, pancreatic duct; E, epithelium of duct; RER, rough endoplasmic reticulum; L, lumen of acinus; N, nucleus of acinar cell; V, vein (Fig. A only); Z, zymogen granules; *, centroacinar cell. Figure A, 1,800 X; Figure B, 2,800 X

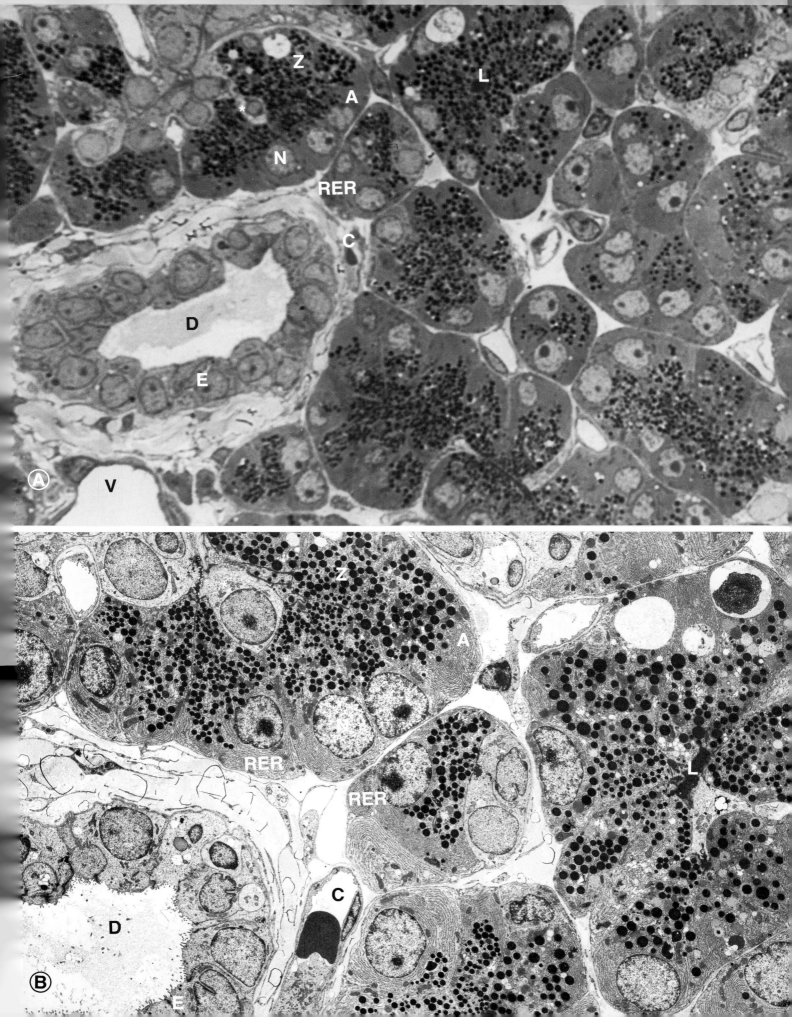

Plate 14-2

The Liver

The liver is a vital organ, essential for life. Its thousands of functions center mostly around taking up molecules and macromolecules from the blood, enzymatically modifying them, and eventually returning them to the bloodstream in different forms for distribution to and use by the rest of the body's cells and tissues. After a meal high in sugar, for example, the liver extracts glucose from the blood, converts it into glycogen for storage, and maintains stores of glycogen within its cells (the hepatocytes) for future use. When blood sugar levels fall below normal limits, however, liver cells convert glycogen into glucose and release it back into the bloodstream.

The liver enzymatically modifies the biochemistry of many substances, such as carbohydrates, proteins, lipids, and steroids. In addition, the liver manufactures and secretes bile—a fluid that, when released into the small intestine by the gallbladder, functions in fat digestion. In all of these processes save bile secretion, interaction between liver cells and blood is crucial. The necessary interactions between liver cells and circulating blood provide the central principle around which the microanatomy of the liver is organized.

The hepatocyte, or liver cell, is the individual unit of structure of the liver. As illustrated in Figure A, hepatocytes (H) are strung together in cords to form a simple cuboidal epithelium. Each cord of cells borders on a blood vessel, a sinusoid, which is a large, leaky capillary with big holes in its endothelial lining that permit free passage of plasma through its wall. The sinusoids (S) all converge on a central vein (CV) that receives blood from the sinusoids (arrows) and carries it away to large vessels that, in turn, return it to the heart.

The blood flowing from the sinusoids toward the central vein comes from two sources, the portal vein and the hepatic artery, illustrated in Figures B and C. The portal vein (PV) bears blood collected from the gut and the spleen and delivers it for filtering and processing to the hepatocytes via the sinusoids. The hepatic artery (HA) brings in fresh oxygenated blood to nourish the liver cells. Within the liver, the portal vein and the hepatic artery usually run side by side—along with the bile duct—to form a structure called the portal triad. The liver, which in humans weighs 3 lbs, includes far more vessels than the single examples illustrated at right; there are thousands of central veins and many more thousands of portal triads. Central veins and portal triads are grouped into extremely efficient histologic units of structure called lobules. (See the overview for a diagram and a description of the liver lobule.)

Blood flows through the liver rapidly. In humans, about 1 L of blood percolates through the liver sinusoids every minute. Given a total blood volume of 7 L, this flow rate is highly significant and underlines the importance of the liver to life.

Where, in this scheme, does the production and flow of bile fit? Hepatocytes make bile from bile salts that are by-products of hemoglobin catabolism. Hepatocytes release bile into tiny channels, called bile canaliculi (*) (Figure A), that are spaces between each hepatocyte and its neighbor. Bile flows from the hepatocytes outward toward the bile ducts that are located at the periphery of the liver lobule in the portal triad (see Figures B and C). The bile ducts, in turn, carry the bile to the gallbladder, which stores bile and releases it into the lumen of the small intestine.

Figure A. Light micrograph of portion of liver lobule showing radial organization of hepatocytes and sinusoids around the central vein. CV, central vein; H, hepatocyte; S, sinusoid; arrows, points of entry of sinusoids into central vein; *, bile canaliculus, 300 X

Figures B and C. Matched pair of light and electron micrographs of serial sections taken through portal triad of monkey liver lobule. BD, bile duct; H, hepatocyte; HA, hepatic artery; PV, portal vein; S, sinusoid. Figure B, 600 X; Figure C, 1,000 X

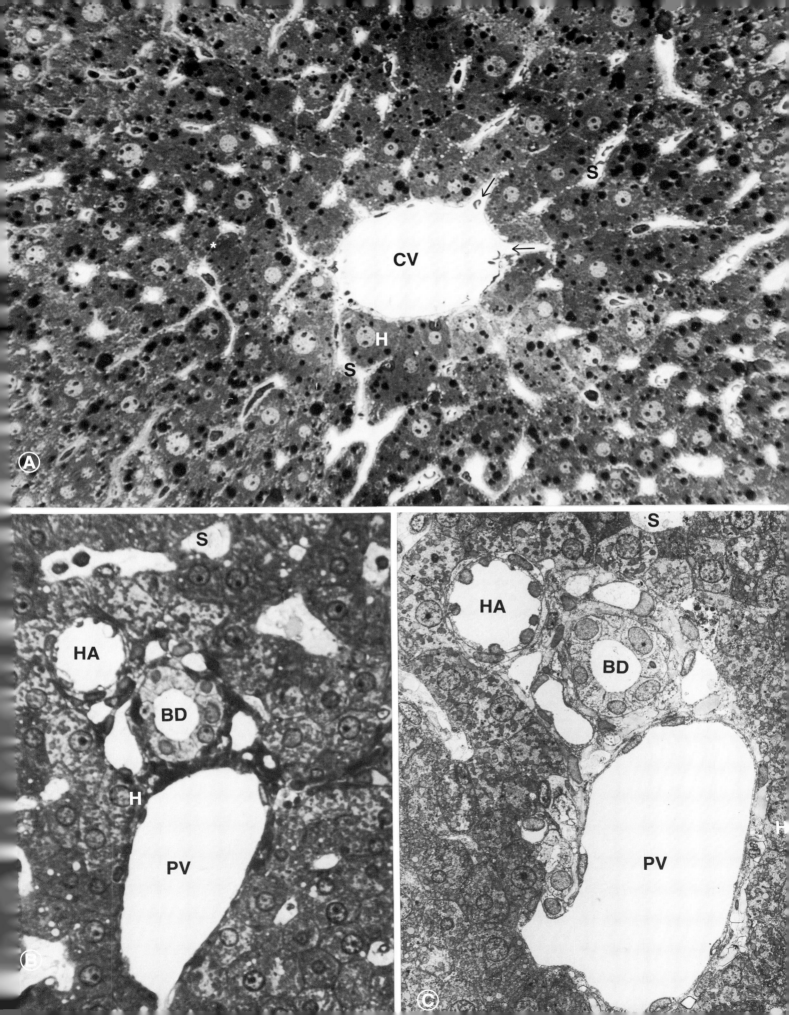

Plate 14–3

The Gallbladder

The gallbladder is a pear-shaped sac attached to the liver. Its primary function is to concentrate and store the bile produced by the hepatocytes of the liver. Under appropriate conditions of stimulation, the gallbladder releases its contents into the small intestine. There, bile emulsifies fats, reducing them to micelles of triglyceride suitable for uptake by the columnar absorptive cells of the intestinal mucosa.

The relationship between the function of the gallbladder and its microanatomic structure is evident in Figures A and B at right, a matched pair of light and electron micrographs of serial thick and thin sections through the gallbladder of the squirrel monkey. The wall of the gallbladder contains a mucosa (MUC), a muscularis externa (ME), and an adventitia (AD). There is no submucosa. The mucosa consists of a simple columnar epithelium (E) that lies atop a well-developed lamina propria (LP) made of loose connective tissue. The muscularis externa, not nearly as powerful as that of the intestine, consists of smooth muscle fibers set in many orientations—some circular, some longitudinal, most oblique. The muscularis externa is surrounded by an envelope of connective tissue, the adventitia.

The epithelial cells that line the mucosa are all alike and are well suited to perform their major function—concentrating bile received from the liver. In many respects, the epithelial cells lining the gallbladder resemble the columnar absorptive cells of the small intestine; they possess a brush border consisting of microvilli (arrow) and they lack the extensive system of rough endoplasmic reticulum and Golgi apparatus generally associated with cells actively engaged in the synthesis of protein for export.

The gallbladder, capable of concentrating bile from 3 to 11 times, does so by removing water. From the level of the nucleus to the basement membrane (arrowhead), the plasma membrane that lines the lateral cell surface is thrown into a prominent and highly convoluted series of lateral infoldings (*). In addition, that same cell surface has, built into its structure, ATP-dependent transport enzymes that pump sodium chloride against an osmotic gradient. When the gallbladder starts to concentrate bile, which it does largely by the process of water resorption, the epithelial cells pump large quantities of sodium chloride into the intercellular spaces between the epithelial cells, creating an osmotic gradient that pulls water out of the bile and into the intercellular spaces. The intercellular spaces greatly distend, as is readily apparent in electron micrographs taken of gallbladders active in water resorption. Water then passes from the intercellular spaces into the lamina propria and enters the bloodstream through the many capillaries (C) that course through the lamina propria. This elaborate biochemical process requires energy, which is supplied in the form of ATP made by mitochondria. Hence, the epithelial cells of the gallbladder contain many mitochondria (M), as seen in Figure B.

Once the bile has been concentrated, it is ready for transport into the lumen of the duodenum. When a person eats a fatty meal, which requires bile for its emulsification, the intestinal mucosa releases a hormone, *cholecystokinin,* into the bloodstream. When cholecystokinin reaches the gallbladder, it stimulates the smooth muscle fibers (S) of the muscularis externa to contract. (For this reason, patients with gallstones are advised to avoid eating fatty meals.) Muscular contraction forces the concentrated bile out of the gallbladder, through the common bile duct, and into the duodenum. In humans, from 0.5 L to 1 L of bile flows from the gallbladder into the duodenum every day.

Figures A and B. Matched pair of light and electron micrographs through the wall of the gallbladder of the monkey. AD, adventitia; C, capillary; E, epithelium; F, fibroblast; L, lumen of gallbladder; LP, lamina propria; M, mitochondrion (Figure B); ME, muscularis externa; MUC, mocosa; S, smooth muscle fiber; *, lateral infoldings; arrow, brush border; arrowhead, location of basement membrane. Figure A, 1,600 X; Figure B, 2,000 X

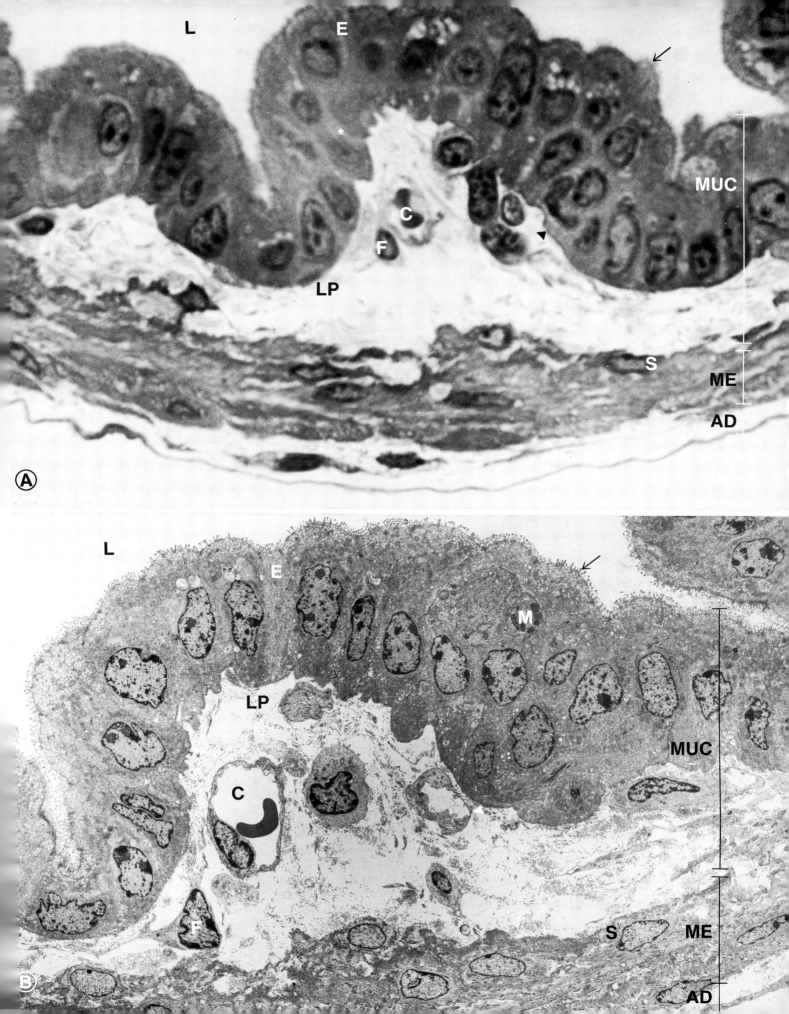

15

The Urinary System

Overview

The urinary system consists of the kidneys, ureters, urinary bladder, and urethra. This chapter focuses on the most complex component of the urinary system, the *kidney.* The kidney is an excretory organ of extreme importance. It cleanses the blood minute by minute, constantly maintaining a delicate balance of elements, compounds, molecules, and macromolecules that, via the general circulation, bathe and feed each of the body's cells. The kidney is so important to life that renal failure is lethal; when the kidneys cease their function, the body does, too.

In humans, the fist-sized kidney contains approximately two million functional units called *nephrons.* To understand the microanatomy of the kidney, one must first understand the microanatomy of the nephron. Unfortunately for the student of histology, it is quite difficult to learn and understand the structure of the nephron from sectioned material alone, because even the most favorably oriented sections through the kidney display complex and confusing images. Why is this the case? The answer lies in the compactness of the kidney. To fit millions of nephrons into a small space it is necessary to coil them and pack them tightly together. Consequently, any given histologic section through a kidney will contain hundreds of circular and elliptical profiles of tubules that represent bits and pieces of thousands of nephrons cut at various points along their length. The objective of this overview, then, is to de-

scribe the structure of the nephron in the simplest manner possible to facilitate interpretation of light and electron micrographs of sections taken through the kidney.

In order to understand biologic structures—or any complicated system, for that matter—it is always best to start with the simple and work up to the complex. In its simplest form, the nephron is basically a hollow tube with an opening at each end. Fluid, called the *glomerular filtrate,* enters at one end and flows out the other. The material that enters the tube is vastly different from the material that leaves it because the fluid's composition is greatly modified as it passes along the length of the tube. This modification is accomplished by cells that line the tubular nephron. Different kinds of cells, posted at different stations along the nephron, perform special biochemical operations on the glomerular filtrate.

Figures 15-1, 15-2, and 15-3 clarify the structure and function of the nephron. Figure 15-1 illustrates the overall layout of a human kidney and the relative position of a typical nephron within it. The kidney is shaped like a common backyard swimming pool. A longitudinal slice through its middle reveals that it has an outer region, called the *cortex,* and an inner region, called the *medulla.* As shown in Figure 15-1, part of the nephron is in the cortex and part is in the medulla. The port of entry to the nephron, called *Bowman's capsule,* is out in the cortex. It receives blood plasma in the form of the

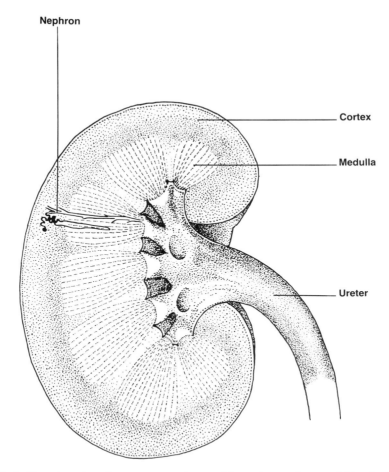

Nephron

Cortex

Medulla

Ureter

FIG. 15–1. Drawing that demonstrates the position of a nephron within the kidney.

glomerular filtrate. The exit from the nephron, the distal end of the *collecting duct,* is located in the medulla. Fully formed urine drips from the tip of the collecting duct into the renal pelvis, where it collects and enters the *ureter.* The ureter then delivers urine to the *urinary bladder* for storage and eventual elimination. Hence, the nephron receives blood plasma in the form of the glomerular filtrate and transforms it into urine.

The blood plasma that enters the nephron and the urine that leaves it are dramatically different in chemical composition. The difference is crucial; should the kidney's nephrons falter in their conversion of blood plasma to urine, toxic elements build up in the blood rapidly, and death is sure to follow unless medical intervention is swift. To understand the transformation of blood to urine by the nephron we

must isolate a nephron from the kidney, uncoil it, lay it out in a straight line, and examine its parts.

Figure 15-2 shows how an uncoiled nephron would look. (The drawing is not made to scale, although the parts are shown in the correct order.) At the top sits the entrance into the nephron, called Bowman's capsule. Bowman's capsule is a complex, microscopic funnel that receives filtered blood plasma—the glomerular filtrate—from a ball of capillaries called the *glomerulus.* (A blood vessel called the afferent arteriole brings blood to the glomerulus; an efferent arteriole carries it away.) After the filtrate has squeezed out of the capillaries and into the *urinary space* within Bowman's capsule, it passes on into the *proximal convoluted tubule.* The proximal convoluted tubule is lined by a simple cuboidal epithelium that, by complex

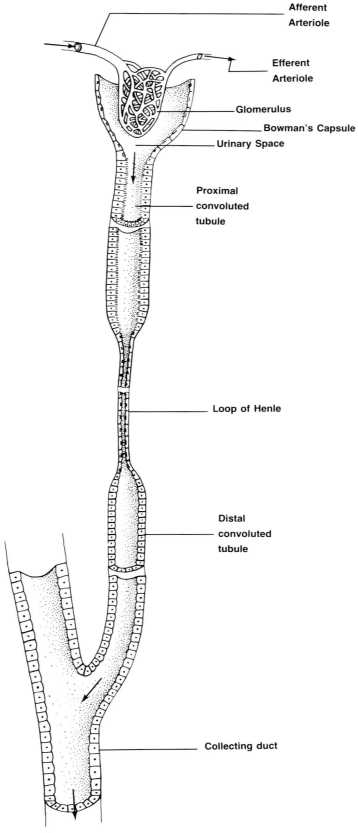

Afferent
Arteriole

Efferent
Arteriole

Glomerulus

Bowman's Capsule

Urinary Space

Proximal
convoluted
tubule

Loop of Henle

Distal
convoluted
tubule

Collecting duct

FIG. 15–2. A cutaway drawing of a nephron, straightened out and shortened, that shows the relative positions of the parts of a nephron along its length.

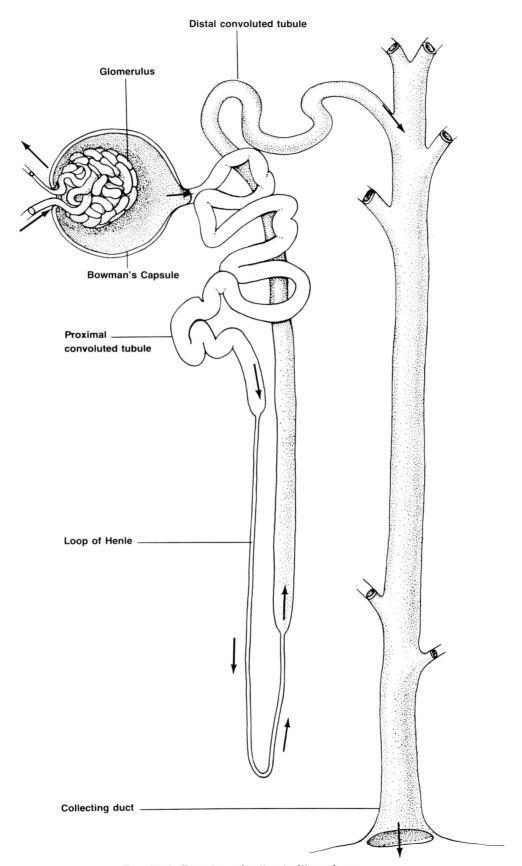

Distal convoluted tubule

Glomerulus

Bowman's Capsule

Proximal convoluted tubule

Loop of Henle

Collecting duct

FIG. 15–3. Drawing of a "typical" nephron.

biochemical processes of active and passive transport, moves most of the filtrate out of the nephron and into the tissue space (called the *interstitial space*) around it. Nearby capillaries then take up the materials from the interstitial space and put them back in the bloodstream for further use by the body.

From this discussion, it is evident that the kidney is not a device that simply filters harmful substances out of the blood. Quite the reverse happens; the kidney recycles useful materials. Bowman's capsule receives a plasma filtrate from the glomerulus; the remainder of the nephron pumps most of the "good" substances back into the bloodstream, leaving urea and harmful nitrogenous wastes behind to be eliminated from the body in the form of urine.

Although much of the work of the nephron is performed by the proximal convoluted tubule, the fluid that leaves it is further modified by the rest of the nephron before it is eliminated from the collecting ducts as urine. Having passed through the proximal convoluted tubule, the fluid passes into a long segment of the nephron called the *loop of Henle.* From there, urine enters the *distal convoluted tubule,* where more salts and water are eliminated, thereby further concentrating the urine. After passing through the distal convoluted tubule, the urine enters the collecting duct, which carries it through the medulla of the kidney and releases it into a container at the base of the kidney—the *renal pelvis*—which, in turn, empties into the ureter, which takes the urine to the bladder.

The actual nephron is coiled back upon itself along its length, as shown in Figure 15-3. It is largely by virtue of this coiling that many nephrons, some two million of them, can be packed into the small volume of a single kidney.

Plate 15–1

Kidney, Part I: The Renal Cortex

Plate 15–1

Kidney, Part I: The Renal Cortex

Figure A illustrates that the cortex of the kidney is an extremely complex histologic structure. To interpret this image, it is necessary to understand the basic structure and function of the nephron, as described in the overview.

The entrance to the nephron is the *renal corpuscle* (RC). When viewed by light microscopy, the renal corpuscle stands out in the cortex as a round, tightly packed mass of cells of types difficult to distinguish from one another. Under the electron microscope, however, the structure of the renal corpuscle appears almost comprehensible (RC, Figure B). As explained and illustrated in the overview, the renal corpuscle consists of two separate parts: the glomerulus and Bowman's capsule. The glomerulus is a ball of capillaries that delivers blood plasma to Bowman's capsule; Bowman's capsule is an elaborate two-layered cup that receives the glomerular filtrate. Figure B shows the *parietal (outer) layer* (arrow) of Bowman's capsule—a thin layer of epithelial cells that lines the capsule itself. Also present is a capillary (C) of the glomerulus, which is surrounded by fuzzy-looking cellular extensions (arrowhead). These tiny cellular extensions that surround the glomerular capillaries are called *pedicles,* parts of cells called *podocytes* that constitute the *visceral (inner) layer* (VL) of Bowman's capsule. These will be examined in more detail in Plate 15–2.

The base of Bowman's capsule is coextensive with the lumen of the first tubular portion of the nephron, the proximal convoluted tubule. When viewed with the light microscope (Figure A), the proximal convoluted tubule (PCT) is a thick-walled, darkly stained tubule. It is lined by a high cuboidal or low columnar epithelium that has a number of dark vertical lines called *basal striations* that extend upward from the basement membrane. The electron micrograph in Figure B reveals that these basal striations are actually many long, thin mitochondria.

In addition to the proximal convoluted tubules, profiles of the distal convoluted tubules (DCT) are evident in the renal cortex (Fig. A). At first, it is easy to confuse the cross-sectional images of proximal and distal tubules. Several key features, listed below, facilitate their individual identification. First, proximal tubules have a prominent brush border (∗) consisting of many microvilli; distal tubules do not. Instead, the apical surfaces of the cells lining the lumen of the distal tubules are smooth and have only a few microvilli. Second, the cytoplasm of the proximal tubules is dense and stains darkly; that of distal tubules is more clear and takes less stain. Third, the epithelial lining of the distal tubules is thinner than that of the proximal tubules. Unfortunately, both types of tubules have basal striations (i.e., mitochondria), which can make them hard to distinguish.

A third type of tubule, the collecting duct (CD), is evident in Figure A. Collecting ducts carry out of the nephron urine received from the distal convoluted tubules. Collecting ducts have a low cuboidal epithelium and a large lumen and are lined by cells with rounded cell surfaces.

Figure A. Light micrograph of the kidney cortex. CD, collecting duct; DCT, distal convoluted tubule; PCT, proximal convoluted tubule; RC, renal corpuscle; ∗, brush border of PCT. 600 X

Figure B. Electron micrograph of the kidney cortex. C, capillary; DCT, distal convoluted tubule; PCT, proximal convoluted tubule; RC, renal corpuscle; US, urinary space; VL, visceral layer of Bowman's capsule; ∗, brush border of lumen of PCT; arrow, parietal layer of Bowman's capsule; arrowhead, pedicles of podocytes. 1,100 X

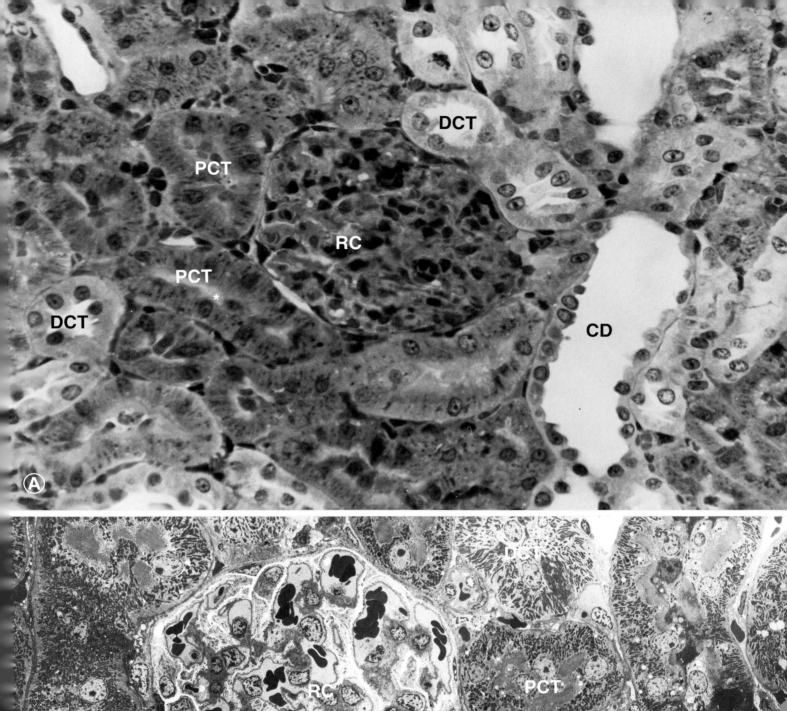

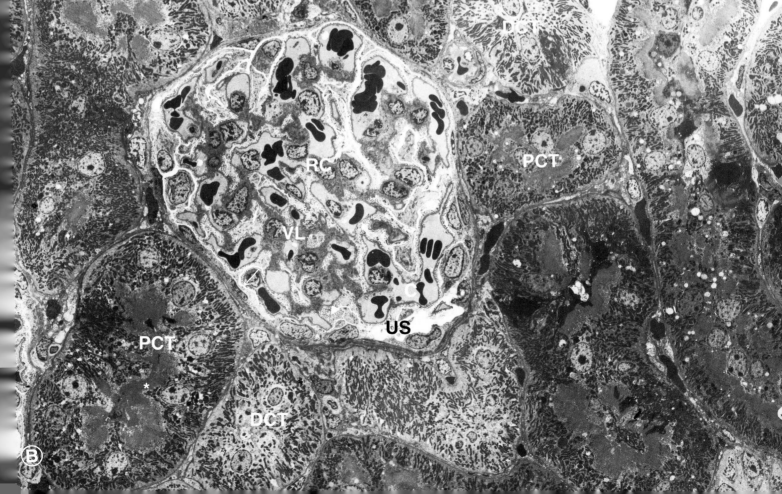

Plate 15–2

Kidney, Part II: The Renal Corpuscle

The renal corpuscle is the site where blood enters the nephron and undergoes the process of glomerular filtration. In order to understand the ultrastructure of the renal corpuscle, first recall that it is made up of two basic parts—the glomerulus and Bowman's capsule. Both structures are illustrated in the electron micrographs at right.

The glomerulus is a tightly coiled ball of capillaries (C) that sits within Bowman's capsule. Bowman's capsule resembles a double-walled chalice that contains the capillaries of the glomerulus. The walls of the chalice are extremely thin. The outer wall is made up of a simple squamous epithelium called the parietal layer (PL); the inner wall, called the visceral layer, is made of a monolayer of intricately sculpted, thin cells called podocytes (P) (Figure A). The podocytes send out fine foot-processes (arrow, Figure A) that, in turn, send out even thinner extensions of cytoplasm, called pedicles (arrowhead, Figure B).

The pedicles wrap tightly around the fenestrated capillaries of the glomerulus in the same way you might wrap your fingers around a leaky garden hose. In this case, the leaky hose would be a fenestrated capillary; your wrist, a foot-process of a podocyte; your fingers, the pedicles. Just as water would leak out through holes in the hose and squeeze through the spaces between your fingers, so does blood plasma leak out of holes in the glomerular capillaries and squeeze in between the pedicles of the podocytes. In this process of microfiltration, large molecules and blood cells are left behind in the blood space (BS) within the capillary; smaller molecules and ions pass along with the plasma through the holes in the capillary wall, through the slits between the pedicles, and move on out into the urinary space (US) of Bowman's capsule to form the glomerular filtrate. Because the urinary space of Bowman's capsule is continuous with the lumen of the proximal convoluted tubule (PCT), it is easy to see that the glomerular filtrate, once produced within the renal corpuscle, continues on through the lumen of the tubular nephron for further biochemical processing—the end product, of course, being urine.

Portions of proximal and distal convoluted tubules are shown in cross section in the micrographs at left. As often happens in histologic preparation of kidneys, the lumens of the tubules have collapsed. The proximal tubules have many radially oriented, basally located mitochondria that provide ATP for the highly bioenergetic processes of active transport of materials out of the tubule. The inner surface of the proximal convoluted tubule is modified to form an elaborate brush border (BB) consisting of thousands of tightly packed microvilli. This structure contrasts greatly with the lumenal surface of the distal convoluted tubule (DCT) shown in Figure B. Here, no microvilli are evident; instead, the cell surface appears rounded.

Figure A. Electron micrograph of the cortex of the kidney. BB, brush border of proximal convoluted tubule; BS, blood space; C, capillary; E, erythrocyte; P, podocyte; PCT, proximal convoluted tubule; PL, parietal layer of Bowman's capsule; RC, renal corpuscle; US, urinary space; arrow, foot-process extending from podocyte to capillary; arrowhead, basement membrane surrounding renal corpuscle. 2,000 X

Figure B. Electron micrograph of same kidney cortex shown at higher magnification. BB, brush border lining collapsed lumen of proximal convoluted tubule; BS, blood space; C, capillary; DCT, distal convoluted tubule; E, erythrocyte; PCT, proximal convoluted tubule; PL, parietal layer of Bowman's capsule; US, urinary space; arrowhead, pedicles of podocytes; *, collapsed lumen of distal convoluted tubule with no brush border. 3,000 X

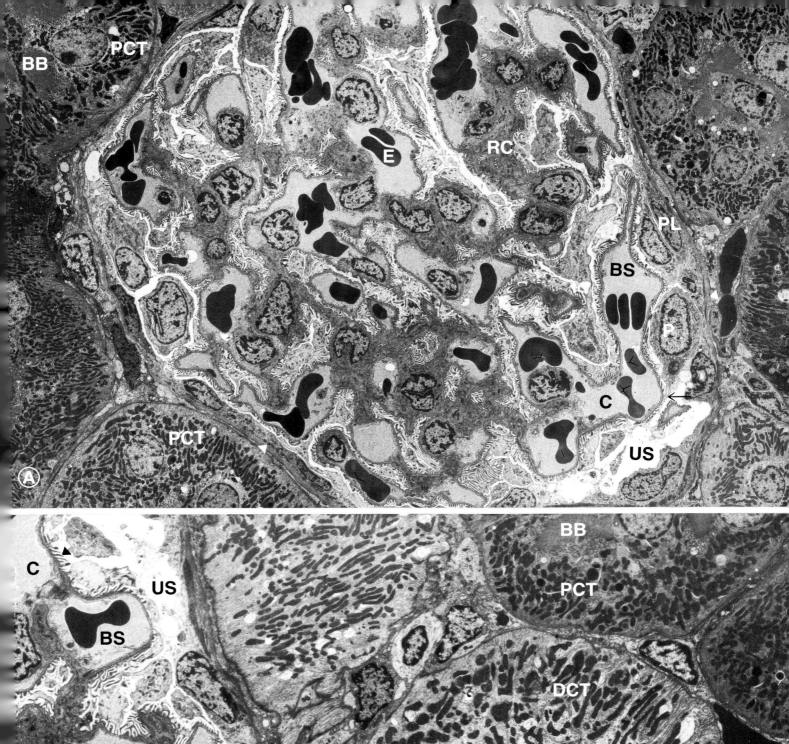

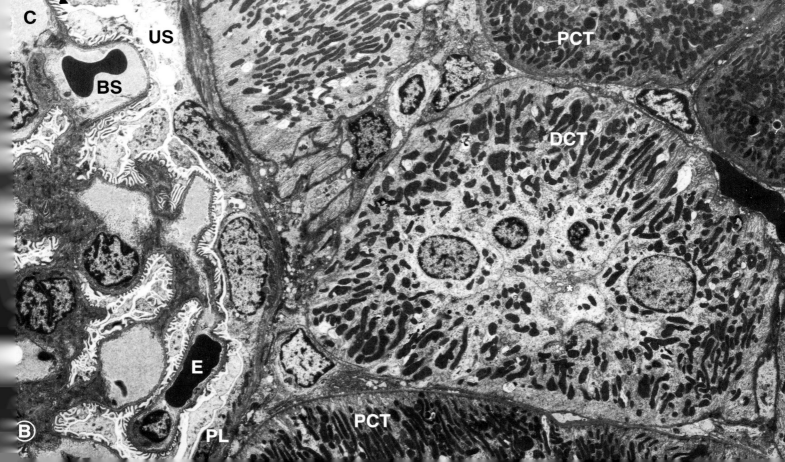

Plate 15–3

Kidney, Part III: The Renal Medulla

The microanatomy of the renal medulla differs dramatically from that of the renal cortex. In the medulla, the renal corpuscle, proximal convoluted tubule, and distal convoluted tubule are absent. Instead, the collecting ducts, loops of Henle, and capillaries called the *vasa recta* are present. These components of the nephron are illustrated by electron microscopy in Figures A, B, and C at right. (To prepare yourself to understand these images, refer to the drawings of the kidney and nephron in the overview to this chapter).

Figure A is an electron micrograph of a longitudinal thin section taken through the medulla of the monkey kidney. The field of view includes longitudinal images of collecting ducts (CD), loops of Henle (LH), and capillaries (C) of the vasa recta. The collecting duct is characterized by a large-caliber, open lumen lined by a simple cuboidal epithelium. The epithelium of the collecting duct is distinctive and easy to recognize. Each of the large, clear cells has a rounded cell surface that lacks a true brush border. The cells have round, euchromatic, centrally located nuclei. The lateral surfaces of neighboring cells form extensive interdigitations with one another (arrow), forming a dense zone so prominent that it is even detectable by light microscopy.

The loop of Henle is radically different in structure and function from the collecting duct. Its open lumen is lined by a very thin simple squamous epithelium that is about twice as thick as the endothelium lining the adjacent capillaries (C). Loops of Henle and capillaries are easily distinguished from one another by the presence of blood cells in capillaries. Under normal conditions, the loops of Henle have only urine in them and are free from erythrocytes.

All of the structures named above are shown in cross section in Figure B. Here the differences in wall structure between the collecting ducts (CD), thin loops of Henle (LH), and capillaries (C) are immediately apparent. Also evident are the connective tissue spaces (CT) that lie between each of the fluid-bearing tubes. These connective tissue spaces are of great functional significance, for not only do they contain collagen fibers that bind the soft tissues of the kidney together, but they also provide space in which fluids can accumulate during the vital exchange of ions, water, and metabolites between nephron and bloodstream.

The lower recesses of the medulla of the kidney are shown in Figure C. Here, the end of a collecting duct (CD) has been cut in longitudinal section as it opens into the renal pelvis (P). As described in the overview, urine drips out of the collecting ducts and into the renal pelvis, where it collects before passing through the ureter en route to the bladder.

Figure A. Electron micrograph of longitudinal section through the medulla of the kidney of the squirrel monkey. C, capillary; CD, collecting duct; CT, connective tissue; LH, loop of Henle; arrow, interdigitated lateral borders of adjoining collecting duct cells; *, basement membrane of collecting duct. 2,300 X

Figure B. Electron micrograph of cross section through medulla of the same monkey kidney. C, capillary; CD, collecting duct; CT, connective tissue; LH, loop of Henle. 1,500 X

Figure C. Longitudinal section through tip of collecting duct of the same monkey kidney. C, capillary; CD, collecting duct; CT, connective tissue; P, renal pelvis. 900 X

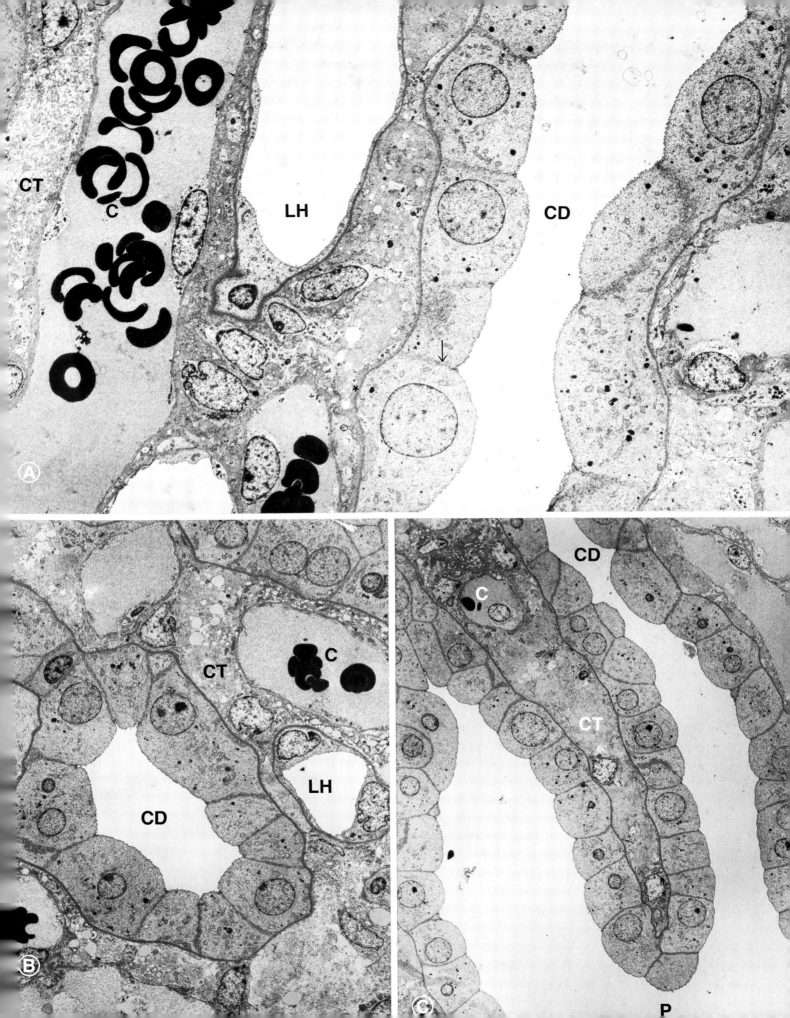

Plate 15–4

The Urinary Bladder

When urine has been formed and collects in the pelvis of the kidneys, it passes through the ureters and enters the urinary bladder, wherein it is stored until one finds an appropriate time and place for its release into the environment. The urinary bladder, then, is a storage tank, and a rather remarkable one at that. It is particularly unusual in two ways. First, it is a highly elastic container faced with a serious physical problem: it must repeatedly undergo formidable volumetric changes. When full, it is a large, turgid, tight-skinned sphere that can hold upwards of 1 L of urine. When empty, it is a flaccid, folded sac lying limp on the pelvic floor. This conformational change can occur with astonishing rapidity. Second, the bladder is faced with a serious physiologic problem: urine is highly hypertonic to cytoplasm, and the epithelial cells lining the lumen must somehow protect themselves from instant death at the hands of osmotic extraction.

The bladder solves these physical and physiologic problems with a number of structures built into its wall. Figures A and B at right are a matched pair of light and electron micrographs of serial thick and thin cross sections taken through the wall of the bladder of the squirrel monkey. This bladder was partially filled with urine at the time of tissue preparation.

The lumen (L) of the bladder is lined by an unusual type of epithelium called *transitional epithelium* (TE). Unique to the conduits and containers of the urinary tract, transitional epithelium is so named because it undergoes a marked morphologic transition in response to the degree to which the epithelium is stretched—which, in turn, depends on the degree to which the container that it lines is filled. Consequently, transitional epithelium has several layers of cells, and the number of layers one can count at any time depends on how slack or taut the epithelium happens to be. In the empty bladder, for example, the epithelium seems to consist of more than five layers of chubby, cuboidal cells. In the full bladder, on the other hand, the epithelium seems to consist of two layers of thin, attenuated cells. In Figures A and B, the transitional epithelium averages three cells thick. The superficial cells, which contain many mitochondria (∗), have a characteristically convex free surface (arrow). This surface, which borders on the lumen (L), consists of a highly modified, thickened plasma membrane, too small to see at this low magnification, that protects the epithelium from extraction by the highly hypertonic urine.

Beneath the epithelium lies the lamina propria (LP). The lamina propria rests directly on the thick muscularis (M), which comprises the bulk of the wall of the bladder. There is no muscularis mucosae or submucosa. The muscularis consists of a very strong, elastic, distensible, and powerful combination of smooth muscle (SM, SM′ in Figure A) and connective tissue (CT). The connective tissue consists of collagenous and elastic fibers, intertwined among the smooth muscle fibers, that run in many directions. Although the smooth muscles, too, run in all directions, a semblance of the "layering" present in the ureter remains; that is, the inner fibers tend to be longitudinally oriented (SM), the middle fibers tend to be circularly oriented (SM′), and the outermost fibers—not shown here—tend to be longitudinally oriented. Since this is a cross section through the bladder, the smooth muscle fibers of the middle circular layer are cut in longitudinal section (SM′, Figure A). The wall of the bladder, then, is a very strong web that is capable not only of withstanding great distension without bursting, but of generating powerful muscular contractions as well.

Figures A and B. Matched pair of light and electron micrographs of serial cross sections through the wall of the bladder of the squirrel monkey. A, artery; C, capillary; CT, connective tissue; L, lumen of bladder; LP, lamina propria; M, muscularis; SM, smooth muscle cut in cross section; SM′ (Figure A), smooth muscle cut in longitudinal section; TE, transitional epithelium; V, vein; ∗, mitochondria; arrow, surface of epithelium. 600 X

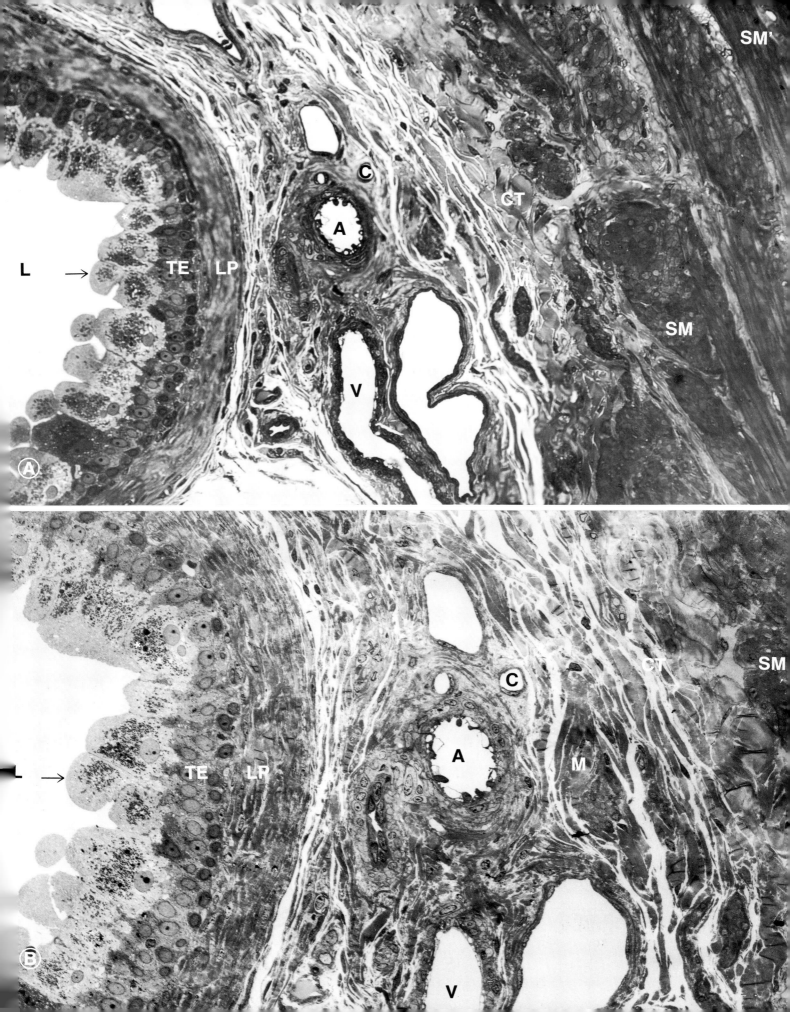

16

Organs Of The Immune System

Overview

This chapter describes the microanatomy of the *lymph nodes, spleen,* and *thymus*—the major organs of an extremely important network of cells, tissues, and organs called the *immune system.* The tissues and organs of the immune system are notable in that they make widespread use of reticular fibers. Each reticular fiber consists of a core of collagen fibrils coated with an amorphous, glycoprotein-rich substance similar to material found in the basement membrane. Recent electron-microscopic studies have shown that each reticular fiber, unlike other connective tissue fibers, is covered by a thin cytoplasmic extension of the reticular cell itself. (Reticular cells are similar in many ways to the fibroblasts that secrete collagen).

In order to understand the structure and function of the organs of the immune system, having a basic knowledge of the cells that participate in the immune response is helpful. Immunology is a highly complex and rapidly evolving field; a detailed discussion of immunology is beyond the scope of this atlas. The following discussion is intended to supply the basics of the subject in order to facilitate learning the histologic organization of the major organs of the immune system.

The immune system distinguishes "self" from "nonself"; it recognizes and destroys (or inactivates) foreign invaders. These invaders, called *antigens,* are potentially harmful bacteria, viruses, fungi, foreign macromolecules, or fragments of unwanted cells and tissues. Lymphocytes are central to the immune response; they recognize antigens. The recognition, moreover, is highly specific; each lymphocyte recognizes one specific kind of antigen. The cells directly involved in the immune response include, among others, lymphocytes, macrophages, and neutrophils. (Neutrophils, you recall, are also called polymorphonuclear leukocytes, or "polys"). Of these, the lymphocytes are the most difficult to understand. It is believed that all lymphocytes can trace their ancestry to the bone marrow. One major class of lymphocyte, the T-lymphocyte, travels to the thymus to mature; the other broad class of lymphocyte, the B-lymphocyte, does not. The functions of the lymphocytes, outlined below, are quite different.

Let us imagine that an antigen find its way into the body. If it encounters a T-lymphocyte with receptors that specifically recognize that particular antigen, that T cell will bind to the antigen and become activated. Activated T cells can proliferate, thus producing more lymphocytes with specific receptors for that antigen. They can then differentiate into large lymphocytes that release *lymphokines*—factors that attract and activate macrophages, which then come and destroy the antigen. The antigen may, however, contact another type of T-lymphocyte—a so-called *killer T cell*—that directly destroys the antigen.

If the antigen should encounter a B-lymphocyte instead of a T-lymphocyte, a different course of events will follow. The B-lymphocyte has receptors that recognize one kind of antigen. Upon contacting that antigen, the B cell becomes activated, proliferates, and differentiates into a plasma cell. Plasma cells make and release antibodies—highly specific macromolecules that bind to the antigen, neutralize it, and form an antigen-antibody complex. In certain cases, these antibody-antigen complexes are quite large and can impede blood flow. Consequently, their presence triggers a highly complex response in which a series of blood proteins called *complement* is activated. Activated complement attracts neutrophils, which become highly phagocytic and ingest the antigen-antibody complexes.

For the immune system to be effective, then, the cells involved in the immune response must be present in many regions of the body where undesirable foreign antigens are likely to gain entrance. Consequently, the *reticuloendothelial system,* a network of connective tissues that contains cells of the immune system, has evolved. The reticuloendothelial system is widespread and diffuse, present along all areas of exposure to the outside world such as the submucosa of the respiratory system and the lamina propria of the alimentary canal. In these regions, local invasion of antigen often triggers local proliferation of lymphocytes. As a result, the presence of lymphoid nodules in regions such as the lamina propria of the gut are quite common and can serve as indicators of the health of the individual.

Because the reticuloendothelial system is so widespread, the question arises as to why specific organs of the immune system, such as the lymph nodes and the spleen, are necessary. The answer lies in the fact that humans, like most vertebrate animals, consist largely of water. Consequently, it seems logical that humans would make use of fluid transport systems to move nutrients and wastes throughout the body. Two of these fluid transport systems, blood and lymph, are encased within vessels that constitute two separate vascular systems— the blood vascular system and the lymph vascular system.

Because many substances are harmful to humans, it is highly probable that harmful substances will find their way into the blood and lymph vascular systems. As a result, humans have evolved a separate filtration system for each vascular system. Circulating lymph is filtered by lymph nodes, and circulating blood, by the spleen. Lymph nodes and spleen are far more than simple filters, however. They are elaborate networks of cells and connective tissues that hold cells of the immune system directly in the path of circulating blood or lymph in order to maximize the possibility of contact between harmful substances—foreign antigens—with the very cells or antibodies that will destroy them.

Because both the lymph node and the spleen are connective tissue networks loaded with immune cells, their organization will, of necessity, be loose and free from distinct layers. This condition makes their histologic organization difficult to understand. Students of microanatomy tend to have more difficulty in understanding the histologic organization of the organs of the immune system than of any other system. The diffuse nature of the immune system, which is so effective in function, is difficult to visualize in sectioned material. The following set of light and electron micrographs should simplify that task.

Plate 16–1

The Lymph Node, Part I

Lymph nodes are large masses (up to 2.5 cm) of lymphoid tissue that take station at intervals along major lymph vessels. Lymph enters one side of the node by way of several small *afferent lymphatic vessels,* percolates through a series of leaky *lymphatic sinuses,* and exits the other side of the node through a single *efferent lymphatic vessel.* In its journey through a major lymph vessel, lymph must filter through many lymph nodes arranged at intervals along the length of the vessel.

Lymph nodes perform several important functions. Within a given node, lymphocytes may leave the general blood circulation through holes in the walls of leaky venules and enter the lymphatic circulation. Similarly, newly produced lymphocytes, born in the node, may enter the lymphatic circulation. These lymphocytes may eventually enter the bloodstream via the subclavian vein, the site at which the lymphatic system empties its contents into the bloodstream. In addition to these functions, lymph nodes harbor many macrophages that phagocytose foreign matter picked up by lymphatic capillaries from the interstitial fluid in the connective tissue spaces.

One of the major functions of the lymph node is to produce new lymphocytes. Under conditions of antigenic stimulation, special regions in the cortex of the node called *primary nodules* become activated. Each primary nodule has a pale-staining core, the *germinal center.* Within the germinal center, large stem cells called *lymphoblasts* multiply. Their progeny are the B-lymphocytes—lymphocytes destined to become antibody-producing plasma cells. B-lymphocytes thus produced in the

lymph node commonly enter lymphatic vessels, are delivered into the blood vascular system at the level of the subclavian vein, and are carried by the bloodstream to various regions of the body, where they differentiate into mature plasma cells. The antibodies made and released by plasma cells are one of the major first lines of defense in the immune response.

The cortex of a monkey lymph node, shown by light microscopy, appears in Figure A. Here, several afferent lymphatic vessels (AL) that bring lymph to the node are evident as they pierce the thin connective tissue capsule (CAP) that envelops the node. Beneath the capsule, out in the cortex, lies a primary nodule (outlined by a dotted line). Note that the primary nodule has a dark periphery and a relatively clear center. The clear central area is the germinal center. The dark periphery of the primary nodule contains B-lymphocytes ready for distribution to areas of need.

Part of the field of view in Figure A is depicted by electron microscopy in Figure B. Here, the thin connective tissue capsule (CAP) is evident, as is part of an afferent lymphatic vessel (AL) that enters the node. Small lymphocytes (L) occupy the periphery of the nodule. Large lymphoblasts (LB), the progenitors of the small lymphocytes, commonly reside in the germinal center of the primary nodule.

The lymph node is held together by a fine network of connective tissue fibers called reticular fibers. Difficult to see by light microscopy without special stains, the reticular fibers are secreted by slender cells called reticulocytes (R) that resemble the collagen-secreting fibroblasts described earlier.

Figures A and B. Matched pair of light and electron micrographs of serial thick and thin sections taken through the cortex of a squirrel monkey lymph node. AL, afferent lymphatic vessel; C, capillary; CAP, connective tissue capsule covering lymph node; L, lymphocyte; LB, lymphoblast; R, reticulocyte; V, venule; arrowhead, mitotic figure (Figure A); dotted line (Figure A), primary nodule. Figure A, 650 X; Figure B, 1,300 X

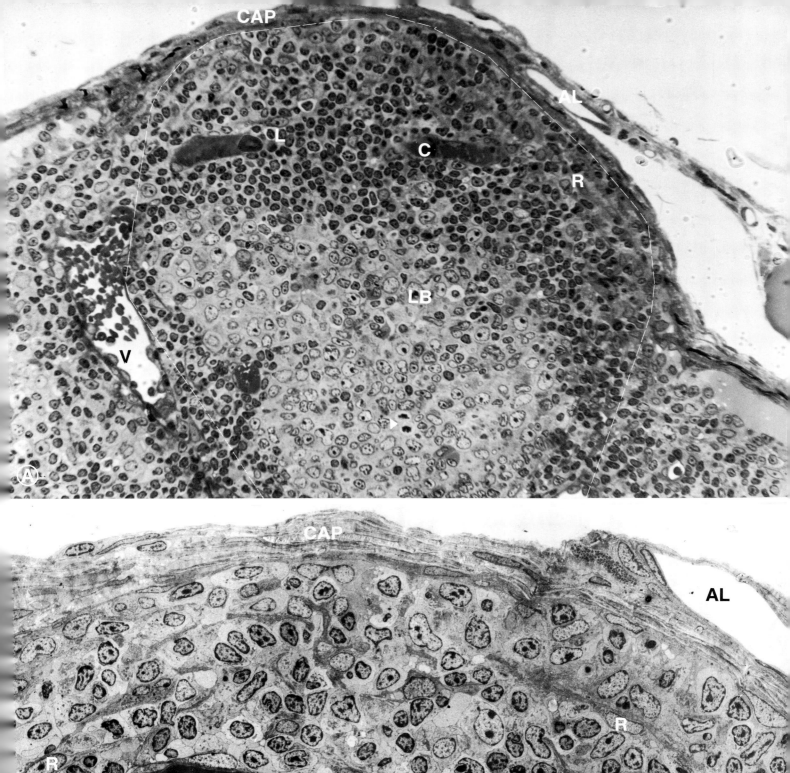
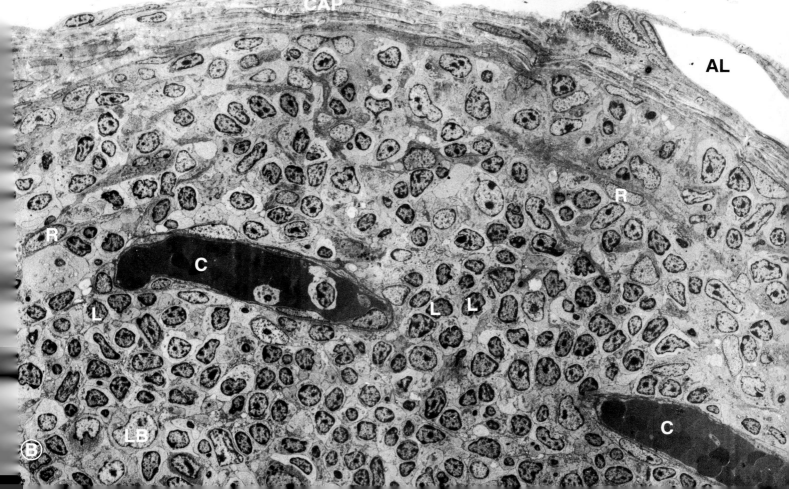

Plate 16–2

The Lymph Node, Part II

Figure A is an electron micrograph of the periphery of a squirrel monkey lymph node depicting the capsule (CAP) and the outer reaches of the cortex. The capsule consists of a thin, densely woven envelope of collagen fibers (Co) that are secreted by fibroblasts (F). Immediately beneath the capsule lies a large lymphatic sinus, the *subcapsular sinus* (SS). The subcapsular sinus, also known as the *cortical sinus* or *marginal sinus,* receives the lymph brought to the node by the afferent lymphatic vessels that pierce the capsule. As with most lymphatic sinuses within the lymph node, the wall of the subcapsular sinus is leaky, more a meshwork of cells and their extensions than a true "wall." Unlike other vessels, which are lined exclusively by endothelial cells, the walls of the subcapsular (and other) lymphatic sinuses are lined by reticulocytes (R) and some macrophages (M) in addition to endothelial cells (E). The endothelial cells found in the walls of lymphatic sinuses are different from the flat, attenuated, squamous endothelial cells found in the walls of arterioles and capillaries. Lymphatic sinuses contain cuboidal endothelial cells, sometimes referred to as *littoral cells.*

Reticular cells, or reticulocytes are connective tissue cells that manufacture and secrete reticular fibers in much the same way as fibroblasts make collagen fibers. (These are different from the immature red blood cells, which are also called reticulocytes.) Unlike collagen, which is often organized into sheets, reticulin is frequently found as thin strands of connective tissue (arrows, Figure B). These strands form the skeleton that supports the lymph node and are often found to extend across the lumen of lymphatic sinuses. When viewed at high magnification with the electron microscope, strands of reticulin appear to be surrounded by thin cytoplasmic extensions of the reticulocyte.

Figure B is an electron micrograph of the cortex of the monkey lymph node. Several blood capillaries (C) are present, as are two postcapillary venules (V1, V2). Postcapillary venules in lymph nodes have wall structures different from those structures found elsewhere; they are lined by cuboidal (instead of squamous) endothelial cells (E). These cuboidal endothelial cells are capable of separating from one another to let whole cells pass through the wall of the leaky venule. Consequently, red blood cells, lymphocytes, and other white blood cells are free to travel in and out between the bloodstream and the inner reaches of the lymph node. The lymph node in this micrograph was fixed by intravascular perfusion that was incomplete; as a result, some blood vessels (such as V1) retain erythrocytes, whereas others (V2, C) have none. Two "marginated" lymphocytes, cells stuck to the vessel wall, are evident in V2.

Between the vessels lies a rich array of cells. Macrophages (M) are abundant, as are reticulin-secreting reticulocytes (R). Numerous lymphocytes (L) are in evidence, as are a few red blood cells (*) that have escaped from the postcapillary venules.

Figure A. Electron micrograph of the capsule and cortex at the periphery of a squirrel monkey lymph node. CAP, collagenous capsule; Co, collagen fibers; E, endothelial (littoral) cell; F, fibroblast; L, lymphocyte; M, macrophage; R, reticulocyte; SS, subcapsular (cortical) sinus. 2,300 X

Figure B. Electron micrograph of a region deep within the cortex of the same lymph node shown in Figure A. C, capillary; E, endothelial cell; L, lymphocyte; M, macrophage; R, reticulocyte; V1, venule with red blood cells; V2, venule with no red blood cells; *, erythrocytes within lymphoid tissue; arrow, reticular fiber. 2,400 X

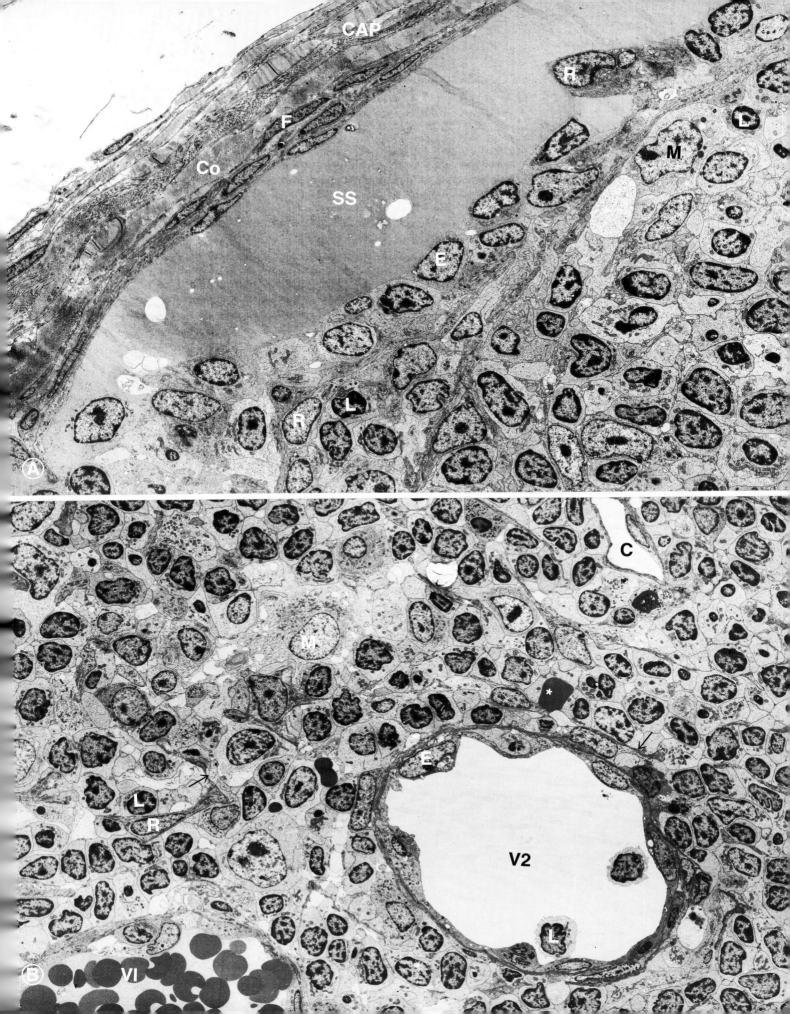

Plate 16–3

The Spleen, Part I: Red Pulp

The spleen is a complex filter placed in the path of the bloodstream. It brings foreign antigens in the blood in direct contact with various cells of the immune system that remove, destroy, or otherwise neutralize those unwanted bits of matter, be they bacteria, cells, or harmful macromolecules. The spleen also removes old erythrocytes from the bloodstream, digests them, and recycles their components for use elsewhere in the body. These functions are accomplished by portions of the spleen grossly described as the *red pulp.* In addition to acting as a filter in the bloodstream, the spleen is a lymphoid organ active in the production of new lymphocytes. These lymphocytes, produced in the region known as the *white pulp,* migrate into the red pulp, where they enter the bloodstream through the walls of leaky venous sinuses.

Figures A and B at right, a matched pair of light and electron micrographs of serial sections taken through the spleen of the monkey, illustrate some of the major splenic structures. At the top of the figures lies the connective tissue capsule (C) that surrounds the spleen. The capsule, coated with a layer of mesothelial cells (M) continuous with the lining of the body cavity, is made of collagen fibers, elastic fibers, and a few smooth muscle cells. The capsule sends into the depths of the spleen a network of *trabeculae* that provides structural support for the organ. Reticular cells associated with the trabeculae send out a fine feltwork of reticular fibers that anchor the loose cells of the spleen. Beneath the capsule lies a portion of the red pulp that contains profiles of several *venous sinuses* (S). These venous sinuses, quite unlike other blood vessels encountered thus far, are central to the workings of the spleen.

The splenic venous sinuses (S) are extremely leaky, highly modified blood vessels endowed with large lumens and discontinuous walls. Unlike other blood vessels, they are not lined by a thin layer of endothelial cells. Instead, each venous sinus is lined by a discontinuous layer of cuboidal cells that, although traditionally referred to as endothelial cells, really resemble modified smooth muscle cells in shape and fine structure. These endothelial cells (E) are fusiform, measure about 100 μm long and are oriented with their long axes parallel to the axis of the venous sinus itself.

The profiles of several venous sinuses are shown by light microscopy in Figure A and by electron microscopy in Figure B. These images clearly show the large lumen of the sinuses (S) and the cuboidal nature of the lining cells (E), and they give an impression of the irregular nature of the wall that makes each sinus so leaky. Because the sinuses are leaky, the tissue between them contains representatives of all the cells found in circulating blood, including erythrocytes, platelets, and white blood cells. The tissue between the venous sinuses is commonly referred to as the *splenic cords* (also called the *cords of Billroth*). In addition to the formed elements of the blood, the splenic cords contain reticular cells, macrophages, and plasma cells. As a result of this configuration, any antigen that strays out of a venous sinus will be subject to direct immunologic attack. In addition, all of the cells of the splenic cords have ready access to the lumen of the venous sinus. Reticular cells send reticular fibers into and across the sinus lumen, creating a cobweblike mesh that entraps passing objects. Macrophages send pseudopodial extensions of their cytoplasm into the sinuses to capture material to be phagocytosed.

The venous sinuses, their contents, and the splenic cords of tissue between them constitute the red pulp. Arteries and the lymphoid tissue associated with them constitute the white pulp. It should be noted that Figures A and B at right show red pulp only. The structure of the red pulp will be examined in more detail in the following plate.

Figures A and B. Matched pair of light and electron micrographs of serial thick and thin sections taken through the spleen of the macaque. C, capsule; E, endothelial cell lining venous sinus; M, mesothelial cell; S, venous sinus; arrow, line formed by dense, actin-like material in foot processes of endothelial cells. Figure A, 1,300 X; Figure B, 2,000 X

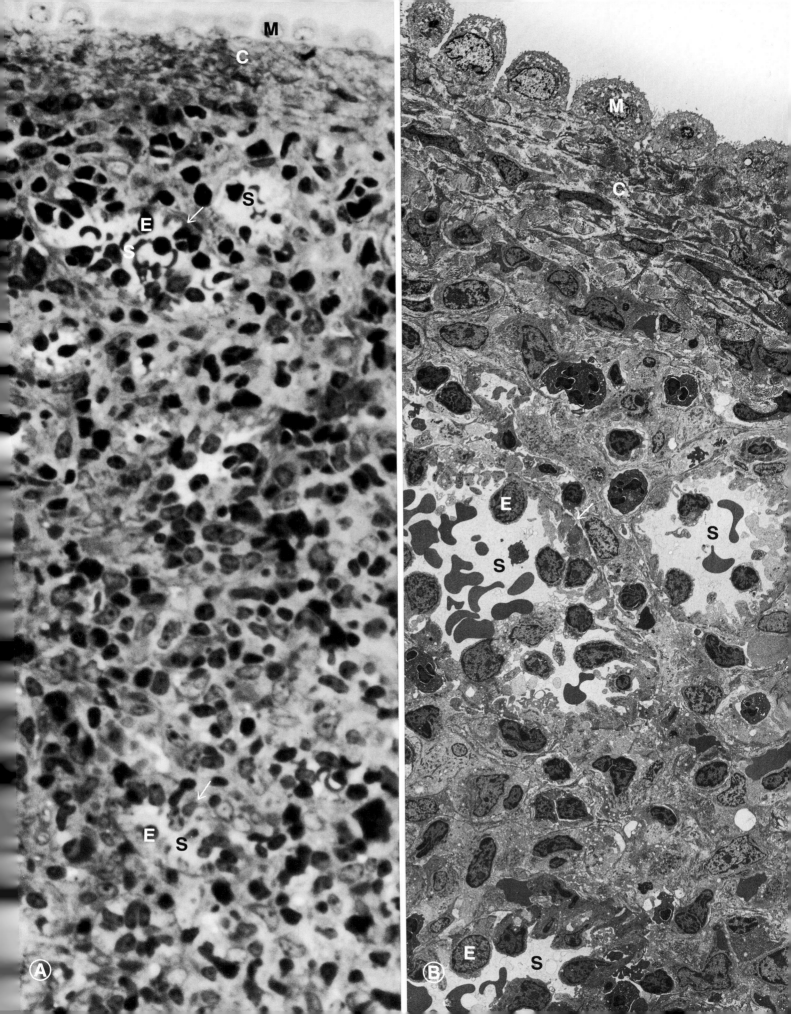

Plate 16–4

The Spleen, Part II: Venous Sinuses

Venous sinuses are large, leaky vessels located in the red pulp that are essential to proper splenic function. Previous discussion of the spleen in this chapter indicated that the venous sinuses are unique in at least two respects. First, the endothelium that lines them is cuboidal; second, large spaces frequently occurring between adjoining endothelial cells permit passage of whole blood, including red and white blood cells, in and out of the sinus itself.

Figure A, a cross section through several venous sinuses (S1, S2, and S3) in the spleen of the macaque, illustrates the special nature of the endothelial cells (E) that line the sinuses. The endothelial cells are long, slender, fusiform cells. They average 100 μm in length and lie with their long axes parallel to the long axis of the venous sinus. Consequently, a cross section through a venous sinus will display cross-sectional images of the endothelial cells that line the sinus. When thus viewed, as in Figure A, the endothelial cells are seen to have a nucleus located close to the lumen. The basal portion of the cell is slender and has a foot-process filled with fine filamentous material that lies at the perimeter of the sinus (arrow). The fine filaments in the foot-process resemble the actin filaments observed in smooth muscle cells. When viewed by electron microscopy, the endothelial cells bear a close resemblance to smooth muscle cells.

The presence of contractile elements within the wall of the venous sinus would, it seems, favor the movement of cells and other blood-borne materials in and out. The sinuses labeled S1 and S3 at right reveal that several red blood cells (Es) are literally caught in the act of escaping, or being squeezed out, through the walls of the venous sinus into the surrounding tissue, the splenic cords. Once out of the vessel and into the splenic cords, macrophages (M) await the now-extravascular red blood cells (Ex), eager to engulf them, digest them, and recycle their contents as bilirubin (a component of bile) and hemosiderin (bearing iron for use in new erythrocytes). In addition to macrophages, plasma cells (P) lie in the splenic cords just outside the boundaries of the venous sinuses. Plasma cells secrete antibodies that combat antigens brought by the blood into the spleen.

The microanatomy of the venous sinuses is made even more apparent when viewed in longitudinal section, as shown in Figure B. Figure B is an electron micrograph of a thin section that caught a curving sinusoid in both longitudinal section (LS) and cross section (XS) at different points along its length. Here, the longitudinal orientation of the endothelial cells (LS) is apparent. The filament-packed foot-processes, cut lengthwise, resemble thin electron-dense strips (arrowheads). The sinusoid is supported by a framework of spirally wound thin strips of basement membrane-like material (arrows) that surround it like the coils of a spring. The actin-containing endothelial cells, acting in concert with the associated skeleton of basement membrane material, may, through cycles of contraction and relaxation, forcibly promote the exchange of materials through the open spaces in the wall of the venous sinus.

Figure A. Electron micrograph of cross sectioned venous sinuses within the spleen of the macaque. E, endothelial cell; Es, erythrocyte escaping from sinus; Ex, extravascular erythrocyte that has escaped from venous sinus; M, macrophage; P, plasma cell; S1, S2, and S3, venous sinuses; *, erythrocyte engulfed by macrophage; arrow, foot-process of endothelial cell tipped with cluster of actin-like filaments; arrowhead, basement membrane wrapped spirally around sinus. 2,000 X

Figure B. Electron micrograph of a macaque's splenic venous sinus cut in longitudinal and cross section at different points along its length. E, endothelial cell; Ex, extravascular erythrocyte; LS, longitudinally sectioned region; M, macrophage; N, neutrophil; XS, cross sectioned region; *, cross section through foot-process of endothelial cell; arrow, cross section through spirally wound strip of basement membrane; arrowhead, longitudinally oriented foot-process of endothelial cell. 2,100 X

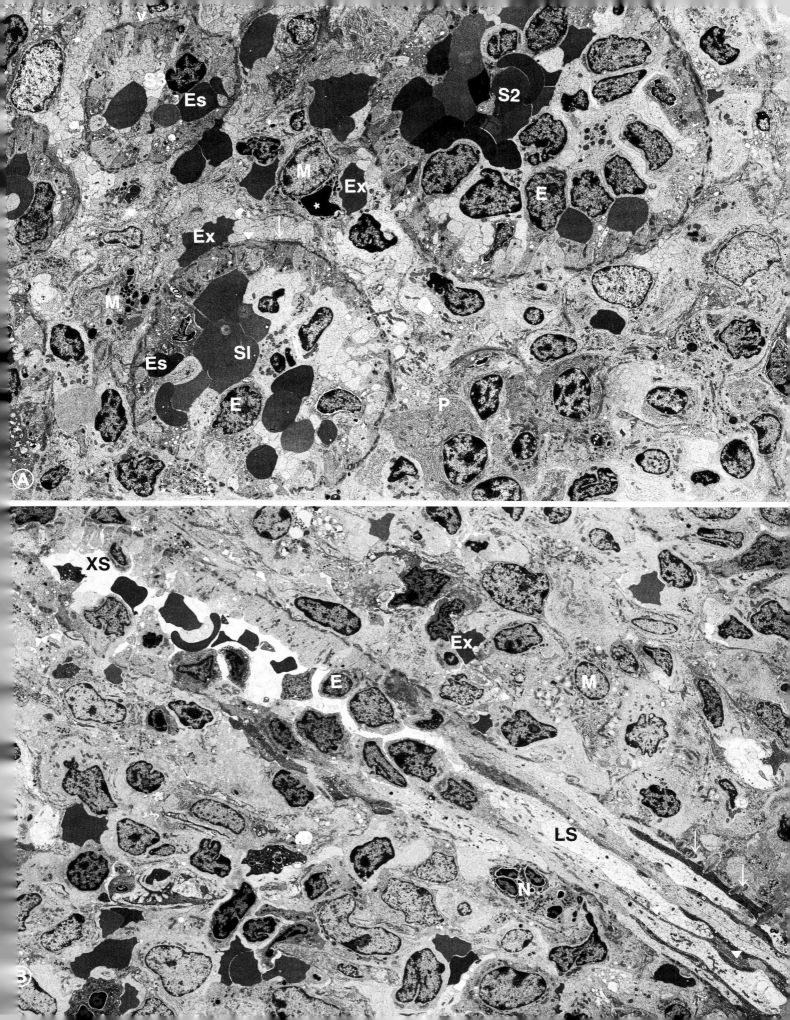

Plate 16–5

The Thymus

Of all the organs of the immune system, the thymus remains the most mysterious. Although much remains to be learned about the functions of the thymus, we do know this; once the stem cell precursors from the bone marrow have taken station in the thymus and have differentiated into thymic lymphocytes, they undergo intense proliferation in the cortex of the lobules of the thymus. Having proliferated, the thymic lymphocytes—still functionally inert—migrate from the cortex to the medulla of the lobules. There, they enter the bloodstream and leave the thymus. The medulla of the thymus is populated by leaky postcapillary venules, similar to those in lymph nodes, that permit passage of lymphocytes through their discontinuous walls. Once in the bloodstream, the lymphocytes that have left the medulla of the thymus acquire immunocompetence, become known as T-lymphocytes (or T cells), and travel through the bloodstream to peripheral lymphoid organs such as the spleen, lymph nodes, appendix, tonsils, or *Peyer's patches* of the ileum of the gut. Once placed in these various outposts of the immune system, T cells become active in the various phases of cell-mediated immunity that so effectively protects the body from foreign invaders.

The microanatomy of the thymus of the squirrel monkey is illustrated at right. Figure A is a light micrograph taken at low magnification. Figure B, an electron micrograph of a serial section taken through the same thymus, illustrates the area enclosed by the rectangle in Figure A. In Figure B it is evident that the thymus is surrounded by a capsule (CAP) of loose connective tissue. A number of connective tissue *septa* (S) extend inward from the capsule; these septa subdivide the thymus into a series of lobules. Each lobule has an outer, darkly staining cortex (CO) and an inner, pale medulla (ME). The thymus contains many different kinds of cells, including lymphocytes (L), macrophages, and epithelial reticular cells (E). The epithelial reticular cells are unique; of endodermal embryonic origin, they are usually stellate. They have a large, clear cell body that sends out numerous protoplasmic extensions that contain tonofilaments for structural support. Despite their misleading name, the epithelial reticular cells are *not* associated with reticular fibers. Their cytoplasmic extensions, which completely line the septa, are intimately associated with lymphocytes.

Lymphocytes—large, medium-sized, and small—are the most numerous cells in the thymus. Large lymphocytes divide and give rise to the small lymphocytes. Many of the small lymphocytes born in the cortex degenerate and die; others migrate to the medulla (ME), wherein they enter the bloodstream. Several dividing cells (arrows) and degenerating cells (D, Figure B) are present in the micrographs at right.

Within the medulla of the lobules of the thymus are structures named *Hassall's corpuscles.* Hassall's corpuscles, illustrated in the insets, consist of conspicuous concentric arrays of squamous epithelial cells. Not found elsewhere in the body, Hassall's corpuscles, whose function remains unknown, provide convenient histologic landmarks by which the thymus may be readily identified in sectioned material.

Figures A and B. Matched pair of light and electron micrographs of serial sections taken through the thymus of the squirrel monkey. CAP, capsule; CO, cortex; D (Figure B),degenerating lymphocyte; E, epithelial reticular cell; F, fat cell; L, lymphocyte; ME (Figure A), medulla, S, connective tissue septum; arrow, mitotic figure of dividing lymphocyte. Inset; Hassall's corpuscle. Figure A, 380 X; Figure B, 900 X; insets, 4,400 X

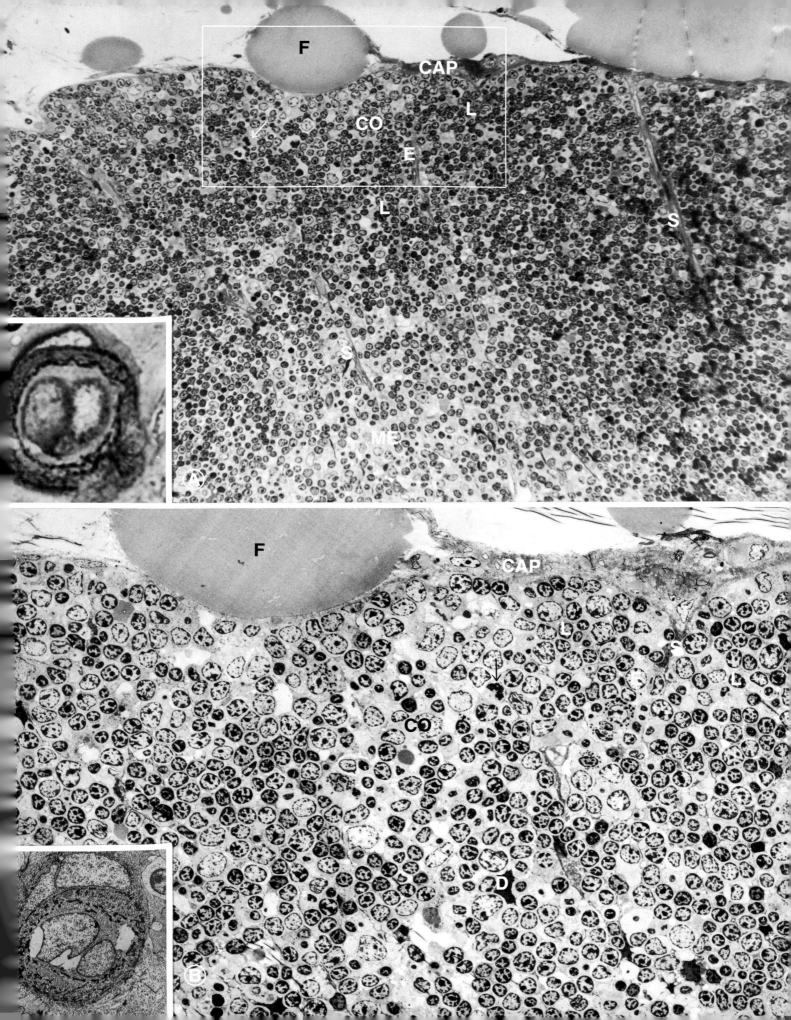

17

The Male Reproductive System

Overview

The micrographs in the preceding chapters have illustrated the diversity of cellular microarchitecture that makes up the various systems of the human body. That such a complex and stunningly beautiful microarchitecture exists is remarkable. What is even more remarkable is the fact that all the 50 trillion cells that make up the human body come from one cell—the fertilized egg.

The present chapter deals with the male reproductive system, the system that produces the sperm that fertilizes the egg. Perhaps the simplest way to describe the male reproductive system is to start with the end product, the mature spermatozoon. The male spermatozoon has been aptly, if somewhat ironically, described as ". . .a nuclear war-head of paternal genes powered by an active tail."[*]

As shown in the drawing in Figure 17–1, a human spermatozoon is a thin cell, some 50 μm long, that has a compact nucleus at one end and a tail at the other. The nucleus, being haploid, contains one half the normal number of chromosomes; the diploid number will, of course, be restored at fertilization, when sperm and egg combine to pool their genetic material. The genetic material within the spermatozoon is highly supercoiled, compact, and compressed. This nuclear condensation not only streamlines the sperm, but protects the genes during their long and hazardous journey to the egg. Of the 100 million spermatozoa that enter the female reproductive tract at a given time, only one reaches, penetrates, and fertilizes the egg.

Behind the discus-shaped nucleus lies the tail, which is divided into three parts: the *midpiece,* the *principal piece,* and the *endpiece.* The core of the sperm tail is the *axoneme*—a motile "9 + 2" complex of microtubules and associated proteins, identical to the axoneme of motile cilia, that is capable of propagating waves along its length in response to the hydrolysis of ATP. The thick midpiece of the sperm carries a "battery pack" of mitochondria tightly spiraled around the axoneme to produce the ATP required for the motility of its flagellar tail. The *seminal fluid* in which the sperm are suspended is rich in fructose, which is thought to serve as a substrate for ATP production by the midpiece mitochondria.

The entire male reproductive system is established for the production of prodigious numbers of spermatozoa and the seminal fluid in which they are suspended upon ejaculation.

[*]Passmore, H., and Robson, J.S.: A Companion to Medical Studies. Vol. 1. London, Blackwell Scientific Publications, 1974.

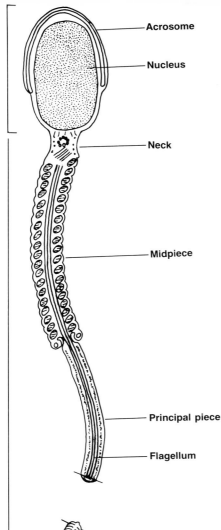

Head
— Acrosome
— Nucleus

Neck

Tail

Midpiece

Principal piece

Flagellum

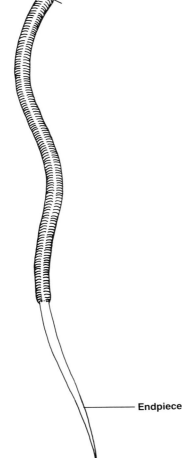

Endpiece

The general layout of the male reproductive system is illustrated in Figure 17–2. The *testicles,* or *testes,* are both endocrine and exocrine organs. The endocrine portion consists of *interstitial cells* (also called *Leydig cells*) that produce testosterone. The exocrine portion consists of *seminiferous tubules* that produce spermatozoa. As shown in Figure 17–2, each testis is subdivided into 250 lobules. Each lobule contains from two to four seminiferous tubules. Each seminiferous tubule is a single tube, some 70 cm long, that is lined by a germinal epithelium that produces spermatozoa. Given these figures, both testes, taken together, contain 1,500 seminiferous tubules whose total length spans 1050 m or 1.05 km. This is an enormous amount of germinal epithelium, and it produces a correspondingly enormous number of spermatozoa. The 100 million spermatozoa in a single ejaculate, isolated and aligned head to tail in a chain, would extend for 5 km. The double-helical DNA molecules from the nucleus of a single spermatozoan, isolated and stretched out, would make a line about 0.5 m long. Were one to perform that operation on all of the 100 million sperm nuclei in one ejaculate, the DNA molecules within the sperm nuclei from one ejaculate alone would stretch for 50,000 km—which would, at the equator, span the globe 1.2 times.

Clearly the male reproductive system makes a lot of spermatozoa. It has to, for not only are the odds quite small of a single spermatozoon reaching the egg, but the odds of the egg being fit for fertilization at the time of sperm arrival also are quite small. Consequently, the male reproductive system knows little rest, and is constantly engaged in the production, maintenance, nutrition, and, in times of sexual inactivity, resorption of large quantities of spermatozoa.

The "production line" in the germinal epithelium, a process known as *spermatogenesis,* starts with stem cells called *spermatogonia.* Under appropriate conditions of hormonal stimulation, spermatogonia divide mitotically and give rise to *primary spermatocytes.* These spermatocytes undergo *meiotic* division, giving

FIG. 17–1. Drawing of a human spermatozoon showing its major components.

rise to *secondary spermatocytes.* Secondary spermatocytes undergo a second meiotic division and produce *spermatids.* Spermatids do not divide; instead, they undergo *spermiogenesis,* a marked and complicated morphogenetic transformation into spermatozoa.

When fully formed spermatozoa are shed from the germinal epithelium into the lumen, they travel along the seminiferous tubule and enter the *epididymis* through a series of intermediate ducts. The epididymis, a 1-cm coiled tube (which if unraveled, would measure 6 m), is closely applied to the outer wall of the testis. As spermatozoa travel through the epididymis, they undergo the process of *capacitation;* that is, they acquire the capacity to move and fertilize the egg. In addition to participating in sperm capacitation, the epididymis resorbs much of the testicular fluid secreted by the seminiferous tubules. Sperm are stored in the large tail, or cauda, of the epididymis and are passed into the *vas deferens* during ejaculation. Sperm are propelled along the length of the vas deferens into the ejaculatory ducts that lead into the urethra, where they are mixed with seminal fluid produced by the *prostate gland* and the *seminal vesicles.* The combination of sperm and seminal fluid is known as *semen;* semen is the substance that enters the female reproductive tract during copulation.

This chapter examines the structure and function of the seminiferous tubules, the epididymis, the vas deferens, the prostate gland, and the seminal vesicles. The microanatomy of the female reproductive system will be described in the next chapter.

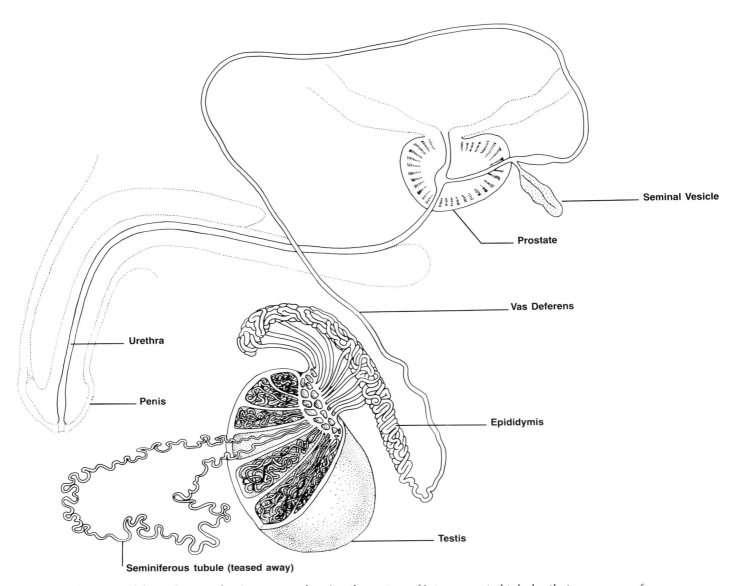

Seminal Vesicle

Prostate

Vas Deferens

Urethra

Penis

Epididymis

Testis

Seminiferous tubule (teased away)

FIG. 17–2. Drawing of the male reproductive system showing the system of interconnected tubules that carry sperm from the testis to the urethra.

Plate 17–1

The Seminiferous Tubule Of The Testis

The testis is both an exocrine and an endocrine organ. The exocrine portion consists of a series of highly coiled seminiferous tubules that make sperm; the endocrine portion consists of specialized cells called interstitial cells (also called Leydig cells) that secrete testosterone. The interstitial cells lie in the connective tissue between adjacent coils of seminiferous tubules.

Each testis is divided into 250 compartments called lobules. Each lobule, in turn, contains from one to four seminiferous tubules. As described in the overview, each seminiferous tubule is quite long; a single one may measure up to 70 cm. Because each long tubule is packed into the confines of a single lobule, the seminiferous tubule is folded back on itself in a highly complex manner. Consequently, a section through the testis reveals the seminiferous tubules as a series of circular profiles.

Figure A is a light micrograph of a cross section through a seminiferous tubule within one of the lobules of the testis. The cells of the spermatogenic lineage are stacked in 4 to 8 layers; although the cells vary in appearance, most are cuboidal, with the exception of the long, thin spermatozoa. The two major classes of cells within the seminiferous tubule are *supporting cells* and *spermatogenic cells.* The supporting cells consist of one type of cell called the *Sertoli cell.* The spermatogenic cells consist of five morphologically distinct classes of cells: spermatogonia, primary spermatocytes, secondary spermatocytes, spermatids, and spermatozoa. At first glance, these cells can be quite difficult to tell apart. Close study of their nuclei, however, reveals distinct differences in nuclear structure—the key to their identification.

In Figure A, the Sertoli cells (S) can be recognized by their large, round, pale nuclei and prominent, centrally located nucleoli. The Sertoli cell nuclei are usually located next to the basement membrane at the periphery of the seminiferous tubule. Sertoli cells span the entire thickness of the epithelium from the basement membrane to the lumen of the tubule. All of the cells of the spermatogenic series are intimately associated with the Sertoli cells and seem to be nourished by them.

The spermatogonia (G), whose nuclei are also located at the periphery of the tubule, undergo mitotic division and give rise to the primary spermatocytes (P). Primary spermatocytes spend much of their time in meiotic prophase and are readily identified as cells with large nuclei that contain condensed chromatin.

Primary spermatocytes divide meiotically to form secondary spermatocytes, which resemble primary spermatocytes but are much smaller. Secondary spermatocytes undergo meiosis very rapidly and give rise to spermatids (ST). Since secondary spermatocytes cycle through their stage so quickly, they are rarely seen; none are present in these micrographs. Spermatids, however, have a long life, are abundant, and are readily identified as small cells, often near the lumen, with small, pale nuclei. Spermatids undergo no further division; instead, they undergo spermiogenesis, in which they are morphogenetically transformed into spermatozoa (arrow).

Many of these cells are readily apparent in Figure B, an electron micrograph of a cross section through a portion of a seminiferous tubule. Compare the appearances of spermatogonia (G), Sertoli cells (S), primary spermatocytes (P), and spermatids (ST) in this electron micrograph with those of the same cells in Figure A. Careful examination of Figure B will reveal some of the key features of spermiogenesis. In some of the spermatids, for example, the forming *acrosome* (∗)—a large lysosome on the head of the sperm that helps it to penetrate the egg—can be seen as a large vesicle, derived from the Golgi complex, that is closely applied to the spermatid's nucleus. In addition, the mitochondria that will wrap themselves around the midpiece can be seen taking station in the cytoplasm of the spermatid.

Figure A. Light micrograph of a cross section through the testis of the cat. Figure B. Electron micrograph through part of a seminiferous tubule from the same testis. C, capillary; CT (Figure A), connective tissue; G, spermatogonium; I, interstitial cell (Leydig cell); P, primary spermatocyte; S, Sertoli cell; ST, spermatids; arrow, developing spermatozoa; ∗ (Figure B), developing acrosome. Figure A, 400 X; Figure B, 1,900 X

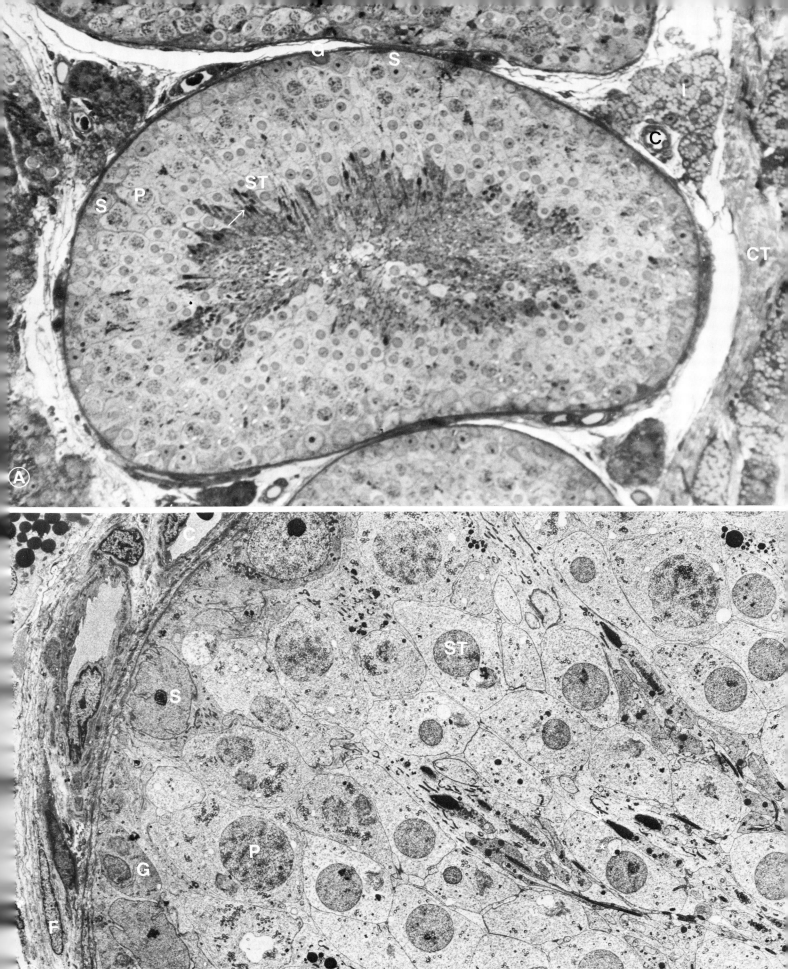

Plate 17–2

The Epididymis

When spermatogenesis is complete, fully formed spermatozoa leave the seminiferous tubules, pass through a series of short ducts, and enter the epididymis. The epididymis is one long, thin tube that is tightly coiled and closely applied to the posterior surface of the testis. When seen with the naked eye, the epididymis is a whitish structure, some 7 cm long, that consists of a head (the caput), body (the corpus), and tail (the cauda). Stretched out, the epididymis would be a single tube that measures over 6 m long. Consequently, spermatozoa entering the epididymis at the head and exiting into the vas deferens at the tail take a long journey. During that journey, sperm become both motile and fertile. Although it is widely believed that the epididymis participates in sperm's maturation and contributes to the development of their motility and fertility, the precise mechanisms by which these functions are accomplished are still unknown. Large numbers of spermatozoa are stored in the lumen of the epididymis prior to ejaculation, and it is believed that the epididymis actively resorbs fragments of cytoplasm eliminated during spermatogenesis and resorbs entire spermatozoa in times of sexual inactivity.

When viewed with the light microscope at low magnification, a section through the epididymis presents a large number of circular profiles that represent cut portions of the supercoiled tube, or duct, of the epididymis. Figure A, a light micrograph taken at intermediate magnification, shows a cross section through one of these coils. Here, the lumen (L) of the epididymis contains many spermatozoa. The epididymis is lined by a pseudostratified columnar epithelium (E) that contains two types of cells: principal cells and basal cells. The principal cells (P) are tall, columnar cells topped by many long, thin microvilli (arrow) called *stereocilia.* The basal cells are small, round cells that lie next to the basement membrane. The basal cells undergo mitotic division and serve as stem cells; the progeny of basal cells grow, differentiate, and replace worn-out principal cells. The epithelium is surrounded by several layers of circularly arranged smooth muscle fibers (SM). These smooth muscle fibers contract rhythmically and slowly propel the spermatozoa along the length of the epididymis from its head toward its tail. The smooth muscle fibers are surrounded by loose connective tissue (CT) that serves to bind together the coils of the epididymis.

Figure B is an electron micrograph of a thin section through the same epididymis shown in Figure A. Here, the lumen (L) containing the spermatozoa is at the top of the field; the smooth muscle (SM) surrounding the epithelium is at the bottom. The pseudostratified columnar epithelium rests atop the basement membrane (BM). Both cell types of the epithelium are evident in this low-magnification electron micrograph. The small, round basal cells (B) may be seen next to the basement membrane. The remainder of the cells are the principal cells (P)—tall, slender, columnar cells topped by hundreds of long, thin microvilli (arrow). The nuclei (N) of the principal cells, located at the basal pole of the cell, are long and thin and display an unusual folded appearance. Just above the nucleus of each principal cell lies a very well developed Golgi apparatus (G). Large numbers of electron-dense vesicles (Ly) lie above and below the Golgi. These vesicles are believed to be lysosomes—organelles directly involved in the intracellular digestion of material taken up from the lumen of the epididymis by pinocytosis.

Figure A. Light micrograph of a cross section through the duct of the epididymis of the squirrel monkey. B, basal cell; CT, connective tissue; E, epithelium; L, lumen filled with spermatozoa; P, principal cell; SM, smooth muscle; arrow, stereocilia. 800 X

Figure B. Electron micrograph of the same epididymis shown in Figure A. B, basal cell; BM, basement membrane; G, Golgi apparatus; L, lumen; Ly, lysosome; N, nucleus of principal cell; P, principal cell; SM, smooth muscle; arrow, long microvilli (stereocilia). 1,500 X

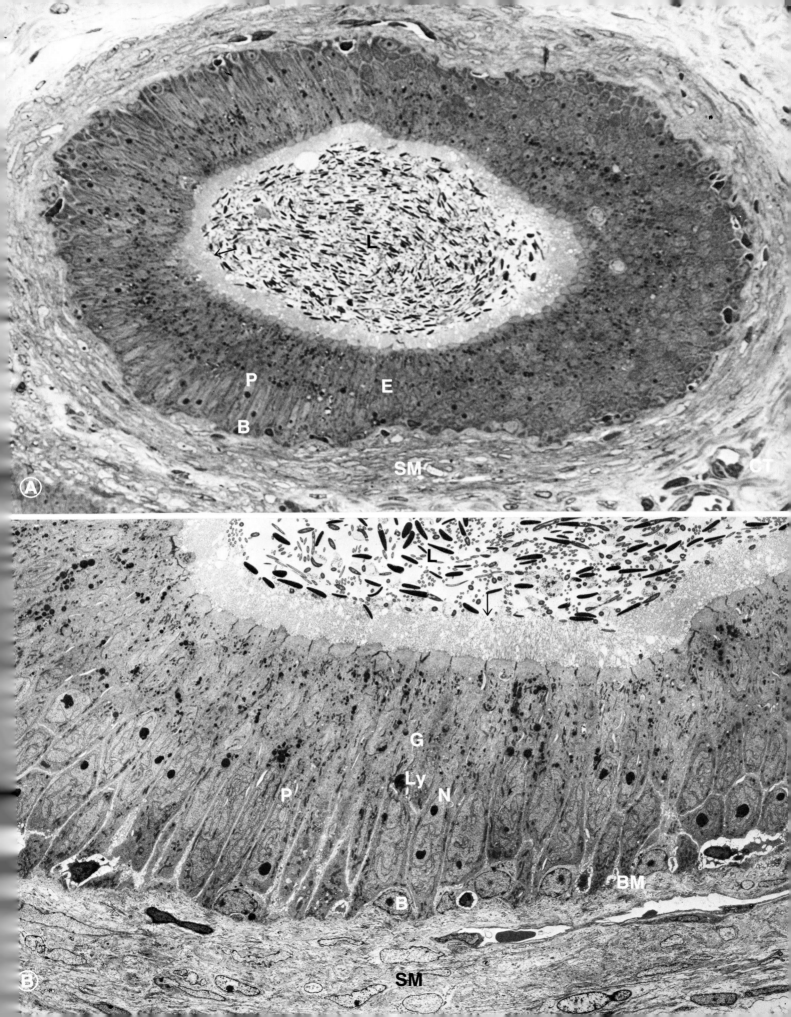

Plate 17–3

The Vas Deferens

The vas deferens, also called the *ductus deferens,* is a thick, highly muscular tube, 45 cm long and 2.5 mm wide, that connects the testis with the urethra. It begins at the tail of the epididymis, passes into the spermatic cord, and ultimately joins the urethra in the vicinity of the bladder and the prostate gland. The diagram in Figure 17–1 clarifies the position of the vas deferens in the male reproductive system.

The purpose of the vas deferens is to propel live spermatozoa, some 100 million per ejaculate, from their site of storage in the epididymis to the urethra. At the moment of ejaculation, sperm delivered by the vas to the urethra are mixed with seminal fluid delivered by the prostate and seminal vesicles to form semen. To reach the urethra from the testis, sperm must travel some 45 cm. Consequently, the vas deferens must move sperm along its length rather rapidly. To accomplish this task, the 1-mm-thick wall of the vas deferens is richly endowed with smooth muscle fibers and elastic fibers. During the process of ejaculation, the smooth muscles, stimulated by the autonomic nervous system, contract in a wavelike manner, rapidly squeezing the sperm up the length of the tube through its narrow lumen.

Figures A and B are a pair of light and electron micrographs of cross sections taken through the vas deferens of the squirrel monkey. Here, the small, star-shaped lumen (L) is lined by a pseudostratified columnar epithelium (E). As in the epididymis, the epithelium contains small, round basal cells (B) and tall columnar cells. The columnar cells are topped by long, slender microvilli, called stereocilia (S). (The term "stereocilia" is misleading, for stereocilia are not cilia at all, but elongated microvilli.) Just beneath the epithelium lies a lamina propria (LP) rich in elastic fibers. The lamina propria binds the epithelium to the underlying layer of smooth muscle (SM). Classically, the smooth muscle is believed to be arranged in three layers: an inner longitudinal layer, a powerful middle circular layer, and an outer longitudinal layer. In the micrographs at right, this arrangement is not apparent; most of the smooth muscle fibers here are caught in oblique section, indicating that many of them are wound in a spiral fashion around the lumen in the core of the vas deferens.

Figures A and B. Light and electron micrographs of cross sections through the vas deferens of the squirrel monkey. B, basal cell; E, pseudostratified columnar epithelium; L, lumen; LP, lamina propria; S, stereocilia (long microvilli); SM, smooth muscle. Figure A, 500 X; Figure B, 900 X

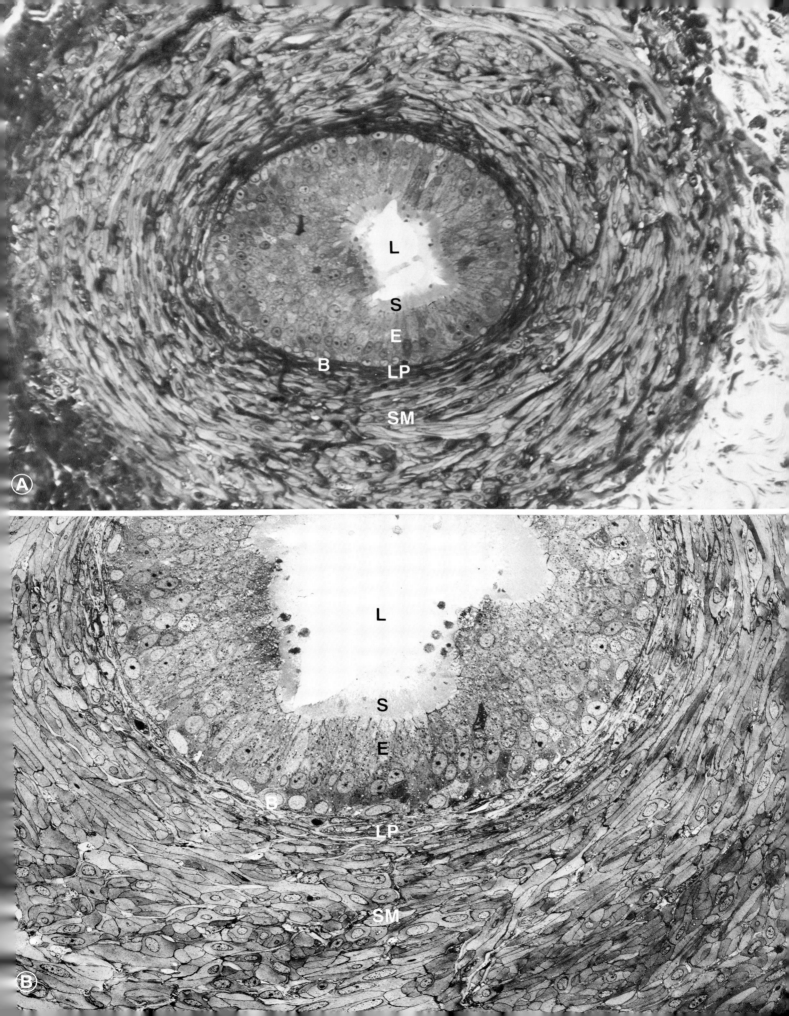

Plate 17–4

The Prostate Gland

When mating occurs, live spermatozoa that are ejaculated from the male reproductive tract are suspended in seminal fluid. The average volume of a single ejaculate, which contains on the order of 100 million spermatozoa, is about 3.5 ml. The ejaculated material, semen, contains 10% spermatozoa and 90% seminal fluid. The seminal fluid consists of the combined secretions of the seminiferous tubules, epididymis, prostate gland, seminal vesicles, and small glands called the bulbourethral glands.

The bulk of the seminal fluid is elaborated by the prostate gland, a chestnut-shaped organ some 3 cm in diameter that surrounds the base of the urethra and the neck of the urinary bladder. The prostate gland is a collection of 30 to 50 branched tubulo-acinar glands, embedded within a dense fibromuscular stroma, that empty their secretions into the urethra. These tubuloacinar glands secrete *prostatic fluid* and store it until the moment of ejaculation. Prostatic fluid is a viscous material that has many ingredients, including acid phosphatase, citric acid, and *prostaglandins.* Prostaglandins, which are a class of long-chain hydroxy fatty acids, have many functions, including the stimulation of rhythmic contractions of uterine smooth muscle. Consequently, the seminal fluid, which contains prostaglandins, not only provides a fluid medium in which sperm can swim and live for long periods of time, but it also promotes muscular contractions of the female reproductive tract that accelerate the delivery of spermatozoa to the waiting egg.

Figures A and B are a matched pair of light and electron micrographs of serial thick and thin sections taken through the prostate gland of the squirrel monkey. Figure A, taken at relatively low magnification, provides a survey view of several of the tubuloacinar glands (G) and the fibromuscular stroma (S) that surrounds them. In the center of the field, two acini of one of the glands contain dense inclusions called *prostatic concretions* (C). Commonly found in middle-aged and older males, prostatic concretions are thought to represent portions of the secretory substance that with time have become crystallized or mineralized.

The cells of the secretory acini are shown at higher magnification by electron microscopy in Figure B. Here, each acinus appears as a grape-shaped cluster of cells with a centrally located lumen (L). The acinus is lined by a row of cells that vary in height from cuboidal to low columnar. The size and shape of the secretory cells can vary considerably. Their structure depends on their secretory activity, which, in turn, is strongly influenced by levels of testosterone in the circulating blood.

The nuclei of the secretory cells in Figures A and B (N) occupy the base of the cell. The apical pole of the cell, in most cases, is filled with clear, round secretory vesicles (V). The "empty" appearance of the secretory vesicles suggests that their contents were extracted during specimen preparation. Because fatty or oily substances are frequently extracted by the organic solvents utilized in specimen preparation, and because prostaglandins are long-chain hydroxy fatty acids, it seems likely that the "empty" vesicles may, in life, have been filled with material rich in prostaglandins.

Many smooth muscle fibers (SM) are evident in the connective tissue surrounding the tubuloacinar glands. At the moment of ejaculation, these smooth muscle fibers, which are under the control of the autonomic nervous system, are stimulated to contract, thus forcing prostatic fluid out of the acini, into the ducts of the glands, and out into the urethra. Here, prostatic fluid mixes with spermatozoa delivered by the vas deferens and fluid secreted by the seminal vesicles to form semen.

Figures A and B. Matched pair of light and electron micrographs of serial thick and thin sections of the prostate gland of the squirrel monkey. C, prostatic concretion; G, acinus of tubuloacinar gland; L, lumen of acinus; N, nucleus of secretory cell; S, fibromuscular stroma; SM, smooth muscle; V, secretory vesicles in apical pole of secretory cell. Figure A, 700 X; Figure B, 1,100 X

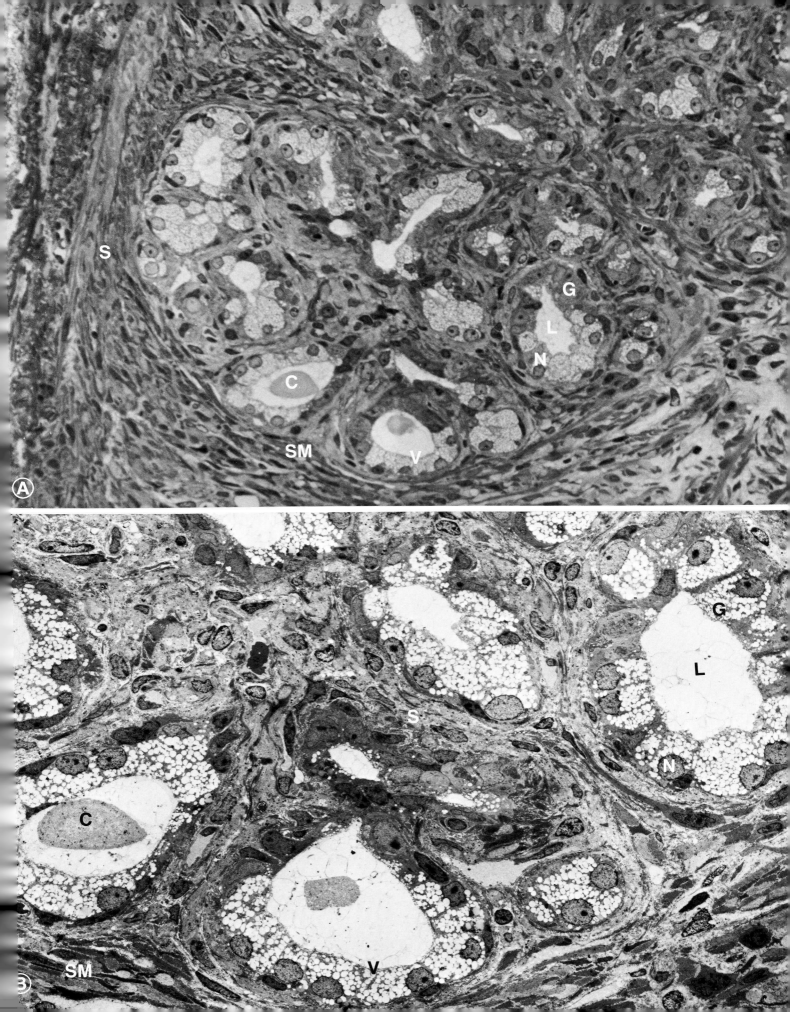

Plate 17–5

The Seminal Vesicles

The seminal vesicles are a pair of highly infolded, saclike bodies, each about 5 cm long, that empty their contents into the vas deferens near the point at which the vas deferens joins the urethra. Spermatozoa depend on the hydrolysis of ATP for their motility, and the seminal vesicles contribute to the semen a yellow, viscous, sticky fluid rich in fructose. Fructose, a substrate for the biochemical production of ATP, serves as fuel for swimming spermatozoa suspended in semen. The ATP required by the sperm flagellum is generated largely by the elongated mitochondria wound around the flagellar axoneme in the vicinity of the midpiece of the sperm (see Figure 17–1). Hence, the contribution of the seminal vesicles to the seminal fluid is of considerable physiologic importance.

Figure A is a light micrograph of a section taken through the seminal vesicle of a squirrel monkey. Here, the lumen (L) is divided into a number of compartments by the extensively folded mucosa. The mucosa of the seminal vesicle consists of a pseudostratified epithelium that rests on a bed of loose connective tissue (Co). The pseudostratified epithelium consists of either cuboidal or columnar epithelial cells (E) and small, round basal cells (arrowhead). The basal cells are so small that they are difficult to detect at this magnification. The structure of the epithelium of the seminal vesicle depends on a number of variables, including the hormonal status and the age of the individual. Under conditions of high testosterone, the cells tend to en-

large and become columnar. When testosterone levels fall, the cells become less active and shrink, becoming cuboidal. Consequently, histologic sections of seminal vesicles derived from different individuals may exhibit considerable variations in epithelial microanatomy.

Figure B is a matching electron micrograph of a serial thin section taken through the same seminal vesicle depicted in Figure A. In this image, the star-shaped lumen (L) is bordered by many folds of the mucosa. Although the epithelium appears to be simple cuboidal at first glance, close study reveals the presence of small basal cells (arrowhead) next to the basement membrane. The small, round basal cells are squeezed in between the bases of the larger cuboidal cells (E), thus placing the epithelium in the pseudostratified category. The cuboidal epithelial cells contain several kinds of cytoplasmic inclusions evident at this relatively low magnification, including pigment granules (arrow) and secretory vesicles (S). The epithelium is supported by loose connective tissue that contains collagen fibrils (Co) and elastic fibers (which require special stains to be seen). A number of small capillaries (C) and nerve fibers pass through the network of connective tissue that supports the epithelium. The mucosa lies on top of a thick layer of smooth muscle (not shown in these micrographs) that contracts during ejaculation, thus squeezing the contents of the seminal vesicles out into the vas deferens, which, in turn, carries the fluid out into the urethra during ejaculation.

Figures A and B. Matched pair of light and electron micrographs of serial thick and thin sections taken through the seminal vesicle of the squirrel monkey. C, capillary; Co, collagen fibrils; E, cuboidal epithelial cells; L, lumen; S, secretory vesicles in apical portion of cuboidal epithelial cell; arrow (Figure B), pigment granules; arrowhead, basal cell. 800 X

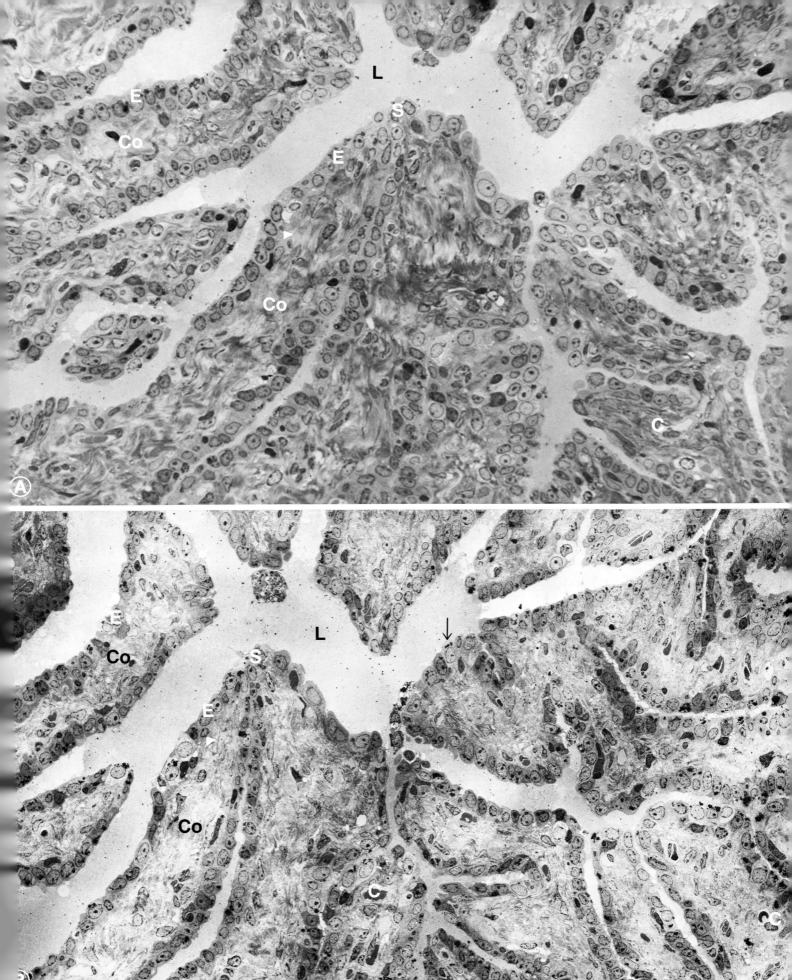

18

The Female Reproductive System

Overview

The female reproductive system performs a number of important functions. First, it produces the egg, or *ovum,* and provides for its maturation. Second, it places the mature egg so that it is available for fertilization by incoming spermatozoa. Third, it provides a warm, safe, secure, and nutritious environment in which the fertilized egg can grow and develop. Fourth, the female reproductive system is an integral part of the endocrine system.

The female reproductive system accomplishes these life-giving acts with three major organs: the *ovary,* the *oviduct,* and the *uterus.* These organs, each of which has several histologic subdivisions, are packaged into a compact and efficient system. Figure 18-1 shows the major components of the female reproductive system. The ovary at left is seen in surface view; the one at right is shown in longitudinal section to reveal the developing follicles within. Close by the ovaries lie the paired oviducts. The oviduct—also called the *uterine tube* or *fallopian tube*—receives the egg when it is *ovulated,* or released from the ovary, and moves the egg through its lumen toward the uterus. Normally, when fertilization occurs, it takes place in the oviduct. The fertilized egg is then transported to the uterus, where it is implanted. Once implantation has occurred, human development continues at a rapid rate, and the uterus undergoes a dramatic increase in size as the baby grows. At term, the baby is pushed through the vaginal canal by uterine contractions and enters the "outside world."

This chapter illustrates the microanatomy of the three major organs of the female reproductive system—the ovary, oviduct, and uterus—by light and electron microscopy.

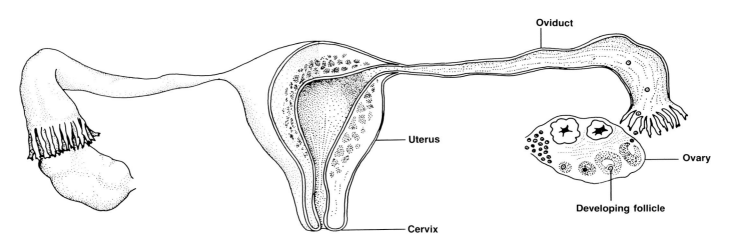

FIG. 18–1. Drawing of the major internal parts of the female reproductive system.

Plate 18–1

The Ovary

Human life begins with the union of two cells, a sperm and an egg. The sperm and egg must first be produced by two adults of the species. The preceding chapter on the male reproductive system began by illustrating the testis, the organ of sperm production. This chapter begins by illustrating the ovary, the organ of egg production.

The human female is born with about 400,000 primordial germ cells that can develop into egg cells, or *oocytes.* Of these, only about 450 are ovulated (at the rate of one per month for some 35 to 40 years) and made available for fertilization. The transition from early germ cell to mature oocyte is dramatic, and much of that transition occurs within the cortex of the ovary itself. The oocyte—a large, round cell that serves as a repository for genetic material and contains many of the cytoplasmic components necessary for early development—cannot grow alone. To undergo its maturation, the oocyte requires assistance from other cells. Consequently, each oocyte and its helper cells are organized into a functional unit called a follicle. The structure and function of the ovarian follicle change dramatically during the process of oocyte maturation. Some of these changes are illustrated in the first three plates of this chapter.

Plate 18–1 at right is a low-magnification light micrograph of a section taken through the ovary of the monkey. The ovary is a large, almond-shaped structure, measuring about 5 cm long, 2 cm wide, and 1 cm thick. Because of its large size, only a small portion of the ovary can be shown in a single photo-micrograph. In the plate, part of the lateral margin of the ovary is covered by a simple cuboidal epithelium known as the *germinal epithelium* (GE). The name is unfortunate because it incorrectly implies that the epithelium participates in germ cell formation. However, the germinal epithelium actually is a continuation of the layer of cells that lines the peritoneal cavity. Beneath the germinal epithelium lies a tough connective tissue coat, the *tunica albuginea* (TA). The tunical albuginea outlines the outer part of the ovary, the cortex, in which the developing follicles lie. The core of the ovary, called the medulla (M), is made up of connective tissue through which blood vessels (V) pass.

Several follicles in different stages of development are evident in Plate 18–1. Numerous *primary follicles* (PF) are clustered at the periphery of the cortex near the tunica albuginea. Each primary follicle consists of a central oocyte (*) surrounded by a single layer of cuboidal epithelial cells. Each of these epithelial cells is called a *follicular cell* (or *follicle cell*). As the follicle develops, the oocyte increases in size, and the follicular cells multiply by mitosis. Soon, the primary follicle has enlarged to become a *secondary follicle* (SF), an oocyte surrounded by several layers of follicular cells. When the follicular cells become arranged in layers, they are known by a new name—*granulosa cells.* Compare the images of primary follicles and secondary follicles in the photomicrograph at right for a visual image of their microanatomy.

Light micrograph of section through part of the ovary of the squirrel monkey. C, cortex; CT, connective tissue in the medulla; GE, germinal epithelium that covers the ovary; M, medulla; PF, primary follicle; SF, secondary follicle; TA, tunica albuginea; V, blood vessel in medulla; *, oocyte. 325 X

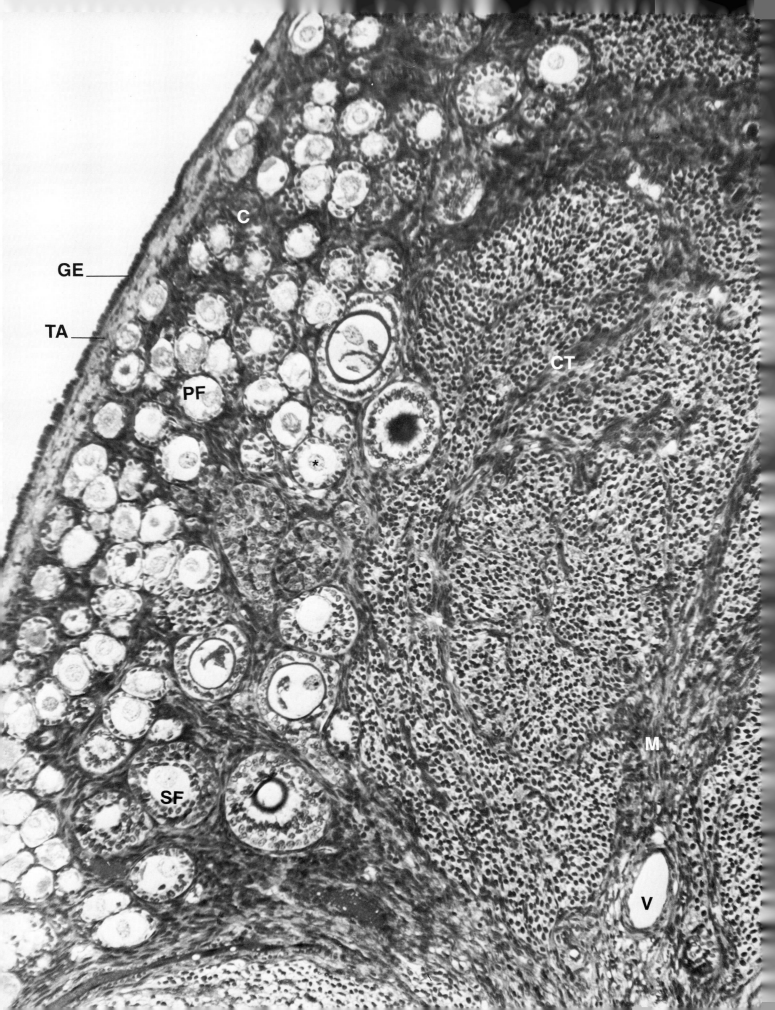

Plate 18–2

The Ovary:
Primary And Secondary Follicles

The follicles present in the ovaries of a newborn female are called *primordial follicles.* A primordial follicle consists of an oocyte surrounded by a monolayer of squamous epithelial cells. Under appropriate conditions of hormonal stimulation, which normally occur at puberty, the primordial follicles become activated and start to grow. The oocyte enlarges, and the squamous cells that surround it swell and become cuboidal. These structural changes herald the transformation of a primordial follicle into a primary follicle. The primary follicle, then, consists of an oocyte surrounded by a single layer of plump cuboidal follicle cells.

Several primary follicles are illustrated in the low-magnification electron micrograph in Figure A. Here, the oocyte (O) appears as a large, spherical, pale cell with its nucleus (N) set slightly off-center. The oocyte is surrounded by a monolayer of cuboidal follicle cells (F). The follicle cells, in turn, are surrounded by a sheath consisting of several layers of flattened connective tissue cells (C). It is important to understand the relative positions of these three elements of the ovarian follicle, for they provide the building blocks for future follicular development.

During the course of normal follicular development, the oocyte will grow, the follicle cells will multiply by mitosis to form a population of granulosa cells, and the connective tissue will become a complex, extensive sheath called the *theca folliculi.*

Some of these changes are apparent in Figure B, a low-magnification electron micrograph of a secondary follicle. When primary follicles continue to grow, the oocyte enlarges considerably. While this enlargement is apparent, it is nowhere as obvious as in the dramatic changes displayed by the follicle cells. In the secondary follicle shown at right the number of follicular cells has greatly increased, forming a large, stratified population of granulosa cells (G) around the oocyte (O).

The granulosa cells secrete fluid, often called *follicular fluid* (or *liquor folliculi*), that is initially secreted into spaces between the adjacent granulosa cells (*). Eventually, these spaces fuse, and the follicular fluid becomes contained within a single large cavity called the *antrum.* An antrum (A) at an early stage of formation is evident in Figure B. Meanwhile, the connective tissue cells in the sheath around the granulosa cells have multiplied, secreted considerable amounts of collagen, and are now known as the theca folliculi (T). The theca folliculi is divided into two portions—an inner, highly cellular region, called the *theca interna,* and an outer, more fibrous region, the *theca externa.* Whereas no visible boundary exists between the theca interna and the theca externa, a distinct boundary—in the form of a basement membrane—separates the granulosa cells from the theca interna. The position of the basement membrane is outlined by the dotted line in Figure B.

Figure B shows a region of medium electron density that surrounds the oocyte. This polysaccharide-rich coat is the *zona pellucida* (Z). The zona pellucida is invaded by cytoplasmic extensions from the granulosa cells and by microvilli from the oocyte. At the time of ovulation, when the follicle ruptures and the egg is released, the oocyte is still surrounded by the zona pellucida and a coating of granulosa cells. These accompany the oocyte on its journey down the oviduct.

Figure A. Electron micrograph of part of the cortex of the ovary of the mouse containing several primary follicles. C, connective tissue cells; F, follicle cells; N, nucleus of oocyte; O, oocyte; S, steroid-secreting cells in the ovarian stroma. 2,050 X

Figure B. Electron micrograph of a secondary follicle within the ovary of the cat. A, antrum; G, granulosa cells; O, oocyte; T, theca folliculi; Z, zona pellucida; *, fluid-filled spaces between granulosa cells; dotted line, boundary between granulosa cells and theca interna. 850 X

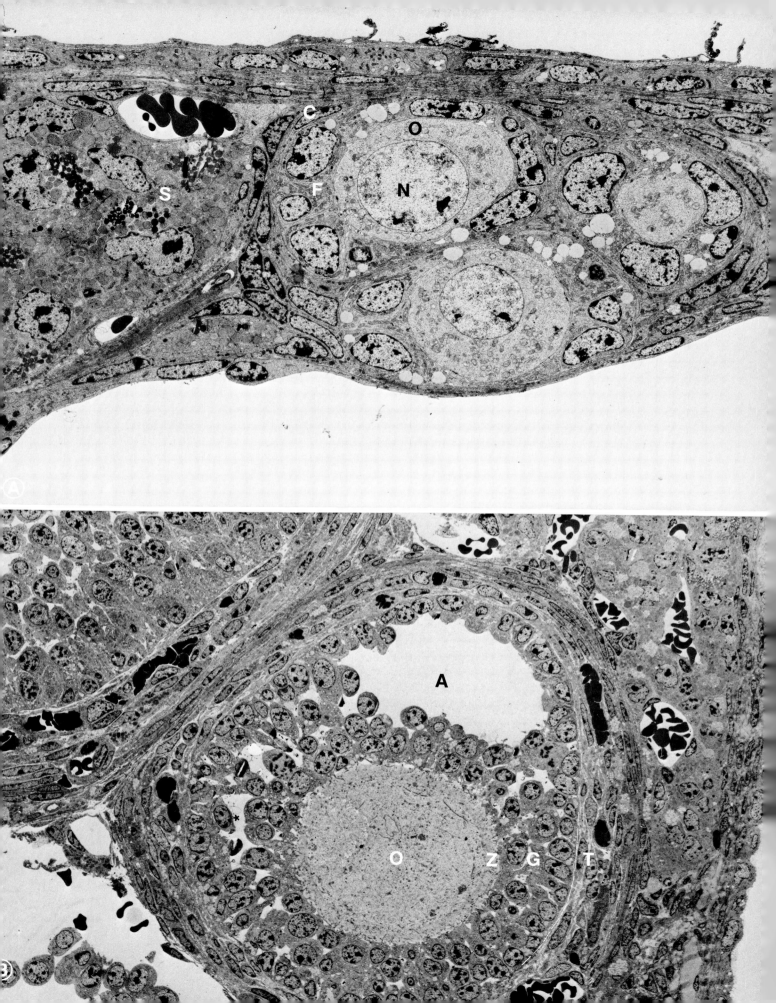

Plate 18–3

The Ovary: The Tertiary Follicle

After menarche, when menstruation begins, some of the secondary follicles in the ovary continue to develop and become *tertiary follicles.* Tertiary follicles are quite large and have a well-developed, fluid-filled cavity, the antrum. In humans, one of the several tertiary follicles will continue to grow and develop into a mature follicle, called the *Graafian follicle.* It is the Graafian follicle that releases the oocyte into the oviduct for fertilization.

Figures A and B at right are a matched pair of light and electron micrographs through an early tertiary follicle. (Classifications of follicular development vary in different texts. Some sources call the structure at right a late secondary follicle; others call it a *growing follicle.*) In this particular follicle, the antrum (A) is well developed, constituting the bulk of the follicular volume. In a mature follicle, the antrum would be continuous; here, it is still traversed by a column of granulosa cells (G') that will eventually move to occupy a peripheral location. The oocyte (O), now surrounded by a prominent zona pellucida (arrow), is situated off to one side. A cloud of granulosa cells, called the *cumulus oophorus* (CO), surrounds the oocyte. The granulosa cells that touch the oocyte have a special name, the *corona radiata.* The cells that form the corona radiata stick tightly to the oocyte and are shed with it at ovulation, forming a noticeable halo. When the sperm arrives to fertilize the ovulated oocyte, it first encounters the corona radiata, then the zona pellucida, before it makes contact with the plasma membrane of the egg cell itself.

Granulosa cells (G) line the antrum and occupy a peripheral location within the tertiary follicle. They sit atop a basement membrane, too small to be seen at this low magnification. The basement membrane separates the granulosa cells from the outer sheath of the follicle, the theca folliculi. As described in the previous plate, the theca folliculi has two structurally and functionally distinct regions: the highly cellular theca interna (TI), which has endocrine functions, and the more fibrous theca externa (TE), which does not. Close examination of Figures A and B will reveal these regions; they are, to be sure, more conspicuous when viewed by electron microscopy (Figure B).

The cells of the theca interna (TI) in Figure B contain large inclusions that look like lipid droplets. These inclusions contain steroid hormones and indicate that the cells of the theca interna are endocrine cells. At this stage, the cells of the theca interna make an estrogen precursor, a steroid molecule called *androstene dione.* Androstene dione is converted by the granulosa cells within the follicle to form *estradiol,* the most potent of all natural estrogens. After ovulation, the function of these cells changes; they become the *theca lutein cells* of the *corpus luteum* and secrete large amounts of *progesterone.* Shortly after the egg is released from the mature Graafian follicle, the entire follicle undergoes a drastic change in structure and function. Instead of being a follicle that supports the development of the egg, it becomes the corpus luteum, an endocrine organ, that secretes progesterone, which prevents maturation and ovulation in other follicles. If the oocyte is fertilized, the corpus luteum persists; if not, it degenerates, and the cycle of follicular development and ovulation begins anew.

Figures A and B. Matched pair of light and electron micrographs of serial sections taken through an early tertiary follicle of the mouse ovary. A, antrum; CO, cumulus oophorus; G, granulosa cells; G', column of granulosa cells that traverse antrum; O, oocyte; N, nucleus of oocyte; TE, theca externa; TI, theca interna; V, blood vessel; arrow, zona pellucida. Figure A, 350 X; Figure B, 600 X

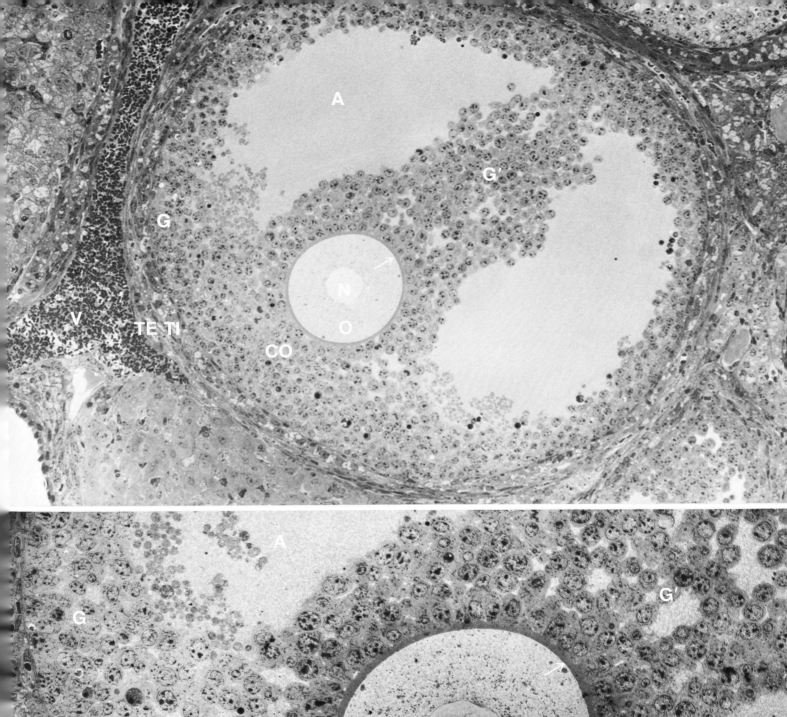

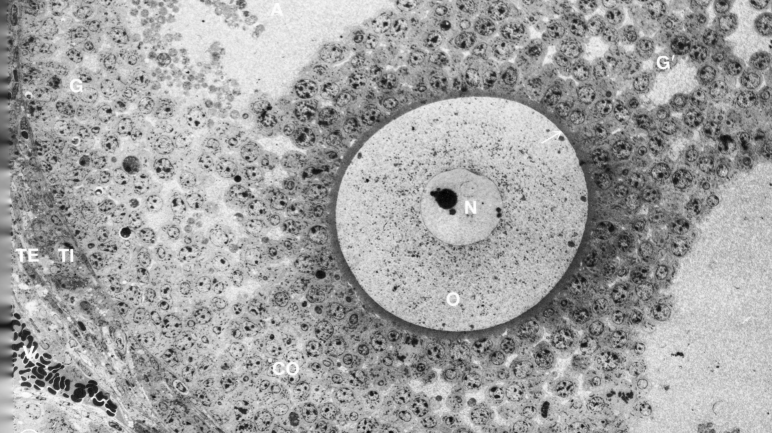

Plate 18–4

The Oviduct

The oviduct is a long, slender, musculomembraneous tube that carries the ovum from its origin in the ovary to its destination in the uterus. The oviduct has three major interrelated functions. First, it must pick up the egg at the moment of its expulsion from the ovary. This is no mean feat, since the ovary and oviduct are not directly attached to one another (see Figure 18-1). Second, it must transport and nourish the egg on its journey to the uterus. Third, it must provide a suitable environment for fertilization of the egg by a single spermatozoon.

The microanatomy of the oviduct is directly related to its function. The oviduct is a complex conduit that is ensheathed by layers of muscle that move the egg. In addition, it is lined by an epithelium that provides a suitable fluid environment not only for the egg, but also for the sperm that fertilizes it. Figures A and B are a matched pair of light and electron micrographs of the wall of the monkey oviduct. The epithelium that lines the oviduct is a simple columnar epithelium that contains *ciliated cells* (C) and *secretory cells* (S). The secretory cells are easily identified in Figure B by the large number of small, electron-dense secretory granules present in the apical cytoplasm. Here, some of the granules just released from the cells are evident in the lumen (L) of the oviduct. The secretory product of these cells forms a viscous fluid that fills the lumen and, in so doing, covers and lubricates the epithelial surface. The fluid is moved toward the uterus not only by the metachronal beating of the cilia of the ciliated cells, but also by the muscular contractions of the smooth muscle in the muscularis (M) upon which the mucosa rests.

The mucosa of the oviduct consists of the epithelium described above and a thin lamina propria (LP) made up of loose connective tissue. Unlike other tubes in the body, such as the gut, the oviduct's mucosa does not contain a muscularis mucosae. In addition, it has no submucosa. Instead, the mucosa—consisting of the epithelium and lamina propria—rests directly on the muscle layers, collectively called the muscularis. The histologic arrangement of the epithelium, lamina propria and muscularis (M) is readily apparent in Figures A and B at right. The mucosa is thrown into an extensive series of branched folds called *folia.* Portions of several folia (F) are evident in the micrographs at right. As in the villus of the intestine, the core of each folium is composed of the lamina propria.

The oviduct, which is some 12 cm long and about twice the diameter of an earthworm, contains four different regions. The distal portion, near the ovary, is called the *infundibulum.* The infundibulum leads to the *ampulla,*the area from which Figures A and B were made. The ampulla leads to a constricted region called the *isthmus.* The isthmus, in turn, enters the uterus. The part of the oviduct that crosses the uterine wall is called the *pars interstitialis.* The folia are most extensive, and the epithelium most well-developed, in the distal portions of the oviduct. As the oviduct nears the uterus, the folia become shorter and flatter, and the epithelium decreases in height.

The microanatomy of the oviduct is greatly influenced by the woman's hormonal status; it will display different structural profiles at different stages of the menstrual cycle. In patients in whom ovariectomy has been performed, for example, the epithelium atrophies. The secretory cells become small and inactive; most of the ciliated cells shed their cilia. Under conditions of hormone replacement with estradiol, however, the epithelium rapidly resumes the condition depicted at right; the ciliated cells regrow their cilia, and the secretory cells become active once again.

Figures A and B. Matched pair of light and electron micrographs of the oviduct of the squirrel monkey. C, ciliated cell; F, folium; L, lumen; LP, lamina propria; M, muscularis; S, secretory cells. Figure A, 500 X; Figure B, 1,000 X

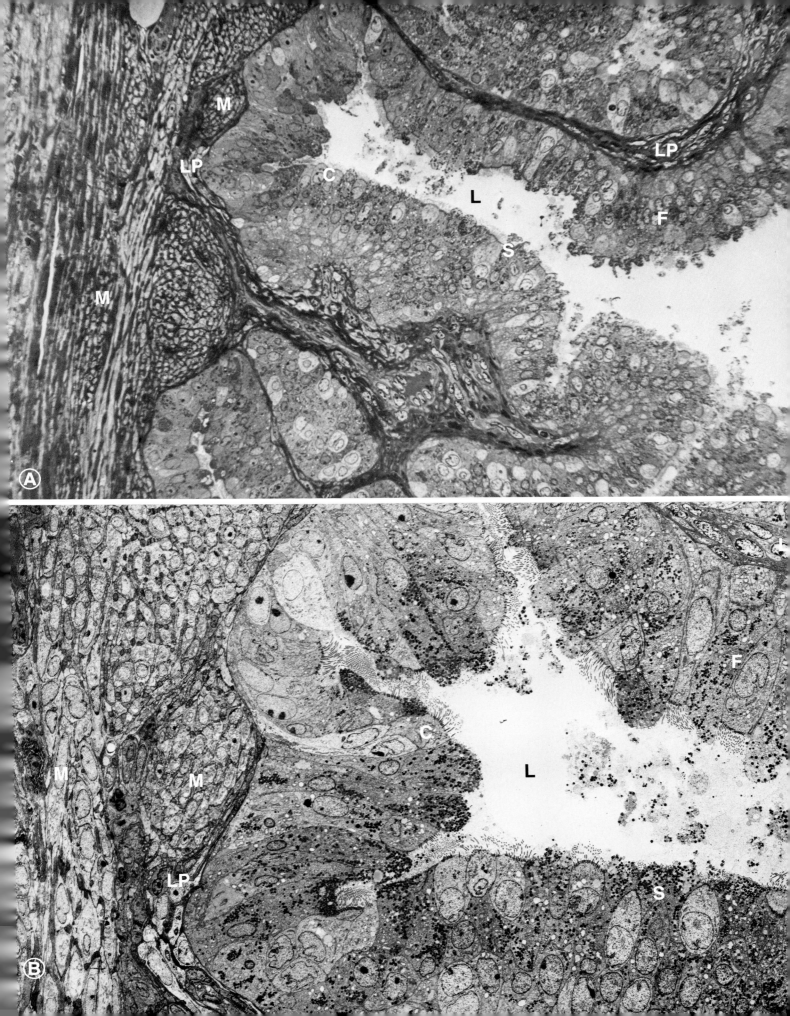

Plate 18–5

The Uterus

After the oocyte has been released from the ovary, it travels down the oviduct. If fertilization occurs, cleavage of the fertilized egg, or *zygote,* follows, and the resultant ball of cells, the *morula,* travels through the oviduct and into the uterus. There, implantation occurs, and the *blastocyst*—the very early embryo—begins to grow.

The uterus is an extremely important organ, for it not only permits attachment and implantation of the blastocyst, but it also establishes a nutritional organ, called the *placenta,* for the developing fetus. The mucosa that lines the inner surface of the uterus, called the *endometrium,* is primed to receive the fertilized egg when ovulation occurs. If fertilization takes place and implantation follows, the uterus becomes the site of embryonic and fetal development. If fertilization and implantation do not occur, however, the uterus abandons its state of readiness and sloughs most of its endometrial lining at menstruation. When a new cycle of follicular maturation in the ovary begins, the uterus renews its lining to prepare for another cycle of ovulation, potential fertilization, and implantation.

Part of the wall of the human uterus is shown at very low magnification by light microscopy in Figure A. The wall of the uterus has the same basic components as the wall of the oviduct described in the previous plate, although the names are different. The mucosa lining the uterus, called the endometrium (ENDO), consists of a simple columnar epithelium that rests on a highly cellular bed of connective tissue. As in the oviduct, no muscularis mucosae or submucosa is present; consequently, the muscularis, here called the *myometrium* (MYO), is situated directly beneath the endometrium. The outer surface of the uterus, not shown here, is covered by a serosal layer (continuous with the peritoneum lining the body cavity) called the *perimetrium.*

The epithelium (EP) that lines the inner uterine wall frequently dives into the underlying connective tissue to form numerous simple tubular *endometrial glands* (G). These glands extend the full thickness of the endometrium. The endometrium changes its structure dramatically during the menstrual cycle. The uterus depicted here is in the *secretory phase,* in which the uterus prepares itself for implantation. Here, the endometrium is very thick, and the glands are coiled into a corkscrew configuration. At this point, the endometrium is divided into two major regions: the *functionalis* (F), which constitutes about 80% of the endometrial thickness and is shed at menstruation, and the *basalis* (B), which is not. During the early phase of the menstrual cycle, the endometrium must rebuild its lost functionalis. This phase of reconstruction is called the *proliferative phase* of the uterus.

The inner surface of the human uterus is shown by electron microscopy in Figure B. Here, the simple columnar epithelium is shown to contain secretory cells (S) and ciliated cells (C). The secretory cells elaborate and release a glycogen-rich, mucous secretion that coats the inner uterine lining. The secretion is moved about by the beating of the motile cilia atop the ciliated cells. The epithelium rests on a highly cellular, richly vascular lamina propria (LP). In this micrograph, an endometrial gland (G) is caught as it opens onto the inner surface of the uterus. This tissue sample, taken shortly before menstruation, contains many free erythrocytes (E) in the lamina propria. Quite a few red blood cells have, at this stage, begun to invade the epithelium itself (arrows). These changes in fine structure indicate that the endometrium is on the verge of being sloughed.

Figure A. Light micrograph of the wall of the human uterus in the secretory phase. B, basalis; ENDO, endometrium; EP, epithelium; F, functionalis; G, endometrial gland; L, lumen of uterus; MYO, myometrium. 95 X

Figure B. Electron micrograph of the wall of a premenstrual human uterus. C, ciliated cell; E, extravascular erythrocyte in lamina propria; G, endometrial gland; LP, lamina propria; S, secretory cell; arrow, erythrocyte free in epithelium. 600 X

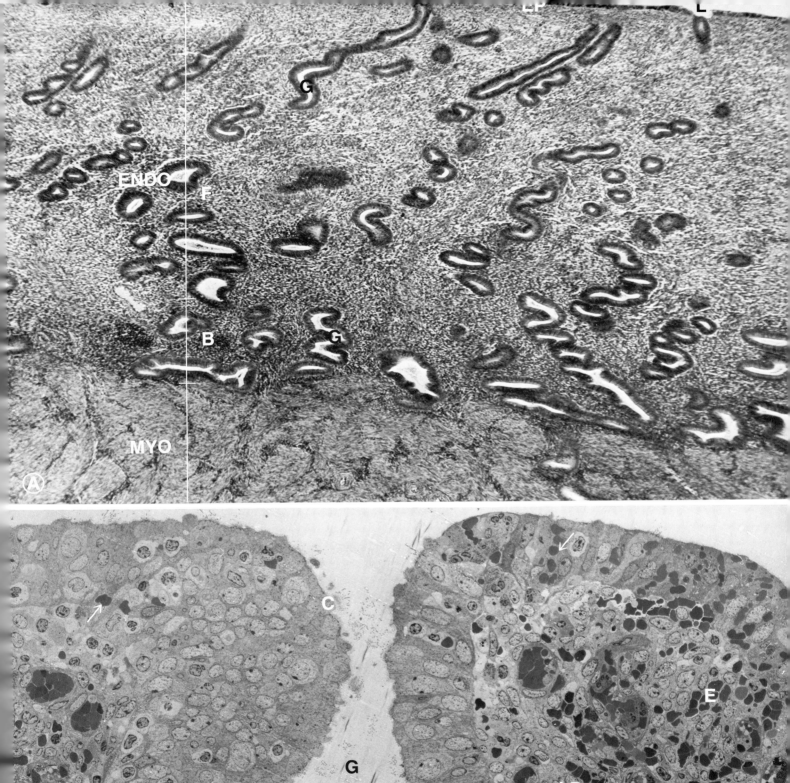

19

The Endocrine System

Overview

This atlas began with a discussion of entropy, the notion that everything tends toward disorder; here, we will consider the effects of entropy at a different level of organization. In Chapter 1, Cells, we discussed the enormous entropic possibilities inherent in a "typical" human cell possessed of some 10 billion individual protein molecules. This chapter deals with the even greater entropic possibilities inherent in a whole human being made up of some 50 trillion individual cells, each of which contains 10 billion protein molecules.

The human organism, composed of 50 trillion cells, copes with the tremendous inherent possibilities for disorder by superb mechanisms for intercellular communication in the nervous system and the endocrine system.

Given that humans are large, watery cellular aggregates, intercellular communication is arranged in two ways. For cells to communicate, they must make contact with one another, either directly, by physical cell-to-cell contact, as in the nervous system, or indirectly, through the common solution in which they all bathe, as in the endocrine system. The nervous system can readily be envisioned as a communication network with myriad branching processes and synaptic contacts all carrying information from place to place in the body. The endocrine system, however, is harder to envision as a communication system because the fluid-borne

molecules that carry information in solution from cell to cell are too small to be seen. In the endocrine system, an endocrine organ—basically a "ductless gland"—secretes a chemical messenger, or *hormone,* directly into the bloodstream. The hormone, rapidly carried through the circulatory system to all parts of the body, has specific effects on cells that have ***specific receptor molecules*** on their cell membranes that bind the hormone. The hormone, then, exerts its effect at some distance from the organ that secreted it. Consequently, the endocrine system has all the virtues of a communication system. Its bits of information, whose effects are far-flung, are blood-borne.

These two communications systems are tied together both anatomically and physiologically; the endocrine system and nervous system have profound effects on one another. Much of their interaction occurs in a part of the brain called the ***hypothalamus,*** in which neurons monitor specific body functions. When a deficit or imbalance of some sort is detected, the hypothalamus secretes ***releasing factors*** into blood vessels, which carry them immediately to the ***pituitary gland.*** The pituitary will in turn secrete a ***trophic hormone*** that will stimulate one of the many glands of the endocrine system to secrete a hormone that will affect the appropriate target cells. Thus, the endocrine system corrects the imbalance originally detected by the nervous system. An example of this sort of hypothalamic regulation of endocrine function is described in detail in the text of Plate 19–4.

The interrelationship between the nervous system and the endocrine system is manifest in the very structure of several endocrine organs themselves, where nerve cells and endocrine cells exist side by side in the same organ. In the *adrenal gland,* for example, the endocrine cells of the *cortex* are wrapped around a medulla made of nervous tissue. In the adrenal gland, cells of the endocrine system and the autonomic nervous system live within the same endocrine gland. In the pituitary, the endocrine cells of the anterior pituitary sit in front of the posterior pituitary, which is made of nervous tissue. In the pituitary, then, cells of the central nervous system and the endocrine system meet and live as near neighbors.

The endocrine system is highly complex, and its organs are many and varied. Some endocrine organs, such as the ovary and testis, have already been discussed. In this chapter, several of the major endocrine organs are illustrated by light and electron microscopy—the *thyroid gland,* the adrenal gland, and the pituitary gland.

Plate 19–1

The Thyroid Gland

The first endocrine organ to be described in this chapter is the thyroid gland—a small, butterfly-shaped organ, weighing less than 45 g, that is essential for the control of the body's metabolic rate. Without the thyroid gland, one would become sluggish, weak, and slow of thought. Fortunately, loss of the thyroid can largely be compensated by administration of its major endocrine product, **thyroid hormone.**

Located in the neck in front of the larynx, the thyroid gland consists of a series of functional units called follicles that range from small to large (nearly 1 mm in diameter). The follicles are filled with a dense, viscous **colloid** that contains **thyroglobulin,** a large, complex protein to which molecules of thyroid hormone are attached. When the epithelial cells of the follicles of the thyroid gland elaborate thyroid hormone, they link the hormone to thyroglobulin molecules. The thyroglobulin is then stored in the colloid in the lumen of the follicles. When the hormone is needed by the body, the epithelial cells begin a series of complicated biochemical maneuvers. First, thyroglobulin is taken up from the lumen of the follicle by pinocytosis; the cells drink the colloid they have made and stored. Next, the thyroglobulin taken into the cells is broken down by lysosomes, and the thyroid hormone is set free. Finally, the thyroid hormone is released from the base of the epithelial cells into nearby blood or lymph capillaries, from whence it is distributed to the tissues of the body.

Just as the thyroid gland has a unique function in the endocrine system, so does it have a unique structure. The thyroid gland is quite easy to identify in sectioned material. In Figure A, a light micrograph, the organization of thyroid tissue into follicles is apparent. The follicles vary in size and being nearly spherical, present a series of circular profiles.

Each follicle consists of a simple cuboidal epithelium (E) that surrounds a lumen filled with colloid (C). The follicles are separated from one another by delicate strands of loose connective tissue that emanate from the capsule that surrounds the gland. The majority of the epithelial cells, called **principal cells,** are concerned with the elaboration and secretion of thyroid hormone. Their structural appearance can change dramatically with their state of function; whereas inactive thyroid glands may have a squamous follicular epithelium, active follicles may have a cuboidal or low columnar epithelium. The principal cells can proliferate (*) by undergoing cell division.

Several follicles of the same thyroid gland are illustrated by electron microscopy in Figure B. The follicle in the center of the field (F1) has been sectioned across its center and displays the typical circular profile of a simple cuboidal epithelium that surrounds a colloid-filled lumen (C). The follicle at the upper left (F2), however, has been cut tangentially; only a small portion of the lumen and colloid are visible. The follicle in the upper right (F3) has been cut tangentially as well; in this case, the knife passed through the epithelium alone and missed the colloid completely, presenting the somewhat misleading appearance of a follicle without a lumen that looks like a solid ball of cells. Although most of the epithelium consists of principal cells, an occasional **parafollicular cell** (P) is evident. Parafollicular cells are neurosecretory cells that release the hormone **calcitonin,** which inhibits bone resorption by osteoclasts and has the effect of lowering blood calcium levels. Parafollicular cells, also called clear cells and C cells, do not reach the lumen of the follicle; instead, they are associated with the many blood and lymph capillaries that are present in the highly vascular thyroid gland.

Figure A. Light micrograph of the thyroid gland. C, colloid in lumen of follicle; Ca, capillary; E, follicular epithelium; P, parafollicular cell; *, dividing epithelial cell. 1,600 X

Figure B. Electron micrograph of the same thyroid gland depicted in Figure A. C, colloid; Ca, blood capillary; E, epithelium; F1, F2, and F3, follicles cut in different planes of section; L, lymph capillary; P, parafollicular cell. 2,800 X

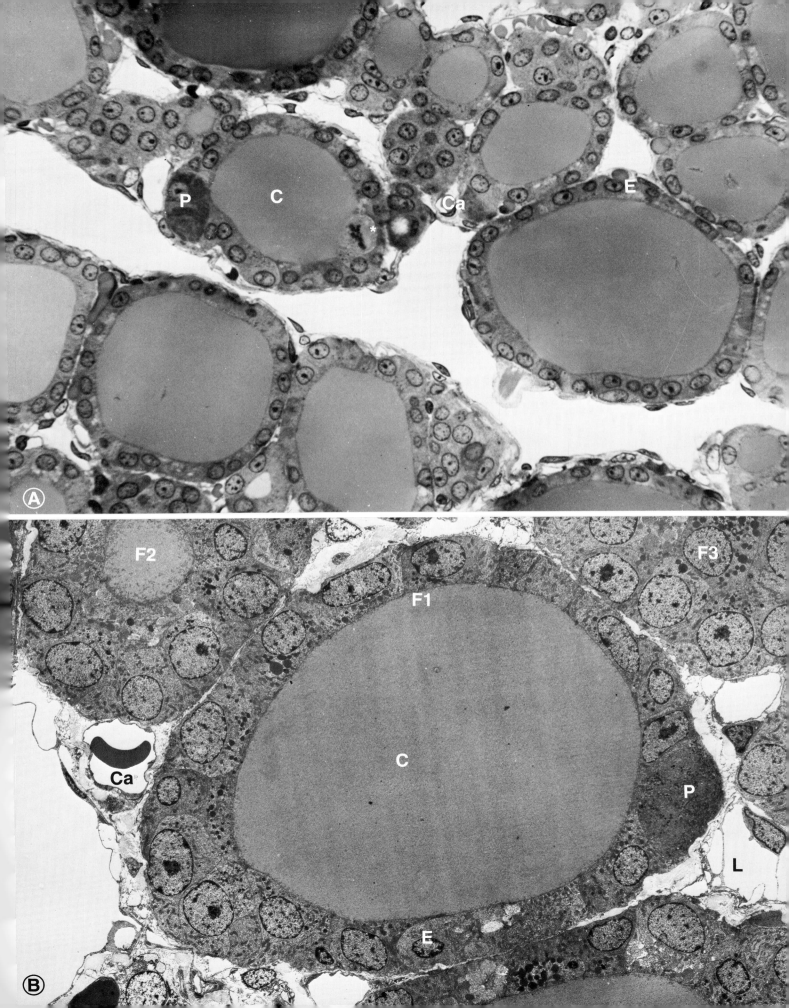

Plate 19–2

The Adrenal Cortex

The adrenal gland is a small, 60-g, half-moon–shaped gland that lies atop the kidney. As with many endocrine glands, its small size belies its importance in the regulation of the body's many homeostatic mechanisms. The adrenal gland is really two glands in one. It consists of an outer cortex that secretes steroid hormones and an inner medulla that secretes the catecholamines *norepinephrine* and *epinephrine.*

Figure A is a light micrograph of a cross section through half of the monkey adrenal gland. All the major histologic subdivisions of the gland are evident at low magnification. Working from the outside in (from the top to the bottom of the micrograph), the gland is covered by a connective tissue capsule (C) that serves to contain the soft underlying endocrine tissues. Beneath the capsule lies the outermost ''layer'' of the adrenal cortex, called the *zona glomerulosa* (ZG). The zona glomerulosa is concerned with the elaboration and secretion of a class of steroid hormones that, taken together, are called *mineralocorticoids*—hormones concerned with salt balance in the blood. Chief among the hormones secreted by the zona glomerulosa is *aldosterone.* Aldosterone promotes resorption of sodium from the glomerular filtrate by the proximal tubules of the kidney. Beneath the zona glomerulosa lies the *zona fasciculata* (ZF), a lightly stained region of the adrenal cortex that secretes *glucocorticoids,* a class of steroid hormones concerned with glycogen metabolism. The major glucocorticoids secreted by the zona fasciculata of the adrenal cortex include *cortisol* and *cortisone.* Beneath the zona fasciculata lies the *zona reticularis,* which produces adrenal *androgens.* The entire adrenal cortex surrounds the *adrenal medulla* (M). The medulla is quite different in structure from the cortex. It consists of a cluster of sympathetic nerve cells, modified to secrete catecholamines, that produce norepinephrine and epinephrine.

As is the case in all endocrine organs, the adrenal gland releases its hormones into the bloodstream, which distributes them to the various target organs throughout the body. Consequently, the adrenal gland, like all endocrine organs, is highly vascular. The capillaries (Ca) in the adrenal gland are not only extremely numerous, they are also quite large. In addition to being vessels of large caliber, the capillaries in the adrenal are *fenestrated capillaries*: their walls are perforated by holes that readily permit the passage of large molecules.

Figure B shows part of the capsule (C), the zona glomerulosa (ZG), and the zona fasciculata (ZF) by electron microscopy. Here, the ovoid, or glomerular, arrangement of cells in the zona glomerulosa is evident. Similarly, the arrangement of cells in the zona fasciculata into parallel cords, or *fascicles,* is obvious. Both of these regions stand in sharp contrast to the zona reticularis, shown in Figure C. Here, the cells are grouped into thin, interconnecting strands, conferring an open, reticular appearance to the region. In all regions of the cortex, the microanatomy of the cells betrays their functional organization as steroid-secreting cells. They have a high content of lipid droplets—membrane-limited vesicles filled with fatty steroid hormones—and they have unique mitochondria with tubular cristae. These and other features of the adrenal gland will be described in more detail on the following plate.

Figure A. Light micrograph of a cross section through the adrenal gland of the squirrel monkey. C, capsule; Ca, fenestrated capillary; M, adrenal medulla; ZF, zona fasciculata; ZG, zona glomerulosa; ZR, zona reticularis. 170 X

Figure B. Electron micrograph through the outer region of the adrenal cortex of the squirrel monkey. C, capsule; Ca, fenestrated capillary; ZF, zona fasciculata; ZG, zona glomerulosa. 850 X

Figure C. Electron micrograph through the inner region of the adrenal cortex of the squirrel monkey. Ca, fenestrated capillary; ZR, zona reticularis. 1,000 X

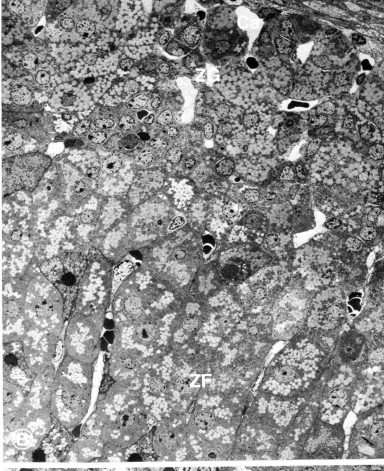
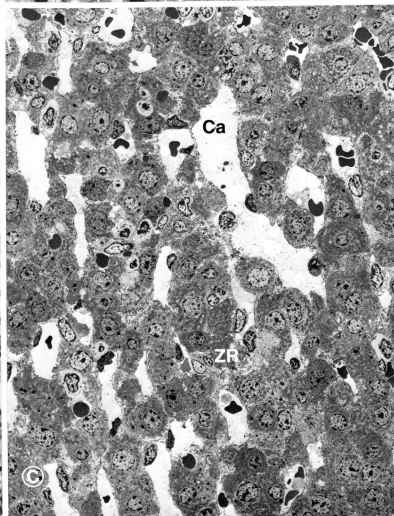

Plate 19–3

Cells Of The Adrenal Gland

A survey of the microanatomy of the adrenal gland was presented in the previous plate; the micrographs at right illustrate some of the specific ultrastructural features of various hormone-secreting endocrine cells from several regions of the adrenal cortex and medulla.

Figure A is an intermediate-magnification electron micrograph of several cells within the zona glomerulosa of the adrenal cortex. The steroid hormone aldosterone is produced by the zona glomerulosa. Consequently, the cytoplasm of the secretory cells is filled with lipid droplets (L) that probably represent packets of steroid hormone awaiting release by exocytosis in the vicinity of nearby capillaries (Ca). A close look at the boundary between the aldosterone-producing cell and its neighboring capillary will reveal a number of short microvilli (∗) on the surface of the endocrine cell. These microvilli are in an ideal position to facilitate exchange of materials across the cell surface. Once the secretory product passes out of the endocrine cell it can very rapidly diffuse into the lumen of the capillary, because this large capillary is a fenestrated capillary, whose wall is perforated to permit rapid entrance and exit of large molecules. One of the fenestrations, hard to see at this magnification, is indicated by the arrow in Figure A.

In addition to these features, the endocrine cell of the zona glomerulosa possesses large numbers of mitochondria (M) with *tubular cristae.* Many steroid-producing cells, such as the cells of the adrenal cortex and the interstitial cells of the testis, contain mitochondria with cristae arranged in a tubular configuration. The functional significance of this highly ordered arrangement of cristae is presently unknown.

Figure B is an electron micrograph of a cell from the zona fasciculata of the adrenal cortex. In having mitochondria (M) with tubular cristae and a large population of lipid droplets (L), it shares features with the cells of the overlying zona glomerulosa. Fine differences exist, however. The lipid droplets, large and dense in the cells shown in Figure A, are small, less dense, and more numerous in the cells in Figure B, perhaps reflecting differences in the quantity and quality of hormone produced by each cell type. The cells of the zona fasciculata produce glucocorticoids such as cortisone, whereas those of the zona glomerulosa produce mineralocorticoids such as aldosterone.

Figure C depicts a portion of the adrenal medulla as viewed by electron microscopy. The adrenal medulla, markedly different in structure from the cortex, actually represents a ganglion of the sympathetic nervous system whose neurons have largely become specialized as neurosecretory cells. The vast majority of cells within the medulla, called *chromaffin cells* (C), are specialized to produce the catecholamines epinephrine and norepinephrine. These cells are filled with tiny, electron-dense, catecholamine-containing granules. Like the adrenal cortex, the adrenal medulla is highly vascular, containing many large fenestrated capillaries (Ca). Occasional ganglion cells (G), large nerve cells not filled with neurosecretory granules, are present. The medulla is held together by fine strands of connective tissue (CT) rich in reticular fibers. Capillaries are often found in association with these wispy strands of connective tissue.

The adrenal gland, then, is really two endocrine glands in one, in that it has an epithelial component (the cortex) and a neural component (the medulla). The pituitary gland, too, as we shall see in the next plate, has an epithelial component (the anterior pituitary) and a neural component (the posterior pituitary).

Figure A. Electron micrograph of cells of the zona glomerulosa of the adrenal cortex of the squirrel monkey. Ca, fenestrated capillary; E, erythrocyte; L, lipid droplet; Ly, lymphocyte; M, mitochondrion; N, nucleus; ∗, microvilli; arrow, fenestration in capillary. 5,300 X

Figure B. Electron micrograph of the zona fasciculata from the same adrenal cortex photographed in Figure A. L, lipid droplet; M, mitochondrion; N, nucleus. 5,600 X

Figure C. Electron micrograph of the medulla of the same adrenal gland photographed in Figures A and B. C, chromaffin cell; Ca, fenestrated capillary; CT, connective tissue strands; G, ganglion cell. 2,300 X

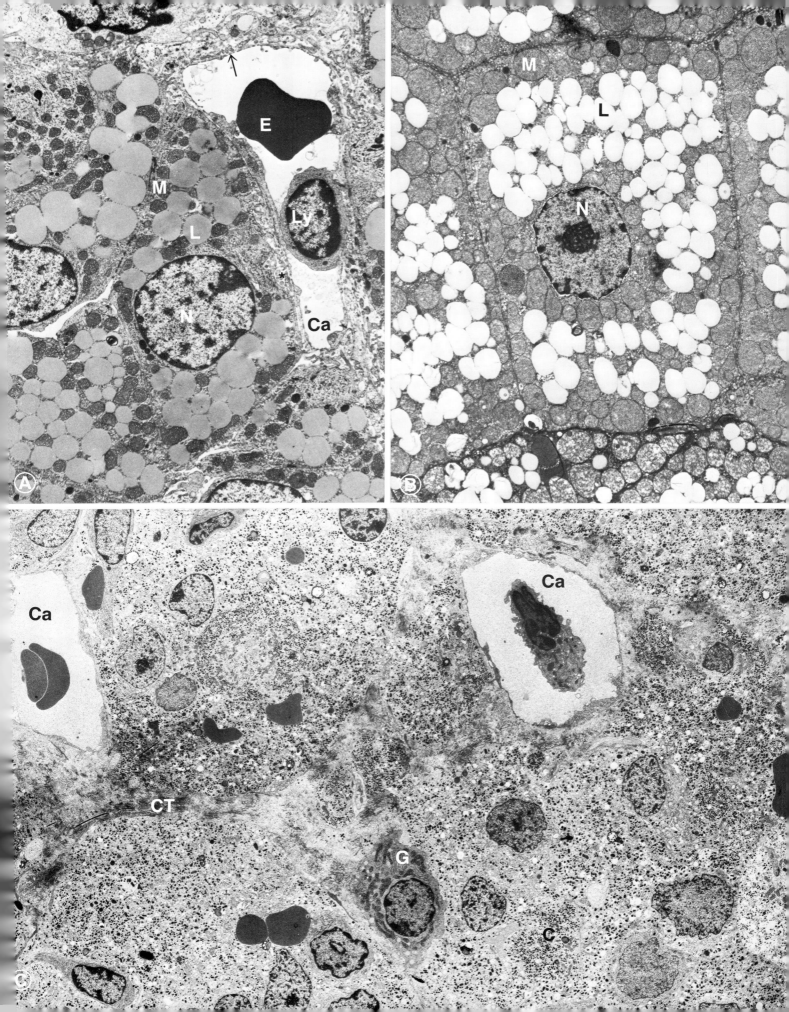

Plate 19–4

The Pituitary Gland

The pituitary gland, or *hypophysis,* is a tiny, pea-sized structure, stationed at the base of the brain, that weighs 0.5 g. Despite its diminutive size, the pituitary gland is of tremendous physiologic importance: it serves as an interface between the two great communication systems of the body, the nervous system and the endocrine system.

An example of the pituitary gland as an interface is the feedback loop involving thyrotropin-releasing factor (TRF), *thyrotropin,* and thyroid hormone. Because thyroid hormone serves to control the body's metabolic rate, levels of thyroid hormone circulating in the blood are critical and must be carefully controlled. When blood levels of thyroid hormone fall, nerve cells in the central nervous system—specific neurosecretory cells in the hypothalamus of the brain—become stimulated to secrete TRF. TRF is released into the bloodstream and travels directly to the pituitary gland through a special system of blood vessels called the *hypothalamic-hypophyseal portal system.* TRF stimulates special cells in the pituitary called *thyrotropes* to secrete the hormone thyrotropin. When released into the bloodstream, thyrotropin travels to the thyroid gland and promotes the secretion of thyroid hormone, which raises the titer of that hormone in the blood to appropriate physiologic levels.

In addition to serving as an interface between the nervous and endocrine systems, the pituitary gland has a dual histologic nature: it has an epithelial component, the *adenohypophysis,* and a neural component, the *neurohypophysis.* Areas of both components are shown in the figure at right, a low-magnification light micrograph of a sagittal section through the monkey pituitary gland. Here, the nervous compo-nent of the gland, the *pars nervosa* (PN), is connected directly with the hypothalamus of the brain by axons that, taken together, form the infundibulum (I)—a slender stalk of nerve tissue that suspends the pituitary gland from the base of the brain. Anterior to the pars nervosa is the *pars distalis* (PD), the largest subdivision of the pituitary gland, commonly referred to as the anterior lobe of the pituitary. In man and primates, the *pars intermedia* (PI) is a thin strip of tissue that lies between the pars distalis and the pars nervosa. Above the pars distalis, a collar of cells of unknown function called the *pars tuberalis* (PT) surrounds the infundibulum (I).

The microanatomic appearance of the pars nervosa is radically different from that of the pars distalis. The pars nervosa consists of axons and their terminals. The cell-bodies of those axons are all in the brain's hypothalamus. These hypothalamic neurons are specialized for neurosecretion, and their neurosecretory products are two hormones—*oxytocin,* which stimulates milk let-down and uterine smooth muscle contraction in females, and *vasopressin,* which promotes water retention by the kidneys. These hormones collect in swollen axon terminals within the pars nervosa. The pars distalis, on the other hand, consists of glandular epithelial cells specialized for the elaboration and secretion of many hormones, including thyrotropin, *growth hormone* (GH), *prolactin, luteinizing hormone* (LH), *follicle-stimulating hormone* (FSH), and *adrenocorticotropic hormone* (ACTH). Specific cell types, identified by immunohistochemistry and often distinguishable by electron microscopy, are responsible for the secretion of specific hormones.

Low-magnification light micrograph of a sagittal section through the pituitary gland of the squirrel monkey. BV, blood vessels of the hypothalamic-hypophyseal portal system; I, infundibulum; PD, pars distalis (anterior lobe); PI, pars intermedia (intermediate lobe); PN, pars nervosa; PT, pars tuberalis. 120 X

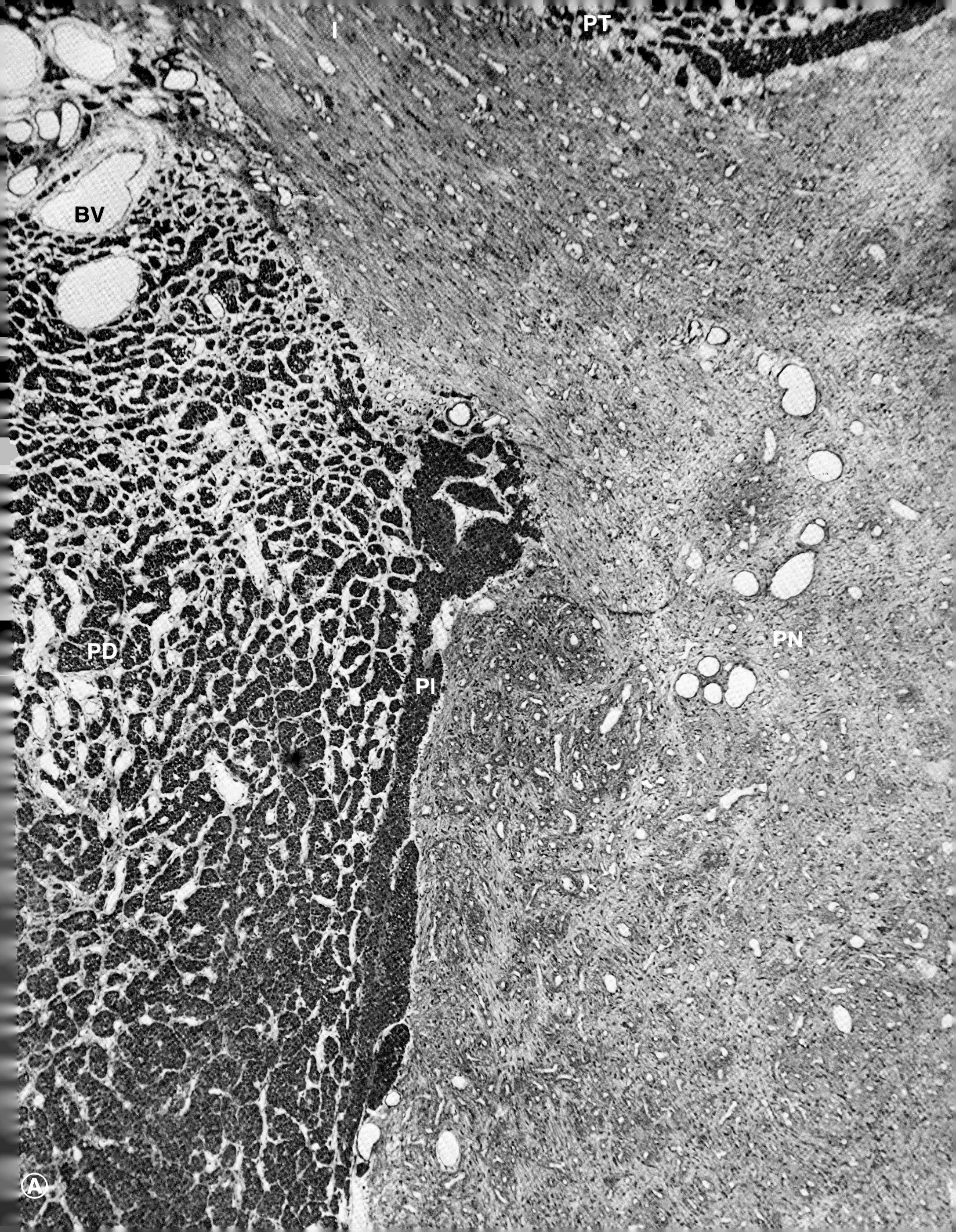
I
PT
BV
PD
PI
PN
A

Plate 19–5

Cells Of The Pituitary Gland

As the previous plate clearly illustrates, the adeno-hypophysis and neurohypophysis look quite different from one another when viewed with the light microscope. The vast structural differences between the two major regions of the pituitary gland are even more striking when examined by electron microscopy.

Figure A is a low-magnification electron micrograph of the pars distalis of the adenohypophysis. The pars distalis secretes six major hormones, including thyrotropin, GH, prolactin, LH, FSH, and ACTH. It is now widely accepted that each hormone is secreted by a single type of cell identifiable by immunohistochemical markers. Standard histologic sections, stained with hematoxylin-eosin, reveal three classes of morphologically distinct cells: *acidophils, basophils,* and *chromophobes,* all named for their staining characteristics. Thin sections, viewed under the electron microscope, reveal several cell types distinguishable by the types of electron-dense secretory granules they contain.

The acidophils of the adenohypophysis contain large (300-nm) granules that stain with eosin; acidophils include cells that secrete growth hormone or prolactin. Basophils, which have small (150-nm) granules that stain with hematoxylin, include cells that secrete either thyrotropin, FSH, LH, or ACTH. Chromophobes are believed to represent acidophils or basophils that have become degranulated after secretion of hormone. In Figure A, several cells (S) contain large, electron-dense granules. Although it is impossible to make a positive identification of these cells, they are in all likelihood *somatotropes*—cells that secrete GH. Of the two cell types that contain large granules, somatotropes are the more numerous. Other endocrine cells (B) have markedly smaller electron-dense granules. These cells correspond to the basophils seen under the light microscope; it is impossible to tell what kind of hormone they elaborate without resorting to antibody-labeling techniques. All of the cells have the ultrastructural characteristics of protein-secreting cells; that is, they have an extensive rough endoplasmic reticulum (RER), a well-developed Golgi apparatus, and numerous electron-dense granules that are actually membrane-limited secretory vesicles filled with the proteinaceous hormone produced by the cell. Many large, fenestrated capillaries (Ca), large enough to be called sinusoids, course between the endocrine cells of the adenohypophysis. The fenestrations in the capillaries facilitate rapid passage of large molecules to and from the endocrine cells.

Figure B is a low-magnification electron micrograph of the neurohypophysis of the same pituitary gland. There is almost no ultrastructural similarity between the adenohypophysis and the neurohypophysis. There are, for example, very few cell bodies in the pars nervosa, because the cell bodies of the neurohypophysis lie in the hypothalamus of the brain. The neurohypophysis, then, is actually a direct extension of the brain itself. Most of its substance consists of axons (A) and swollen axon terminals (AT) (also called Herring bodies) of neurosecretory cells that produce the octapeptide hormones oxytocin and vasopressin. Consequently, the neurohypophysis functions largely as an organ of storage that releases oxytocin and vasopressin into the bloodstream when they are required by the body. Nuclei of several cell bodies, however, are present. These nuclei (N) belong to specialized cells called *pituicytes.* Pituicytes are not endocrine cells; instead, they are similar to glial cells and seem to play a role in the maintenance of the axons of the neurohypophysis.

Figure A. Electron micrograph of the pars distalis of the adenohypophysis. B, basophils with small granules; Ca, fenestrated capillaries; RER, rough endoplasmic reticulum; N, nucleus of somatotrope; S, somatotrope; arrow, large granules in cytoplasm of somatrotrope. 2,600 X

Figure B. Electron micrograph of the pars nervosa of the neurohypophysis from the same pituitary gland shown in Figure A. A, axon; AT, axon terminals filled with neurosecretory vesicles; N, nucleus of pituicyte; P, pituicyte. 5,200 X

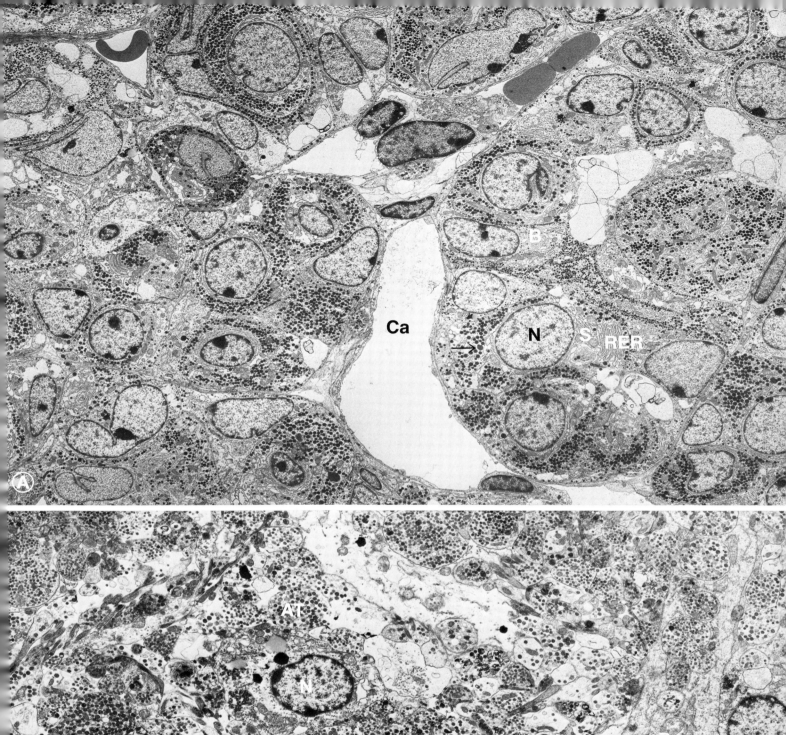
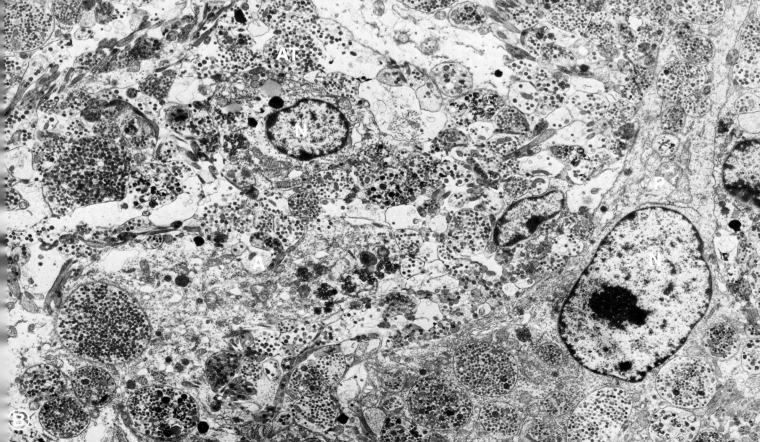

20

The Senses

Overview

Human beings—indeed, all animals—must interact favorably with the environment so that they can survive and reproduce. They must be aware of their surroundings so they can react to circumstances to better their chances for survival. Awareness has been set at a very high priority by natural selection. Consequently, during the course of many millions of years, special cells that are capable of detecting various classes of environmental stimuli have evolved.

Sources of energy from the environment that can serve as effective stimuli take many forms. Among those most commonly detected by different animals are light (the sense of sight), compression waves in air and water (the sense of sound), and specific molecular configurations (the chemical senses—taste and smell). The organs of special sense, the eye, ear, nose, and tongue, are tremendously complex. Each organ would take a book in itself to describe. This chapter concentrates on the special regions of the eye, ear, tongue, and nose that contain the receptor cells active in the detection and sensory transduction of stimuli supplied by the environment.

Sensory transduction is the process by which an environmental stimulus is detected, received, and transduced into bioelectric signals that are carried to the brain in the form of nerve impulses. In the eye, the *retina* contains the photosensitive cells, called *rods* and *cones,* that respond to light. Plate 20–1 shows how the ret-

ina is incorporated into the structure of the eyeball; Plates 20–2 and 20–3 illustrate the cellular elements of the monkey retina that receive incoming rays of light, transduce their energy into neuronal excitation, and transmit nerve impulses to the brain along the optic nerve.

In the ear, the *cochlea,* a tiny spiral of bone and soft tissue, contains exquisitely sensitive mechanoreceptors, the *hair cells,* that respond to vibrational stimuli. Plate 20–4 presents a matched pair of light and electron micrographs that illustrate the *organ of Corti*—the part of the inner ear that contains the hair cells—in its normal position within the cochlea.

In the nose, the *olfactory epithelium* contains chemoreceptors—the *olfactory receptors,* a series of bipolar neurons that are excited by chemical stimulation. Plates 20–5 and 20–6 illustrate the ultrastructure of human olfactory epithelium and its sensory receptors.

In the oral cavity, the tongue contains several types of projections, the papillae, that bear taste buds. Each taste bud is sensitive to sweet, sour, salty, or bitter stimuli. Plate 20–6 presents a low-magnification electron image of a single human taste bud from a circumvallate papilla.

Many other types of sensory receptors exist in addition to those mentioned above. In this chapter we focus on the sensory regions of the eye, ear, nose, and tongue—areas of tissue that will be of greatest interest to students of microanatomy.

Plate 20–1

The Eye: Sclera, Choroid, And Retina

Plate 20–1

The Eye: Sclera, Choroid, And Retina

In order to understand the microanatomy of the retina and its photoreceptors, it is important to see how the retina is incorporated into the structure of the eye itself. This structure is clearly shown in the plate at right, a light micrograph of a cross section through the posterior wall of the eyeball of a large monkey, the pig-tailed macaque. The retina of the macaque is quite similar to that of man, and the specimen at right was preserved unusually well by intravascular perfusion.

In this photomicrograph, the outside of the eyeball is at the top of the figure, and the inside of the eye, filled with *vitreous humor* (V), is at the bottom. Working from the outside in, the outermost part of the posterior wall of the eyeball is protected by pads of fat, here represented by clusters of *fat cells* (F). Close to these protective fat pads are numerous *skeletal muscle fibers* (M)—muscles associated with voluntary movements of the eye. These muscles attach to the *sclera* (S), here seen as a thick, uniform layer of dense regular connective tissue. It is the sclera that gives strength to the wall of the eyeball, and in so doing it does double duty, for not only does it confer strength and shape to the spherical eyeball, but it acts as a tendon that links muscle to eye.

Beneath the sclera lies the *choroid,* (Ch), a highly vascular mass of loose connective tissue that is interposed between the sclera and the retina (R). The choroid is filled with small blood vessels (BV), which, taken together, are called the *choriocapillaris.* The choriocapillaris supplies the oxygen-hungry photoreceptors of the retina with blood.

The retina lies in the lower third of the figure. Many students of histology, when confronted with the task of learning retinal microanatomy, set out to devise mnemonic devices to memorize names of the layers, which at first seem to make little sense. This step is unnecessary, for with an understanding of the cellular basis for retinal organization (described in detail in the next plate), the histologic organization of the retina seems obvious and the reasons for the names become apparent.

In the low-magnification light micrograph in Plate 20–1, the outermost layer of the retina—the layer closest to the outside of the eyeball—is the *pigment epithelium* (PE). The pigment epithelium is closely associated with the layer of rods and cones (LRC), the extensions of the photoreceptors active in sensory transduction. Beneath the layer of rods and cones lies the *outer nuclear layer* (ONL); beneath the outer nuclear layer is the *outer plexiform layer* (OPL). Still working toward the center of the eye, the next layer is the *inner nuclear layer* (INL), which lies atop the *inner plexiform layer* (IPL). The inner plexiform layer is closely apposed to the underlying layer of ganglion cells (LGC), from which emanate axons of the *nerve fiber layer.* The nerve fiber layer (NFL), the innermost layer of the retina, is close to the vitreous humor that fills the eyeball and maintains its turgor. The arrow indicates the path of light through the eye; note that light must pass through all of the layers of the retina before it reaches the photoreceptors.

Light micrograph of a cross section taken through the posterior wall of the eyeball of the pig-tailed macaque. BV, blood vessel in choroid; Ch, choroid; F, fat cell; INL, inner nuclear layer; IPL, inner plexiform layer; LGC, layer of ganglion cells; LRC, layer of rods and cones; M, muscle; NFL, nerve fiber layer; ONL, outer nuclear layer; OPL, outer plexiform layer; PE, pigment epithelium; R, retina; S, sclera; V, vitreous humor; arrow, direction of light path through eye. 325 X

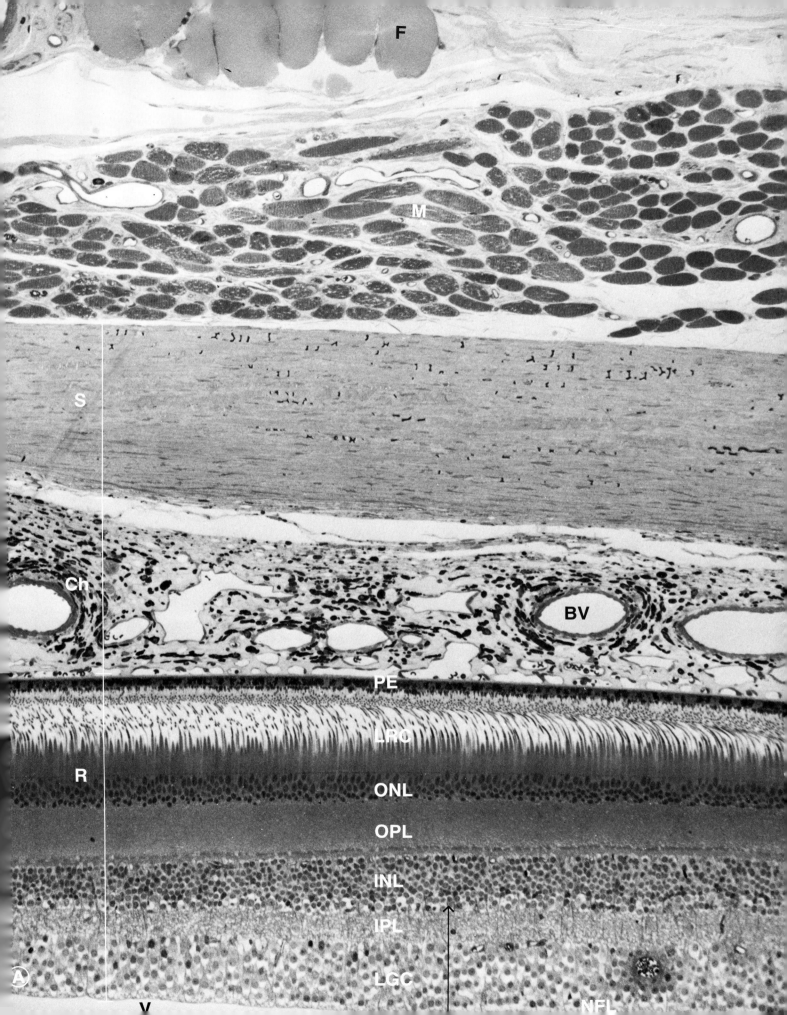

F

M

S

Ch

BV

PE

LRC

R

ONL

OPL

INL

IPL

LGC

V

NFL

A

Plate 20-2

The Eye: The Retina

The cellular basis of retinal organization is clearly shown in the figures at right. Figure B is a light micrograph of a cross section through the monkey retina; Figure C is an electron micrograph of a serial section through the same retina photographed at the same magnification; and Figure A is a schematic drawing of the major types of cells whose relative vertical arrangement generates the histologically distinct layers of the retina. As in the preceding plate, the outside of the retina is toward the top of the micrographs; the inside, toward the bottom. The arrow indicates the direction of the light path through the retina.

In Figure A, the uppermost cell is a *cone photoreceptor.* The outer segment of the cone (OS) is arranged in parallel with the outer segments of thousands of other rods and cones to form the layer of rods and cones (LRC) evident in Figures B and C. The outer segments are membranous extensions of the photoreceptor cell bodies such as that of the cone drawn in Figure A. The apical pole of the cell body is a dense region called the *ellipsoid* (E), which is packed with dark-staining mitochondria. The lower part of the cell body contains the nucleus (N). Taken together, the nuclei of the cell bodies of the rod and cone photoreceptors constitute the outer nuclear layer (ONL, Figures B and C) of the retina. The base of the cone gives rise to an axon (A), which travels inward to meet the dendrite of the next cell in the series—the *bipolar cell.* The synaptic contacts between photoreceptors and bipolar cells are, for the most part, made in the outer plexiform layer (OPL, Figures B and C). The dendrites of the bipolar cell (DB) extend from the cell bodies of the bipolar

cells, which contain centrally located nuclei (NB). The nuclei of the bipolar cells lie in the inner nuclear layer. From there, the axons of the bipolar cells (AB) travel inward to meet the dendrites of the next cell in the series, the ganglion cell. The axons of the bipolar cells and the dendrites of the ganglion cells make synaptic contacts in the inner plexiform layer (IPL, Figures B and C). The cell bodies of the ganglion cells, from which the dendrites grow, are located in the layer of ganglion cells (LGC, Figures B and C). Each ganglion cell gives rise to an axon (AG). The axons of the ganglion cells pass through the nerve fiber layer (NFL, Figures B and C) and coalesce to form the *optic nerve.* The optic nerve travels from the retina to the brain and carries visual information to higher centers within the central nervous system.

There are other types of cells in the retina in addition to those mentioned above. There are horizontal elements called *amacrine cells* and *horizontal cells;* there are glial cells called *Muller cells.* To understand these cells, however, it is advantageous to first learn about the relative positions of the rod and cone photoreceptors, the bipolar cells, and the ganglion cells. Given an understanding of their positions, as drawn in Figure A, one can envision all the classic histologic layers of the retina. With that understanding, a close comparison of the drawing with the light and electron micrographs shown in Figures B and C will not only help in understanding the organization of the retina, but is good preparation for further investigation of the fine structure of retinal photoreceptors as described in Plate 20-3.

Figure A. Drawing of a cone photoreceptor, a bipolar cell, and a ganglion cell showing their relative positions in the retina, which generate the "layers" of the retina shown in Figures B and C. From the top down, structures are: OS, cone outer segment; E, ellipsoid; N, nucleus of cone photoreceptor; A, axon of cone; S1, synapse between cone and bipolar cell; DB, dendrite of bipolar cell; NB, nucleus of bipolar cell; AB, axon of bipolar cell; S2, synapse between bipolar and ganglion cell; NG, nucleus of ganglion cell; AG, axon of ganglion cell. 1,000 X

Figures B and C. Matched pair of light and electron micrographs of the retina of the macaque. A, axon of cone; Ch, choroid; E, ellipsoid; INL, inner nuclear layer; IPL, inner plexiform layer; LGC, layer of ganglion cells; LRC, layer of rods and cones; N, nucleus of cone; NFL, nerve fiber layer; ONL, outer nuclear layer; OPL, outer plexiform layer; PE, pigment epithelium; arrow, light path through retina. 1,000 X

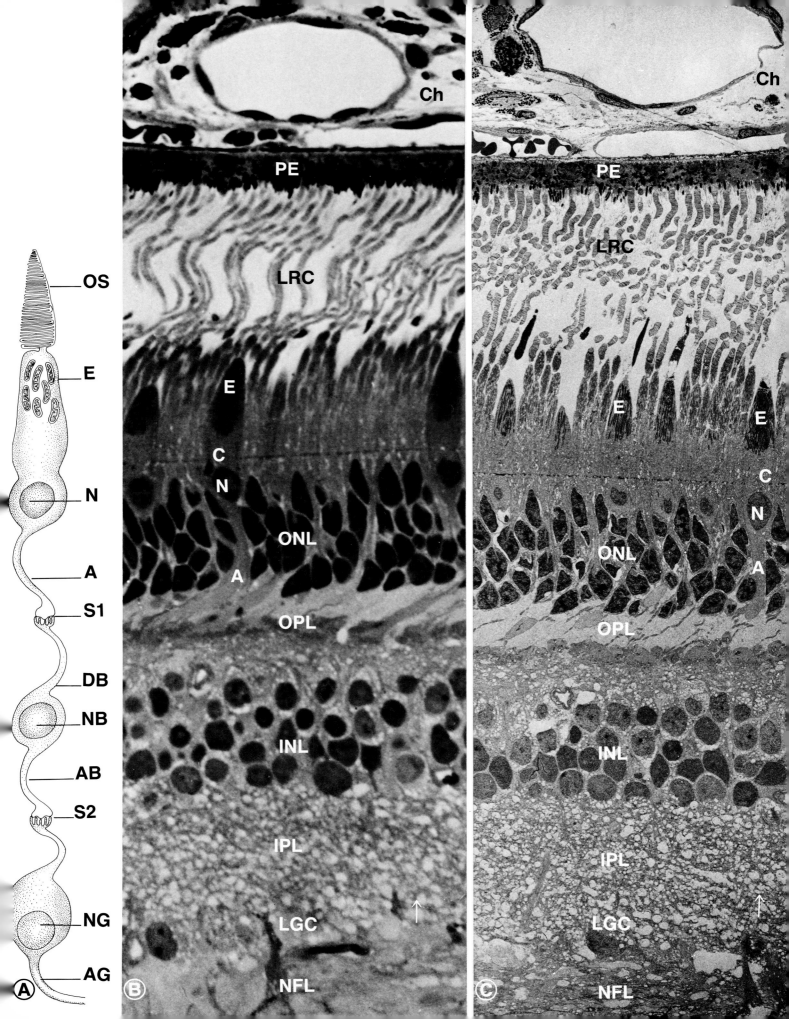

Plate 20–3

The Eye: Photoreceptors Of The Retina

The photoreceptors of the retina—the rods (R) and cones (C)—are illustrated by electron microscopy in Figure A. Rods "see" only black and white and come into play in dim light. Cones are color sensitive and are used for vision in bright light. Although rods and cones differ somewhat in structure and function, they share many cytoarchitectural features.

Each rod or cone is a specialized sensory cell, a bipolar neuron that is composed of two major structurally distinct regions: the *inner segment* (IS) and the *outer segment* (OS). These regions are evident in the longitudinally sectioned cone in Figure A. The inner segment, which contains the nucleus (N), consists of the cell body of the bipolar neuron and its apical pole. Whereas the basal pole of the cell tapers sharply to form an axon (A), the apical pole tapers gradually to form the ellipsoid (E). The ellipsoid of the cone is a football-shaped body, filled with many long mitochondria, that provide ATP for the bioenergetically demanding process of photoelectric sensory transduction that occurs in the outer segment.

The cone's outer segment, like that of adjacent rod photoreceptors (R), consists of a series of stacked cell membranes that are rich in photosensitive pigments. In living tissue, the outer segments, which in these preparations are artificially bent, are oriented parallel to the rays of incoming light (arrow). The membranous lamellae of the photoreceptors are oriented at right angles to the long axis of the outer segment. Consequently, the membranes and their contained photopigments are optimally positioned to be struck and stimulated by photons focused on the retina by the eye's dioptric apparatus.

The distal tips of the rod outer segments are intimately associated with the outermost layer of the retina, the pigment epithelium (PE, Figure B). (When looking at these micrographs, remember that each outer segment is a continuous, linear structure. In Figures A and B, the outer segments were distorted during specimen preparation, and they weave in and out of the plane of section, giving them the misleading appearance of discontinuity and making them look like "islands" of tissue, which they are not). The pigment epithelium serves a vital function in the normal metabolism of rod photoreceptors. The rod outer segments, it seems, are in a continuous state of flux; new stacks of membrane are added at the base of the outer segment, and old, worn-out stacks of membrane are shed from its distal tip. When the worn-out lamellae are ready to be shed from the tips of the outer segments, they are phagocytosed by cells of the pigment epithelium. The shed membranes, taken up by cells of the pigment epithelium, and engulfed by lysosomes, are evident as *residual bodies* (arrowhead, Figure B) in the cytoplasm of the epithelial cells themselves.

One very important feature of photoreceptor fine structure, not apparent in the micrographs at right, is the joining of the inner and outer segments of each rod and cone photoreceptor by a slender stalk, the *connecting cilium.* This modified cilium, which has a "9 + 0" axoneme and arises from a basal body at the tip of the inner segment, gives rise to the outer segment itself. In a sense, then, the outer segment may be regarded as a highly modified ciliary derivative. The presence of the basal body from which the cilium arises is essential for regeneration of rod outer segments that have degenerated in response to adverse conditions such as vitamin A deficiency.

Figure A. Electron micrograph of longitudinal section through photoreceptors of the monkey retina. A, axon of cone; C, cone photoreceptor; E, ellipsoid; IS, inner segment of cone; N, nucleus of cone; OPL, outer plexiform layer; OS, outer segment of cone; R, rod photoreceptor; RN, nucleus of rod; ROS, rod outer segment; arrow, direction of light passing through retina. 2,700 X

Figure B. Electron micrograph of choroid, pigment epithelium, and distal portion of photoreceptors of the monkey retina. Ca, capillary in choroid; M, melanocyte in choroid; PE, pigment epithelium; ROS, rod outer segment; arrow, direction of light passing through retina; arrowhead, residual body in pigment epithelium containing remains of phagocytosed tip of rod outer segment. 5,700 X

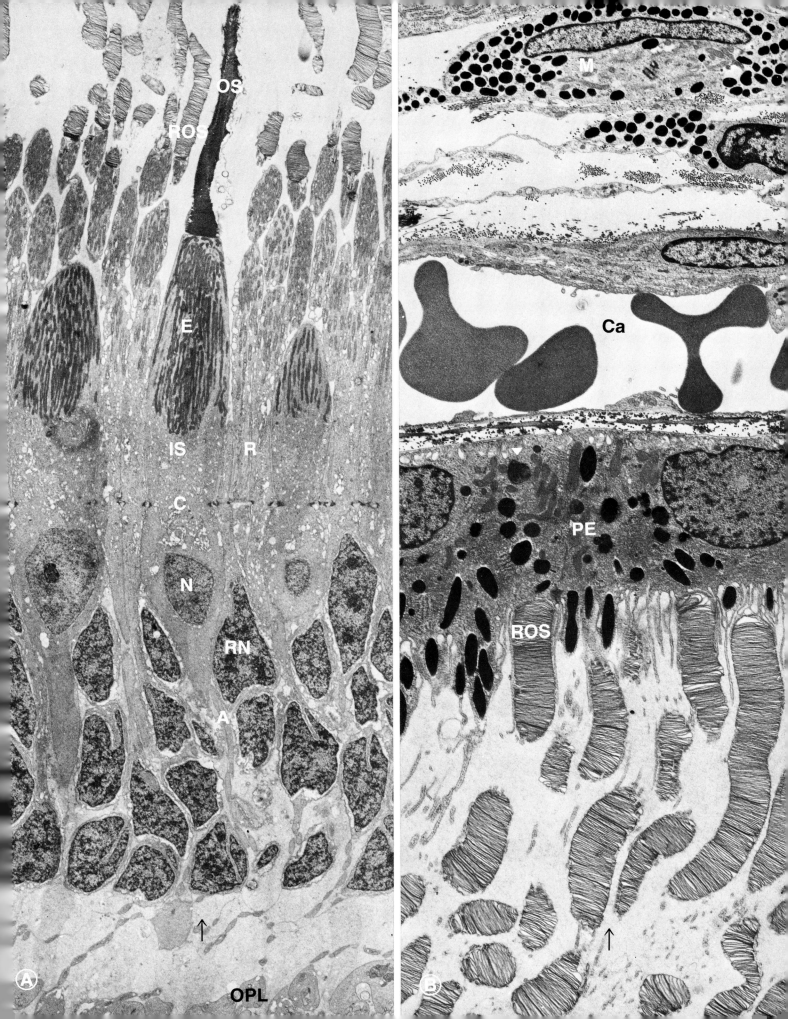

OS

ROS

E

IS   R

C

N

RN

A

OPL

M

Ca

PE

ROS

Plate 20–4

The Ear: The Organ Of Corti

The human ear is tremendously complex; its structure is beyond the scope of this atlas. This plate describes one specific component of the ear, that part crucial to the sensory transduction of sound waves into nerve impulses—the organ of Corti.

Buried deep within the bony recesses of the cochlear spiral, the organ of Corti, the epithelial organ of hearing, is a spirally wound epithelial sheet endowed with exquisitely mechanosensitive vibration detectors called hair cells. These hair cells are excited by extremely small displacements of their stereocilia, which are modified microvilli that project from the hair cell surface and contact an overlying structure called the *tectorial membrane.*

In order to understand the way in which the hair cells are stimulated during sound detection, it is necessary to become familiar with the overall organization of the organ of Corti. Figures A and B at right are a matched pair of light and electron micrographs of serial sections taken through the organ of Corti. The organ is anchored to a bony shelf, the *limbus spiralis* (LS), which projects from the central bony shaft of the cochlea, the modiolus, in the same way as does the spirally wound drill blade of a carpenter's wood-boring bit. An epithelium-lined sheet of connective tissue called the basilar membrane (BM) projects from the base of the limbus spiralis and supports the organ of Corti.

The tectorial membrane (TM) projects from the top of the limbus spiralis and, in living tissue, covers the tip of the stereocilia (arrows) that project from the free surface of the hair cells. During the process of hearing, sound waves ultimately cause the basilar membrane to vibrate, which in turn causes the hair cells and their stereocilia to vibrate as well. However, the tectorial membrane, into which the stereocilia insert, is motionless. Consequently, sound waves cause mechanical stimulation of the hair cells by creating shear forces between the stereocilia (which vibrate) and the tectorial membrane (which does not). The organ of Corti, then, is an elaborate structure whose complex microanatomic architecture is dedicated to the achievement of one major goal: mechanical stimulation of hair cells by sound waves.

The hair cells are arranged into two groups—the inner hair cells (IHC) and the outer hair cells (OHC). Both groups of hair cells are held in place by an elaborately sculpted set of supporting cells, including the inner and outer *pillar cells* (IP, OP) and the inner and outer *phalangeal cells* (IPC, OPC). These supporting cells have thin processes that arch out and around to hold the apical poles of the tall, slender hair cells firmly in place in a manner similar to the flying buttresses that support the walls of a tall, slender Gothic cathedral. These features of supporting cell microanatomy, not readily apparent in sectioned material, have recently been revealed in detail by scanning electron microscopy.

The hair cells are innervated by neurons that travel to the organ of Corti via the cochlear nerve. Myelinated fibers of the cochlear nerve (CN), evident below the limbus spiralis (LS) in Figures A and B, constitute the cochlear branch of VIII, the acoustic nerve, which conveys auditory information to the brain, wherein it is processed to generate our perception of sound.

Figures A and B. Matched pair of light and electron micrographs of sections taken through the organ of Corti. BM, basilar membrane; CD, cochlear duct; CN, cochlear nerve; IHC, inner hair cell; IP, inner pillar cell; IPC, inner phalangeal cell; LS, limbus spiralis; OHC, outer hair cell; OP, outer pillar cell; OPC, outer phalangeal cell; TM, tectorial membrane; arrows, stereocilia atop hair cells. Figure A, 540 X; Figure B, 970 X

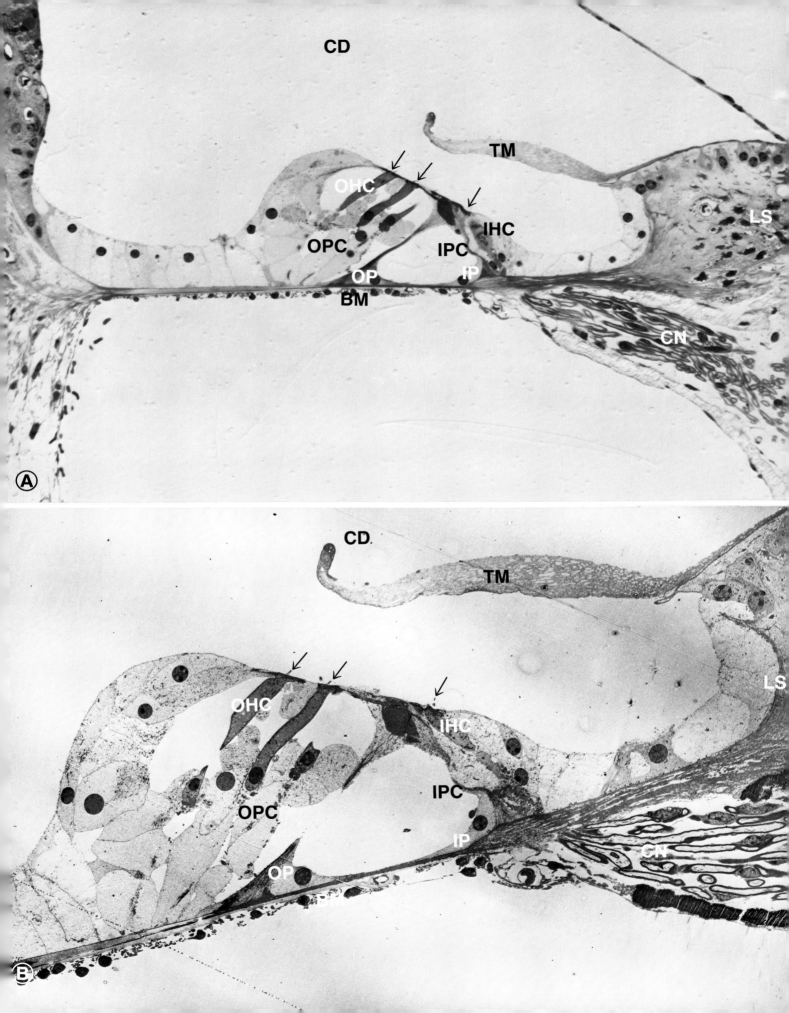

Plate 20-5

The Nose: Respiratory And Olfactory Epithelia

The human nose, an exquisitely sensitive odor detector and discriminator, is equipped with over a million olfactory receptors. Each olfactory receptor is a primary sense cell, a bipolar neuron that sends its dendrite to the site of stimulus reception and its axon to the olfactory bulb in the brain. Because the site of stimulus reception is the free surface of the olfactory epithelium in the nasal cavity, the olfactory receptors are vulnerable—they are truly "naked neurons," exposed to the outside world on one side and the brain on the other. This exposure has interesting clinical implications.

In humans, the olfactory receptors are situated in a small region of olfactory epithelium that is confined to an area of approximately 2 cm^2. The rest of the nasal cavity, it seems, is devoid of olfactory receptors. Respiratory and olfactory epithelia are markedly different in structure and function, as illustrated in the photomicrographs at right.

Figure A is an electron micrograph of the human respiratory epithelium in which there are no olfactory receptors; Figure B is an electron micrograph of the olfactory epithelium itself. In Figure A, it is evident that the respiratory epithelium is lined by a ciliated pseudostratified columnar epithelium that contains three major cell types: ciliated cells (C), goblet cells (G), and basal cells (B). The surface of the ciliated cells bears both cilia and slender microvilli that project well into the mucous layer that lines the nasal cavity (NC). The goblet cells, located in between the ciliated cells, are packed with mucous droplets (M) that extend from the level of the nucleus to the cell surface. The basal cells lie on top of the basement membrane, which, in turn, is supported by the connective tissues of the lamina propria.

The olfactory mucosa, shown in Figure B, is lo-cated in the superior region of the nasal cavity. Much thicker than the respiratory epithelium, it consists of a pseudostratified columnar epithelium and the underlying highly cellular lamina propria (LP). Figure B, a low-power electron micrograph through the human olfactory epithelium, shows the four major cell types: ciliated olfactory receptors (O), microvillar cells (M), supporting (or sustentacular) cells (S), and basal cells (B). In addition, degenerating olfactory receptors (D) are present. All cells, with the exception of basal cells, reach the free surface of the epithelium. In living tissue, the epithelial surface is covered with a blanket of mucus. In Figure B, the mucus was washed away during tissue preparation, exposing the surface specializations of the underlying cells. Here, we find cilia that extend from the olfactory vesicles (arrows) of the ciliated olfactory receptors, and microvilli extend from the microvillar cells (M). When the olfactory epithelium is seen in longitudinal section, as in Figure B, the uppermost nuclei are those of the microvillar cells. Next are the somewhat flattened, heterochromatic nuclei of the supporting cells (N'). Beneath these are the round, largely euchromatic nuclei of the ciliated olfactory receptors (N), seen to be distributed in a broad band that covers half the thickness of the epithelium. Deep to the nuclei of the ciliated olfactory receptors, lying above the basement membrane (BM), are the nuclei of the basal cells (B). The basal cells are capable of undergoing mitotic division and replacing lost ciliated olfactory receptors. Olfactory receptors, unique among human nerve cells, degenerate and are replaced in the normal course of life. Olfactory receptors are the only neurons known that not only "turn over" during normal life, but are replaced following loss from illness or injury.

Figure A. Low-magnification electron micrograph of respiratory epithelium from the human nasal mucosa. B, basal cell; C, ciliated cell; G, goblet cell; Ly, lymphocyte; M, mucus droplets in goblet cell; NC, nasal cavity. 3,500 X

Figure B. Low-power electron micrograph of human olfactory epithelium. B, basal cell; BM, basement membrane; D, degenerating olfactory receptor; LP, lamina propria; M, microvillar cell; N, nucleus of olfactory receptors; N', nucleus of supporting cell; NC, nasal cavity; O, ciliated olfactory receptor; S, supporting cell; arrow, olfactory vesicle bearing olfactory cilia. 1,200 X

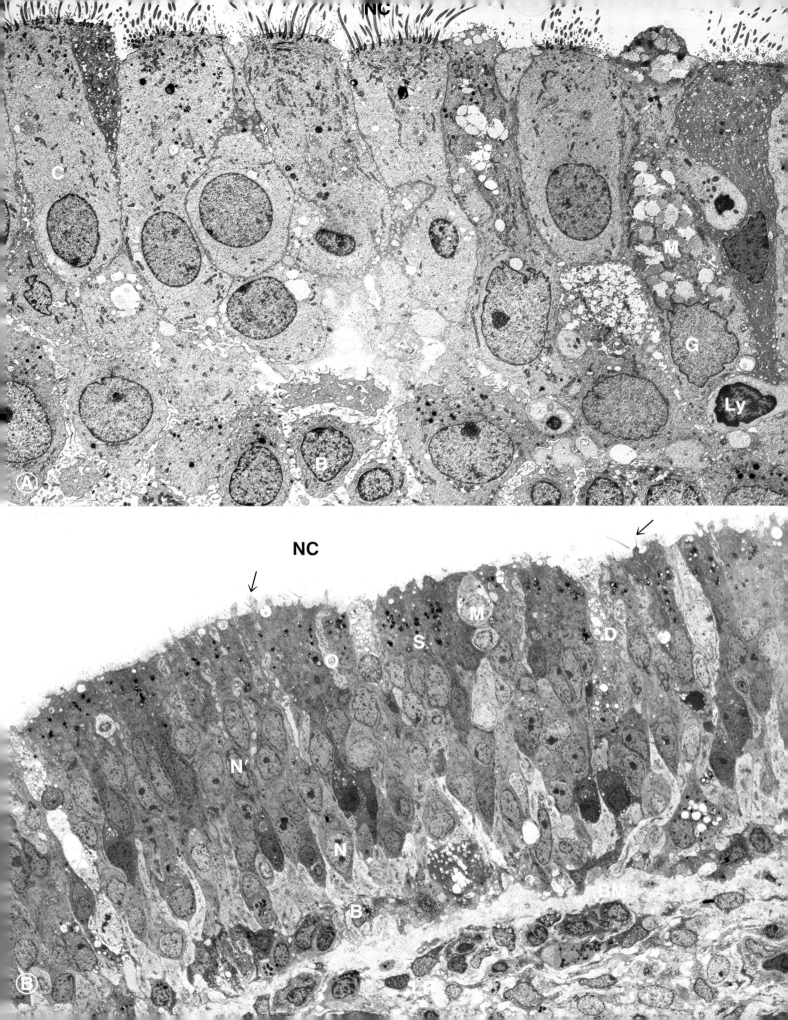

Plate 20-6

The Nose: Olfactory Receptors

Several of the olfactory receptors described in the previous plate are shown at higher magnification in Figure A at right. Here, one of the receptors has been cut along its length from cell body (O) to dendrite tip (arrow). The nucleus (N) lies at the center of the bipolar neuron. Above the nucleus are most of the cytoplasmic organelles typically associated with sensory neurons—elements of the rough endoplasmic reticulum, the Golgi apparatus, and a large population of free ribosomes. The basal pole of the bipolar nerve cell body gives rise to an extremely thin axon (0.1 μm in diameter) that travels through the basement membrane into the underlying lamina propria. Here, it joins with other similar axons and forms one of many tiny nerve bundles—the *fila olfactoria*—that form the *olfactory nerve* that travels to the olfactory bulb in the brain. The apical pole of the bipolar neuron sends a slender dendrite (D) to the free surface of the olfactory epithelium. As the dendrite approaches the surface, it acquires many mitochondria. The dendrite terminal swells to form the *olfactory vesicle*, a structure that projects above the epithelial surface.

Figure B shows the olfactory vesicle (OV) in more detail. Here, it is evident that the olfactory vesicle is stabilized by a network of cytoplasmic microtubules (∗) that enter from the shaft of the dendrite (D) below. Some 10 to 30 *olfactory cilia*, the probable sites of chemosensory transduction, project from basal bodies (B) embedded in the lateral and apical margins of the olfactory vesicle. These olfactory cilia, presumed to be immotile in man, display the typical "9 + 2" pattern of axonemal substructure at the ciliary base. Several micrometers distal to the base, however, the ciliary shaft tapers sharply to form a long, slender filament supported by two to four single microtubules.

In addition to the ciliated olfactory receptors, the human olfactory epithelium contains microvillar cells—cells of unknown function that occupy a superficial position in the olfactory epithelium. These cells, one of which is shown in Figure C, are characterized by a flask-shaped cell body and a round, euchromatic nucleus (N). Several short, stubby microvilli (arrow) project into the mucous layer that lines the nasal cavity (NC). The basal pole of the cell tapers sharply to form a slender cytoplasmic extension (E) that travels toward the basement membrane. Near the microvillar cell sits a degenerating cell (D), a reminder that all of the cells in the olfactory epithelium, including the olfactory receptors themselves, are in a constant state of cellular turnover.

Beneath the olfactory epithelium lies the highly cellular lamina propria, which contains large secretory glands known as Bowman's glands. A cross section through one of the secretory acini of a Bowman's gland is shown in Figure D. The large, pyramidal cells, filled with electron-dense secretory granules (G), suggest that the secretory product of these glands may add a serous component to the mucus that moistens and bathes the free surface of the olfactory epithelium.

Figure A. Electron micrograph of a longitudinal section through several receptors in the human olfactory epithelium. D, dendrite of olfactory receptor; N, nucleus of olfactory receptor; NC, nasal cavity; O, ciliated olfactory receptor; S, supporting cell; arrow, olfactory vesicle. 5,000 X

Figure B. Longitudinal section through an olfactory vesicle atop a ciliated olfactory receptor. B, basal body; C, olfactory cilium; D, dendrite; NC, nasal cavity; OV, olfactory vesicle; ∗, microtubule. 20,500 X

Figure C. Longitudinal section through a microvillar cell in the human olfactory epithelium. D, degenerating cell; E, cytoplasmic extension; N, nucleus of microvillar cell; NC, nasal cavity; arrow, microvilli. 5,100 X

Figure D. Cross section through secretory acinus of Bowman's gland in the lamina propria of the human olfactory epithelium. G, secretory granules; L, lumen; LP, lamina propria. 1,600 X

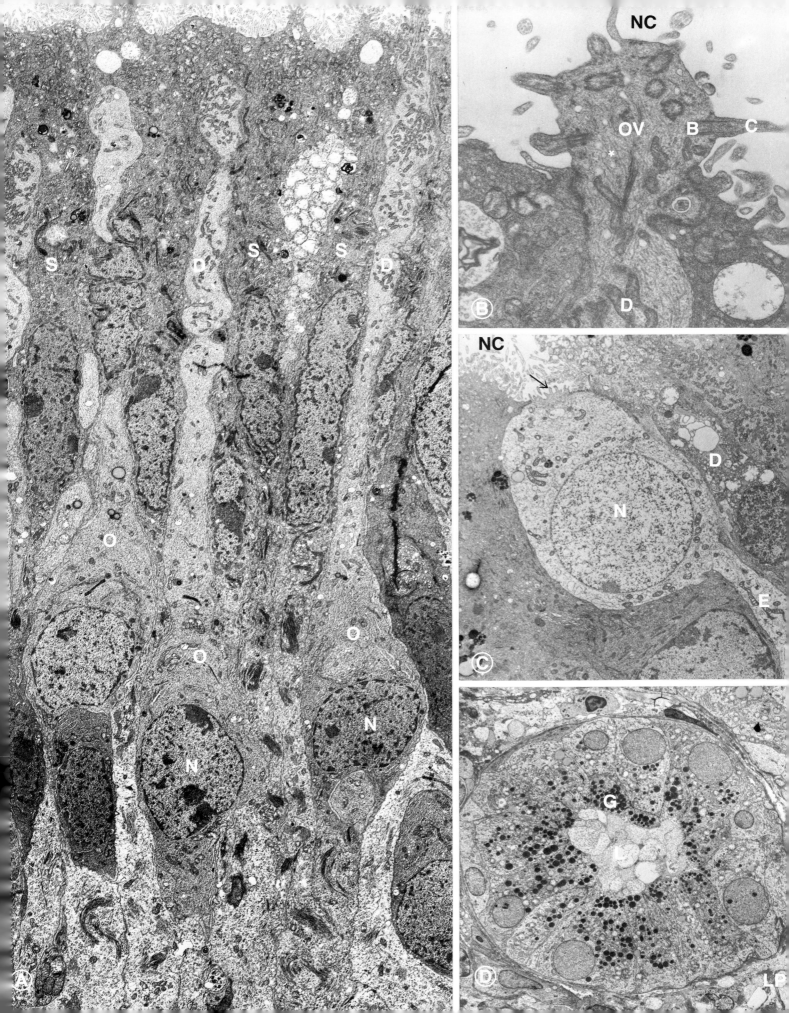

Plate 20–7

The Tongue: The Taste Bud

The microanatomy of the tongue itself was covered in Chapter 12, The Oral Cavity. That section of the atlas introduced the taste bud, the sense organ that houses the chemoreceptors responsible for the detection of dissolved sweet, bitter, sour, and salty substances that come into contact with the tongue.

Figure A is a longitudinal section through a single taste bud within the circumvallate papilla of the human tongue. At the top of the micrograph is the surface of the stratified squamous epithelium (E) that covers the papilla. This free epithelial surface is a mucous membrane that is in direct contact with the oral cavity (OC). A few stray bacteria (*) are evident near the taste pore, the entrance to the taste bud. The taste pore (P, inset) is a narrow channel that, in living tissue, permits fluids to pass from the oral cavity into the apical pole of the taste bud, wherein they make contact with microvilli (arrow, inset) that are extensions of the cell surface of the taste cells themselves. (In Figure A, the taste pore is sectioned slightly off-axis, giving the misleading impression of being covered by epithelium. The inset affords a better view of the taste pore.)

The cells within the taste bud are usually referred to as *light cells* (L) and *dark cells* (D). In Figure A, the origin of these names is evident: the light cells have a relatively electron-lucent cytoplasm, and the dark cells, a more dense cytoplasm. The light cells typically contain a large, round, euchromatic nucleus. The dark cells, on the other hand, have a more heterochromatic nucleus that is somewhat irregular in shape. Numerous profiles of nerve fibers (N) are evident as they course through the taste bud. At present, some controversy exists among specialists in the field as to whether the light and dark cells are indeed different "cell types," or simply represent different morphologic manifestations of a single type of cell caught at different stages of development. In any case, both light and dark cells are long, slender, fusiform cells that extend to the region of the taste pore. At the lumen of the taste pore (see inset), the apical poles of the light and dark cells are thrown into long, irregular folds that resemble thick microvilli (arrow, inset). Above the microvillar surface, the taste pore is often filled with dense, amorphous material that resembles the contents of the electron-dense, membrane-limited vesicles that crowd the apical cytoplasm of the dark cells.

Lateral to the taste bud lies the stratified squamous epithelium that lines the circumvallate papilla. Cells of the stratum spinosum, here pulled apart from one another by shrinkage during fixation, are held together by numerous desmosomes that give the epithelium its characteristic "spiny" appearance.

Figure A. Low-magnification electron micrograph of a longitudinal section taken through a taste bud within a circumvallate papilla of the human tongue. D, dark cell; E, stratified squamous epithelium that covers the circumvallate papilla; L, light cell; N, nerve fiber; OC, oral cavity; *, bacteria in vicinity of taste pore. 4,400 X
Inset. Longitudinal section through a region of the taste pore from the taste bud shown in Figure A. P, taste pore; arrow, microvilli of light and dark cells. 6,700 X

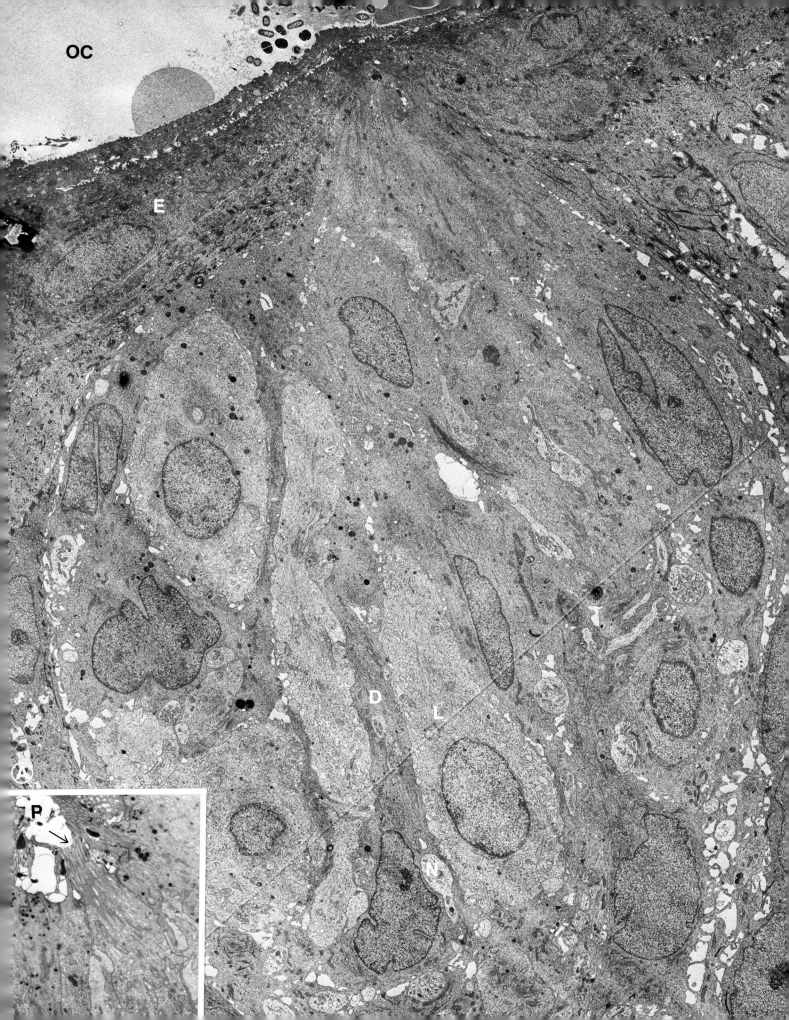

Appendix

Notes on Tissue Preparation

With few exceptions, the tissues photographed for this atlas were prepared in our laboratory in the Department of Cellular and Structural Biology in the University of Colorado School of Medicine, in Denver, Colorado. We have improved methods for obtaining large (1-mm square), flat, contaminant-free thin sections that permit photography of large fields of view at very low magnifications with the transmission electron microscope. In addition, we have devised a method that greatly simplifies mounting these large thin sections on Formvar-coated slot grids and permits the photographing of any field of view uninterrupted by the grid bars present on common support screens. Rather than present a detailed description of these methods here, we refer the reader to the following reference, in which the methods of specimen preparation employed in this atlas are described in considerable depth:
Moran, D. T., and Rowley, J. C. III: Biological specimen preparation for correlative light and electron microscopy. *In* Correlative Microscopy: Instrumentation and Methodology. Edited by M. A. Hayat. New York, Academic Press, 1986, pp. 1–22.

Fresh tissue samples were fixed in one of a variety of buffered paraformaldehyde-glutaraldehyde mixtures, post-fixed in buffered 2% osmium tetroxide, dehydrated in a graded acetone series, and infiltrated with (and embedded in) epoxy resin. Thick section (1 μm thick) for light microscopy and thin sections (500 to 800 Å thick) were cut with a diamond knife mounted in a Porter-Blum MT-2B ultramicrotome. For light microscopy, thick sections were stained with toluidine blue and photographed in a Zeiss Ultraphot II photomicroscope fitted with Zeiss planapochromatic lenses. For electron microscopy, sections were mounted on Formvar-covered "slot" grids, using a new and effective device, the Domino Rack (Sundance Technology, Denver, CO). Once mounted on the slot grids, thin sections were doubly stained with uranyl acetate and lead citrate, and photographed with a Philips EM-300 transmission electron microscope.

We found nerve tissue particularly difficult to preserve and are indebted to several investigators for providing us with well-fixed tissue blocks from various regions of the nervous system. Tissues for Plates 8-1, 8-2, and 8-4 were kindly sent to us by Dr. Cedric Raine of the Albert Einstein College of Medicine; tissues for Plate 8-5 were given to us by Dr. Stephen Roper of Colorado State University; and the negative for Plate 8-4 was generously offered to us by Dr. Tom Mehalick of our department. In addition, the elegant scanning electron micrograph of a macrophage engaged in phagocytosis of an erythrocyte that appears in Plate 4–1 (Figure A) was given to us by Dr. Keith R. Porter of the University of Maryland. We are most grateful to these investigators for supplying us with examples of their work that enrich this atlas and enhance its instructional value.

Glossary

Acidophil. A cell that stains with an acid dye. Example: the acidophils of the anterior pituitary.

Acidophilic. A substance within a cell or tissue that stains with an acid dye (such as eosin).

Acinus (plural: acini). A grape-shaped secretory unit, composed of acinar cells, found in a variety of secretory glands such as the salivary glands and pancreas.

Acrosome. A massive lysosome located on the head of a spermatozoon that facilitates penetration of the egg.

Actin. A filamentous protein, composed of globular subunits, that composes the "thin filaments" of muscle and the microfilaments of motile, nonmuscle cells.

Action Potential. An electrical signal that consists of an ionic current, or "wave of depolarization," that passes across the plasma membrane of certain nerve and muscle cells. Action potentials do not lose strength over distance.

Active Transport. The active "pumping" of small dissolved substances, such as certain ions, sugars, and amino acids, across a biologic membrane against a concentration gradient.

Adenohypophysis (synonym: anterior lobe). That portion of the pituitary gland that contains the pars distalis, the pars tuberalis, and the pars intermedia.

Adipocyte. A fat cell.

Adrenal Cortex. The outer portion of the adrenal gland; it surrounds the adrenal medulla and consists of three regions, the zona glomerulosa, zona fasciculata, and zona reticularis, which secrete steroid hormones.

Adrenal Medulla. The inner portion of the adrenal gland, surrounded by the cortex, that secretes epinephrine and norepinephrine.

Adrenaline. See Epinephrine.

Adrenocorticotropic Hormone (ACTH). A hormone released by the pituitary gland that stimulates the adrenal cortex.

Adventitia. The outer covering, composed of loose connective tissue, that surrounds a variety of organs such as blood vessels and intestines.

Afferent. An adjective describing a structure, be it a blood vessel or a nerve, that carries materials or information in a central direction (inward).

Agranulocyte. A broad category of white blood cell that lacks cytoplasmic granules visible by light microscopy. Includes lymphocytes and monocytes.

Aldosterone. A steroid hormone, secreted by the adrenal cortex, that stimulates cells of the proximal convoluted tubule of the nephron to pump sodium ions back into the bloodstream.

Alveolus (plural: alveoli). A thin-walled, air-filled sac within the lung that permits gas exchange across its wall between air and circulating blood.

Amacrine Cell. A type of interneuron within the retina that connects ganglion cells; one of the "horizontal" components of the retina that promotes intercellular communication.

Ameloblast. An epithelial cell, located within a developing tooth, that secretes enamel.

Amino Acid. An organic acid that is a building block of protein.

Ampulla. A saccular dilation of a canal or duct. Example: the ampulla of the oviduct, which lies between the infundibulum and the isthmus.

Amylase. A starch-digesting enzyme that is a component of saliva.

Androgen. Testosterone; a male sex steroid hormone.

Androstenedione. A precursor of the female steroid hormone, estrogen.

Angstrom Unit (abbreviation: Å). A unit of measure equal to 1/10 of a nanometer; 1/10,000 of a micrometer; 1/10,000,000 of a millimeter; 1/250,000,000 of an inch.

Antibody. A class of protein, secreted by the plasma cell, that binds antigen. Antibodies are immunoglobulins endowed with specific amino acid sequences that bind specifically with the antigens that induced their biosynthesis.

Antigen. A substance, usually foreign, that is recognized by the organism's immune system. Antigens tend to stimulate formation of antibodies that bind to them.

Antrum. The space in the ovarian follicle filled by follicular fluid (liquor folliculi).

Apocrine Sweat Gland. A class of large sweat gland, usually located in the groin and armpits, that produces odoriferous secretions. Unlike eccrine sweat glands, they are not concerned with temperature regulation.

Arrector Pili. A smooth muscle that raises a hair. Example: when a large number of these muscles are stimulated, one gets "goose bumps."

Arteriole. A tiny artery, less than 10 μm in diameter, that leads to a capillary bed.

ATP. Adenosine triphosphate, a molecule that serves as an energy source for many of the cell's biochemical processes.

Atrium (plural: atria). An auricle; a chamber of the heart that receives venous blood.

Auerbach's Plexus. A group of autonomic neurons, located between the muscle layers of the gut, that permit peristaltic contractions.

Autonomic Nervous System. That portion of the nervous system concerned with the involuntary activities of cardiac muscle, smooth muscle, and glands; often subdivided into the sympathetic and parasympathetic nervous systems.

Axon. The cytoplasmic extension of a neuron by which impulses travel (usually) away from the cell body.

Axoneme. The cytoskeletal part of a cilium or flagellum, responsible for motility, that is characterized by a "9 + 2" pattern of microtubular organization.

Axoplasmic Transport. The movement of materials through an axon.

B-Lymphocyte. A class of lymphocyte, thought to be derived from the bone marrow, that can differentiate into an antibody-secreting plasma cell.

Basal Body. An organelle, identical in appearance to a centriole, that contains nine triplets of microtubules and is found at the base of a cilium or flagellum.

Basal Cells. Small stem cells, located at the base of a variety of stratified and pseudostratified epithelia, that undergo mitosis and provide new cells to replace those periodically shed from the epithelium.

Basal Lamina. A filamentous, 800-Å-thin subdivision of the basement membrane.

Basal Striations. Thin, acidophilic, vertical striations, located at the basal pole of many epithelial and glandular cells, that represent long, thin mitochondria positioned to provide ATP for active transport.

Basalis. That part of the endometrium of the uterus that is not shed at menstruation, but remains to participate in the regeneration of the functionalis (which is shed at menstruation).

Basement Membrane. A thin layer that underlies epithelia and separates muscle and nerve fibers from surrounding connective tissue.

Basilar Membrane. A sheet of connective tissue, found within the cochlea of the ear, that supports the mechanoreceptive "hair cells."

Basket Cell. A myoepithelial cell whose contractions express (squeeze) the contents out of secretory cells.

Basophil. A substance within a cell or tissue that stains with basic dyes such as hematoxylin.

Bile. A fluid, secreted by the liver and released into the duodenum, that serves to emulsify fats.

Bile Canaliculus (plural: canaliculi). A thin channel between the plasma membranes of adjacent liver cells through which bile flows en route to a bile duct.

Blastocyst. A very early mammalian embryo.

Blastula. An early stage of the embryo formed by the rearrangement of the cells of the morula; a fluid-filled sphere surrounded by a single layer of cells.

Bowman's Capsule. A simple squamous epithelium, intimately associated with the glomerulus of the nephron, that consists of outer (parietal) and inner (visceral) layers.

Brunner's Glands. Mucoserous glands located within the submucosa of the duodenum.

Brush Border. See Striated border.

Calcitonin. A hormone secreted by parafollicular cells of the thyroid gland that inhibits bone resorption by osteoclasts and lowers blood calcium levels.

Callus. A hard, bonelike material that covers the ends of a fractured bone during the healing process.

Canaliculi. Small channels, or canals, whose margins are frequently defined by cell membranes.

Capacitation. The maturation of spermatozoa, thought to occur within the epididymis, during which sperm acquire fertility and motility.

Cardiac Muscle Cell. See Cardiac muscle fiber.

Cardiac Muscle Fiber. The contractile unit of cardiac muscle; a single branched cardiac muscle cell, usually having one or two nuclei.

Catecholamine. A class of neurosecretory substances including epinephrine and norepinephrine.

Caveolae. Small, membrane-limited invaginations of the cell surface that are especially conspicuous in smooth muscle cells.

Cell Membrane (synonyms: plasma membrane, plasmalemma). An 80-Å-thin biologic membrane that surrounds the cell.

Cementum. A hard, bonelike substance that covers the root of the tooth.

Central Nervous System. The brain and spinal cord.

Central Vein. A blood vessel, located in the center of a liver lobule, that collects blood from the venous sinuses that pass between hepatocytes.

Centriole. An organelle, characterized by nine triplets of microtubules, that sits in the cell center (cytocentrum) of nondividing cells and is found at the poles of the mitotic spindle of dividing animal cells.

Centroacinar Cell. A clear cell, found in the center of secretory acini of the pancreas, that forms the wall of the duct of the acinus.

Chief Cell. A generic term used to describe the major (chief) cell type found within an organ. Example: the enzyme-secreting (zymogenic) cells of the stomach are called chief cells.

Cholecystokinin. A hormone, elaborated by neurosecretory cells of the intestinal mucosa, that has many effects—including contraction of the gallbladder following ingestion of fats.

Cholesterol. The most abundant steroid in animal tissue.

Chondroblast. A young cartilage cell active in the secretion of extracellular matrix.

Chondrocyte. A mature cartilage cell necessary for the maintenance of matrix.

Chondromucoprotein. A generic term referring to the major macromolecular components of cartilage matrix.

Choriocapillaris. A system of small blood vessels in the choroid of the eye.

Choroid. A highly vascular layer of loose connective tissue situated between the sclera and retina in the wall of the eyeball.

Chromaffin Cells. Neurosecretory cells of the adrenal medulla that contain small granules rich in epinephrine and/or norepinephrine.

Chromatin. The genetic material (DNA) of the nucleus and associated proteins.

Chromophobes. Cells of the anterior pituitary that appear clear when stained with H&E. Although their function is unknown, they may represent spent (degranulated) acidophils or basophils.

Chromosome. A structural unit within the nucleus into which the genetic material and associated proteins are packaged. Chromosomes, of which 46 exist in man, stain heavily with basic dyes.

Chyme. The mass of partially digested food that passes from the stomach into the duodenum.

Cilium. A long, thin organelle, usually motile, that extends from the free surface of many cells. The cilium, which arises from a basal body, consists of a supporting axoneme surrounded by an extension of the plasma membrane.

Circumvallate Papilla. A large, circular structure, located near the base of the tongue, that contains many taste buds.

Cisternae. Flattened, membrane-limited sacs found in the rough endoplasmic reticulum and the Golgi apparatus.

Clara Cell. A nonciliated, club-shaped cell, probably secretory in function, found in the epithelium of the terminal bronchiole.

Collagen. A fibrous protein, unusually rich in the amino acid hydroxyproline, that is an essential constituent of connective tissue.

Collagenous Fibers. Connective tissue fibers, visible with the light microscope, that consist of aggregations of collagen fibrils.

Collecting Duct. A large duct in the nephron that collects urine for eventual excretion.

Colloid. A viscous, gel-like substance such as the material within the follicles of the thyroid gland.

Columnar Epithelium. An epithelium characterized by surface cells taller than they are wide. Example: the epithelium of the small intestine.

Compact Bone. The dense bone that forms the walls of hollow long bones and the outer and inner tables of flat skull bones.

Complement. A series of proteins in blood plasma, associated with the immune response, that when activated attracts neutrophils that become phagocytic.

Cone. A class of retinal photoreceptor that participates in color vision.

Cords of Billroth. See Splenic cords.

Corium. See Dermis.

Corona Radiata. A "radiating crown" of cells and extracellular material that adhere to the perimeter of the ovulated egg.

Corpus Luteum. A large, yellowish, progesterone-secreting body, found in the ovary, formed from an ovarian follicle following rupture and release of the egg.

Cortical Sinus. See Subcapsular sinus.

Cortisol (synonym: hydrocortisone). A steroid hormone; one of the major glucocorticoids secreted by the zona fasciculata of the adrenal cortex.

Cortisone. A glucocorticoid (a class of steroid), secreted by the adrenal cortex, often used as an anti-inflammatory drug.

Cristae. Little baffles formed from infoldings of the inner mitochondrial membrane.

Crown. The exposed part of a tooth above the gumline.

Crypts of Lieberkühn (synonym: intestinal glands). Simple tubular glands, extending below the lumenal surface of the intestine, lined by epithelium coextensive with that covering the intestinal villi.

Cuboidal Epithelium. An epithelium characterized by surface cells approximately equal in height and width. Example: the epithelium of the thyroid gland.

Cumulus Oophorus. A group or "cloud" of granulosa cells that surround the oocyte in a growing (tertiary) follicle or a Graafian follicle.

Cytokinesis. Part of the process of cell division in which the cytoplasm of one cell is subdivided to give rise to two daughter cells. Usually accompanies mitosis (nuclear division).

Cytoplasm. The contents of the cell exclusive of the nucleus.

Cytoskeleton. A generic term that describes a wide variety of fibrous and tubular elements, such as microfilaments and microtubules, that support the structure and maintain the shape of the cell.

Dark Cells. A class of dark-staining cell within the taste bud to which no definite functions have yet been ascribed.

Dendrite. One of many slender cytoplasmic extensions of a neuron that carry electrical excitation toward the cell body.

Dense Irregular Connective Tissue. Connective tissue consisting of cells and densely packed, nonparallel fibers.

Dense Regular Connective Tissue. Connective tissue consisting of cells and densely packed, parallel fibers.

Dentin. A hard, bony substance that constitutes the bulk of the tooth; dentin is covered by enamel in the crown and by cementum in the root.

Dermis (synonym: corium). The connective tissue that underlies the epidermis of the skin.

Desmosome (synonym: macula adherens). An intercellular junction that provides a "spot weld" between the plasma membranes of neighboring cells.

Diastole. That phase of the heartbeat during which the left ventricle (which pumps blood to the body but not the lungs) relaxes.

Distal Convoluted Tubule. That portion of the nephron that connects the loop of Henle with the collecting duct.

DNA. Deoxyribonucleic acid; the genetic material.

Ductus Deferens. See Vas deferens.

Dust Cell. See Pulmonary alveolar macrophage.

Dynein Arm. A small projection from the microtubular doublets of the ciliary axoneme that provides the motive force for ciliary motility.

Eccrine Sweat Gland. A class of sweat gland associated with temperature regulation.

Efferent. An adjective describing a structure, be it a blood vessel, nerve, or duct, that carries materials or information in a peripheral direction (outward).

Elastic Cartilage. A resilient cartilage, similar in histologic structure to hyaline cartilage; its matrix is rich in elastic fibers. Example: cartilage found in the external ear.

Elastic Fiber. A class of connective tissue fiber, made largely of the protein elastin, that can recoil elastically after being stretched. Example: elastic fibers are abundant in the arterial walls.

Elastin. The protein component of elastic fibers.

Enamel. The hardest substance in the human body, found covering the crown of the tooth.

Endocardium. The lining of the chambers of the heart; the innermost tunica of the heart that contains endothelium and some loose connective tissue.

Endometrial Glands. Secretory glands within the lining of the uterus, or endometrium.

Endometrium. The inner lining of the uterus into which the trophoblast implants; failing implantation, the endometrium is shed at menstruation.

Endomysium. The thin connective tissue sheath surrounding a muscle fiber.

Endoneurium. A delicate sheath of connective tissue that surrounds a single axon or other extension of a single neuron.

Endoplasmic Reticulum. A system of intracellular membranes that comes in two varieties: rough ER (with ribosomes) and smooth ER (without ribosomes).

Endothelium. A layer of flat cells that line the inner surfaces of blood and lymph vessels and the heart.

Enterochromaffin Cells. Neurosecretory cells in the gastric and intestinal glands that frequently release serotonin, a substance that promotes smooth muscle contraction.

Entropy. The tendency of everything to fall into disorder.

Enzyme. A protein molecule that serves as a catalyst in a biochemical reaction.

Eosinophil. A class of white blood cell, thought to be active in the phagocytosis of antigen-antibody complexes, that contains conspicuous cytoplasmic granules (specialized lysosomes called specific granules) that stain red with eosin.

Epicardium. The outermost region of the wall of the heart.

Epidermis. The keratinized stratified squamous epithelium that covers the skin.

Epididymis (synonym: ductus epididymidis). A thin coiled tube connected to the posterior surface of the testis that carries sperm, made in the seminiferous tubules, to the vas deferens. The epididymis contributes to the maturity and acquisition of motility (capacitation) of spermatozoa.

Epinephrine (synonym: adrenaline). The major hormone released by the adrenal medulla. A catecholamine, epinephrine is also a neurotransmitter in the sympathetic nervous system.

Epineurium. A sheath of connective tissue that surrounds a whole nerve, such as the sciatic nerve.

Erythrocyte. A red blood cell.

Estradiol. The most potent of all naturally occurring estrogens.

Estrogen. A class of female steroid sex hormone.

Euchromatin. Fine, light-staining strands of dispersed chromatin present in the interphase nucleus.

Excitable Membrane. A kind of plasma membrane, found on nerve and muscle cells, capable of conducting an action potential. Most axons are covered by excitable membrane; most dendrites are not.

Exocrine Gland. A gland that releases its secretion into a duct.

Exocytosis. An active transport process by which secretory granules are released from a cell.

Extracellular Matrix. That material, found outside of (between) cells and produced by cells, that gives tissues much of their character.

Fallopian Tube. See Uterine tube.

Fascicle. A generic term meaning bundle, as in a bundle (fascicle) of muscle or nerve fibers surrounded by a common connective tissue sheath.

Fenestrated Capillary. A capillary with small holes in its wall that permit the passage of certain macromolecules, but not cells, across the capillary's wall.

Fiber. A long, thin structure, made either of cells (as in nerve fiber, muscle fiber) or by cells (as in collagen fiber).

Fibril. A thin, filamentous structure, often made of protein, that is a component of a fiber. Example: a collagen fiber, visible by light microscopy, is made up of tiny fibrils visible only by electron microscopy.

Fibroblast. A connective tissue cell that makes collagen.

Fibrocartilage. A cartilage rich in collagenous fibers that has relatively few chondrocytes and lacks a perichondrium. Example: cartilage found in the intervertebral disks.

Fila Olfactoria. Bundles of olfactory receptors' axons that coalesce to form the olfactory nerve (Cranial Nerve I).

Filiform Papillae. Tiny projections atop the tongue, devoid of taste buds, that give the tongue its feltlike texture.

Flagellum. A long, thin, whiplike, motile extension of the surface of certain cells (such as spermatozoa); it has an axoneme like that of a motile cilium.

Folia. A broad, thin, leaflike structure. Example: the branched folds of the mucosa of the oviduct.

Follicle. A generic anatomic term for a small sac. Examples: thyroid follicle; hair follicle.

Follicle-Stimulating Hormone (FSH). A hormone secreted by the anterior pituitary that stimulates development of the ovarian follicle.

Follicular Cells (synonym: follicle cells). The cells that surround the ovum during development and maturation of the ovarian follicle.

Follicular Fluid. See Liquor folliculi.

Formed Elements of the Blood. The cells and platelets of blood; the elements of the blood that remain when the plasma is removed.

Fructose. A simple sugar found in fruits and honey; a product of sucrose hydrolysis.

Functionalis. That part of the endometrium of the uterus that is shed at menstruation.

Fungiform Papillae. Small, mushroom-shaped projections atop the tongue that usually bear one or more taste buds.

Ganglion. A cluster of nerve cell bodies in the peripheral nervous system.

Gap Junction (synonym: nexus). A point of contact between adjacent cells that allows ions (hence electric currents) and certain small molecules to pass from one cell to another.

Gastric Gland. An invagination of the surface epithelium of the stomach that contains parietal (HCl-secreting) cells and chief (enzyme-secreting) cells, among others.

Gastric Juice. The digestive fluid found in the stomach that consists of secretions of gastric glands; it contains proteolytic enzymes and hydrochloric acid.

Gastric Pits. Funnel-shaped indentations in the mucosa of the stomach that lead to the gastric glands.

Gastrin. A hormone secreted by the mucosa of the pyloric region of the stomach that stimulates parietal cells within gastric glands to produce HCl.

Gastrocnemius. The calf muscle of the leg.

Germinal Center. The central region of an activated lymph nodule (within a lymph node or other lymphoid tissue, such as the tonsil) that is mitotically active in the production of new lymphocytes.

Germinal Epithelium. The simple cuboidal epithelium that lines the outer surface of the ovary. Despite its misleading name, it does not produce germ cells.

Glomerular Filtrate. The solution remaining after blood has passed through the walls of the fenestrated capillaries of the glomerulus, through the slits created by podocytes, and into the urinary space of Bowman's capsule; it contains no blood cells.

Glomerulus. A ball of capillaries, surrounded by Bowman's capsule, in the renal corpuscle of the nephron.

Glucagon. A hormone secreted by alpha cells of the islets of Langerhans in the pancreas that mobilizes liver glycogen. An insulin antagonist.

Glucocorticoid. A class of steroid hormone, secreted by the adrenal cortex, that affects carbohydrate metabolism. Often used clinically as an anti-inflammatory agent.

Glucose. A simple sugar, the most common form in which carbohydrate is absorbed by mammals.

Glycogen. The major storage form of sugars in mammalian cells. Readily converted into glucose.

Glycoprotein. A macromolecule made of protein and carbohydrate components.

Goblet Cell. A mucus-secreting epithelial cell named for its shape.

Golgi Apparatus (synonym: Golgi complex). A stack of flattened, membrane-limited sacs and vesicles, found in most cells, that is intimately involved in the process of secretion and in the production of cytoplasmic organelles.

Golgi Complex. See Golgi apparatus.

Graafian Follicle. A large, mature ovarian follicle that contains the ripe egg ready for ovulation.

Granulocyte. A class of white blood cell that contains cytoplasmic granules visible by light microscopy. Includes neutrophils, eosinophils, and basophils.

Granulosa Cell. One of the cells of the epithelial lining of a growing or mature ovarian follicle.

Greater Alveolar Cell. See Pneumocyte type II.

Ground Substance (synonym: matrix). The amorphous (as opposed to the fibrillar) component of the intercellular matrix.

Growing Follicle. See Tertiary follicle.

Growth Hormone (synonyms: somatotrophic hormone; somatotropin; STH). A polypeptide hormone, secreted by the anterior pituitary, that has several functions including the regulation of growth.

Haploid. A cell with half the normal number of chromosomes. Example: sperm and egg cells are haploid.

Hassall's Corpuscle. A conspicuous structure of unknown function, peculiar to the thymus, that resembles a ball of concentrically wrapped flat epithelial cells.

Haversian System (synonym: osteon). The structural unit of organization of compact bone found in the cortex of long bones of large animals.

Hemoglobin. The oxygen-bearing protein molecule of the red blood cell.

Hemosiderin. A yellow-brown insoluble protein produced by the phagocytic digestion of hemoglobin-packed red blood cells.

Heparin. An anticoagulant released by degranulation of mast cells.

Hepatic Artery. An artery that brings fresh, oxygenated blood to a liver lobule.

Hepatocyte. The liver cell; the major cell type that constitutes the mass of the liver.

Heterochromatin. Densely staining material, found in the interphase nucleus, that consists of supercoiled DNA and associated proteins.

Histamine. A biologically active compound that, among other functions, causes increase in capillary permeability, bronchial constriction, and vasodilation.

Holocrine Secretion. A secretory process in which whole cells are the secretory product. Example: holocrine secretion occurs in sebaceous glands.

Horizontal Cell. A small interneuron in the vertebrate retina thought to interconnect spatially separated photoreceptors.

Howship's Lacuna. A depression in bone, created by the erosive action of an osteoclast, in which the osteoclast sits.

Hyaline Cartilage. A glassy, smooth cartilage found in structures such as the trachea and the articular surfaces of joints.

Hydrocortisone. See Cortisol.

Hydrolysis. A chemical process by which a compound is cleaved into several simpler compounds.

Hydroxyapatite. The major crystalline component of mineralized bone matrix.

Hypertrophy. Growth or enlargement of a unit such as a cell or organ.

Hypophysis. The pituitary gland.

Hypothalamic-Hypophyseal Portal System. A special system of blood vessels that carry materials from the hypothalamus to the pituitary gland.

Hypothalamus. A basal part of the forebrain that contains vital autonomic regulatory centers and, among many other functions, secretes "releasing factors" that stimulate release of hormones from the pituitary gland.

Immunoglobulin. A class of serum proteins, found in blood plasma, that includes antibodies.

Implantation. The attachment of the fertilized ovum (blastocyst) to the endometrium (lining of the uterus).

Infundibulum. A funnel or funnel-shaped structure or passage; a generic term that applies to structures found in a variety of organs such as the kidney, oviduct, and pituitary gland.

Inner Nuclear Layer. A histologically distinct region of the retina that contains the nuclei of the bipolar, amacrine, and horizontal cells.

Inner Plexiform Layer. A histologically distinct region of the retina, situated between the inner nuclear layer and the layer of ganglion cells, that contains nerve fibers and synapses.

Inner Segment. That part of the rod or cone photoreceptor that includes the cell body and ellipsoid, but not the outer segment.

Insulin. A hormone secreted by beta cells of the pancreatic islets of Langerhans that promotes passage of glucose into cells.

Interalveolar Septum. The thin wall that separates adjacent airsacs (alveoli) of the lung.

Intercalated Disk. A series of intercellular junctions that interconnect branches of adjacent cardiac muscle fibers.

Intercalated Duct. The tiny duct that connects an acinus with a secretory duct in a gland such as the pancreas or the salivary gland.

Intermediate Junction (synonym: zonula adherens). An intercellular junction, often part of a "junctional complex," that surrounds the apical pole of many epithelial cells and helps them to adhere to one another.

Internal Elastic Membrane. A perforated sheet of elastic tissue found between the inner layer (tunica intima) and middle layer (tunica media) of arteries.

Interstitial Cells (synonym: Leydig cells). Large, foamy-appearing, androgen-secreting endocrine cells found between seminiferous tubules in the testis.

Interstitial Fluid. Tissue fluid found in the spaces between and around cells.

Interstitial Space. The space between and around cells normally filled with interstitial fluid.

Intestinal Glands. See Crypts of Lieberkühn.

Islets of Langerhans. Groups of endocrine cells, located in the pancreas, that produce the hormones insulin and glucagon.

Isthmus. A narrow anatomic passage that connects two larger structures or cavities. Example: the isthmus of the oviduct projects from the uterus.

Junctional Complex. A group of intercellular junctions, located at the apical poles of cells in an epithelial sheet, that bind the cells together and control passage of materials between them. Includes the tight junction (zonula occludens), intermediate junction (zonula adherens), desmosome (macula adherens), and often the gap junction (nexus).

Keratin. A tough, fibrous, waterproof protein found in skin, nails, and hair.

Keratinocyte. An epidermal cell that makes keratin.

Keratohyalin Granules. Dense granules found in the stratum granulosum of the epidermis.

Killer T Cell. A T-lymphocyte that has become actively phagocytic; it recognizes and destroys specific antigens and participates in cell-mediated immunity.

Kupffer Cells. Phagocytic cells found in the lining of liver sinusoids.

Lacteal. A lymphatic capillary in the core of a villus of the small intestine.

Lacuna (plural: lacunae). A small space, cavity, or depression in a tissue or organ.

Lamella (plural: lamellae). A thin sheet or layer.

Lamina Propria. A highly cellular loose connective tissue, located beneath the epithelium, that provides a supporting framework for the epithelium of mucous membranes.

Layer of Ganglion Cells. A histologically distinct region of the retina containing the ganglion cells, whose axons coalesce to form the optic nerve that connects the retina with the brain.

Leukocyte. A white blood cell.

Leydig Cell. See Interstitial cells.

Ligament. A tough strap of dense regular connective tissue that connects adjacent structures. Example: ligaments connect adjacent bones in a joint.

Light Cells. A class of light-staining cell within the taste bud to which no definite functions have yet been ascribed.

Limbus Spiralis. A structure within the cochlea of the inner ear; a bony spiral, extending inward from the modiolus, that supports the organ of Corti.

Lipase. A class of enzyme that splits fats.

Lipids. Molecules—including fats and waxes—that are soluble in nonpolar organic solvents.

Lipofuscin Granules. Pigment-containing granules, found in a variety of cells and especially common in old neurons, that represent remnants of lysosomes filled with indigestible material. Also called wear-and-tear granules.

Liquor Folliculi (synonym: follicular fluid). Fluid that fills the antrum of growing and mature ovarian follicles.

Littoral Cell. A type of cell that lines the lymphatic sinuses of lymph nodes and blood sinuses of bone marrow.

Lobule. A generic term referring to a unit of histologic organization that is often a subunit of a lobe. Example: liver lobule.

Loop of Henle. A thin tube of the nephron that connects the proximal and distal tubules.

Luteinizing Hormone (LH). A hormone secreted by the anterior pituitary that stimulates development of the corpus luteum from an ovarian follicle following ovulation.

Lymphoblast. A large, immature lymphocyte often found in the germinal center of a lymphatic nodule.

Lymphocyte. A small white blood cell, classified as an agranulocyte. It is involved in the immune response in several ways, depending, in part, on whether it arises in the thymus (T-lymphocyte) or the bone marrow (B-lymphocyte).

Lymphokines. Substances released by sensitized lymphocytes (those that have contacted specific antigens) that stimulate activity of monocytes and macrophages.

Lysosome. A small, membrane-limited cytoplasmic organelle, filled with a wide array of hydrolytic enzymes, that fuse with and destroy unwanted foreign material or senescent intracellular components.

Lysozyme. An enzyme that destroys bacterial cell walls.

Macromolecule. A generic term referring to large and complex biologic molecules. Examples: proteins, polysaccharides, nucleic acids.

Macrophage. A large, ameboid, phagocytic cell.

Macula Adherens. See Desmosome.

Marginal Sinus. See Subcapsular sinus.

Mast Cell. A large connective tissue cell characterized by conspicuous cytoplasmic granules thought to contain heparin, an anticoagulant, and histamine, which increases capillary permeability.

Matrix. See Ground substance.

Medulla. A general term referring to a region deep within an organ. Examples: the medulla of the kidney; the adrenal medulla.

Megakaryocyte. A large, multinucleate cell, found in the bone marrow, from which cytoplasmic fragments break off and become platelets.

Meiosis. A highly complex series of "cell divisions" that include a reduction division in which the number of chromosomes is halved during sperm and egg (gamete) formation.

Meissner's Corpuscle. A class of mechanoreceptor, found in the skin and some mucous membranes, thought to be sensitive to light touch.

Meissner's Plexus. A plexus of autonomic neurons, located in the submucosa of the gut, that affects contraction of smooth muscle fibers in the muscularis mucosae.

Melanin. A dark pigment that gives coloration to skin, hair, and other body parts.

Melanocyte. A cell that makes the dark pigment called melanin.

Menarche. The onset of menstruation in the female at puberty.

Merkel's Cell. A type of cell located in the epidermis of the skin thought to participate in mechanoreception.

Meromyosin. A product of the tryptic digestion of the myosin molecule, further classified as heavy meromyosin and light meromyosin.

Mesenchyme. Embryonic connective tissue that can give rise to such structures as connective tissues, blood, lymphatics, cartilage, and bone.

Mesothelial Cell. A type of flattened cell that lines the body cavity and many of the organs found within the body.

Metachronal Wave. The coordinated wave of ciliary beating of a field of ciliated cells.

Metaphase. That stage of cell division in which the chromosomes are aligned along the equatorial metaphase plate (prior to their migration to opposite poles at anaphase).

Microfilament. A thin cytoplasmic filament, some 50 Å in diameter, often composed of actin and associated with cell motility. An important component of the cytoskeleton.

Micrometer (abbreviation: μm). A unit of measure, formerly called the micron, equal to 1/1000 of a millimeter.

Microtubule. A thin tube in the cytoplasm whose wall is made up of proteinaceous subunits called tubulin. Microtubules make up the framework of the mitotic spindle, are a vital part of the cytoskeleton, and are often associated with motility.

Microvilli (singular: microvillus). Tiny, membrane-limited, finger-shaped projections of the apical surface of many cells. Supported by core filaments made of actin, microvilli greatly increase the surface area available for secretion and absorption.

Mineralocorticoids. Steroid hormones, secreted by the adrenal cortex, that affect salt balance. Example: aldosterone.

Mitochondria (singular: mitochondrion). Long, slender, membrane-limited cytoplasmic organelles that are active in the production of ATP.

Mitosis. The process of nuclear division in which the nucleus divides to form two daughter nuclei, each with an identical complement of chromosomes. Mitosis usually is accompanied by cytoplasmic division (cytokinesis) that gives rise to two daughter cells. The major phases of mitosis are prophase (chromosomal condensation), metaphase (alignment of chromosomes on the equator of the mitotic spindle), anaphase (migration of one of each pair of chromosomes to opposite poles of the mitotic spindle), and telophase (formation of daughter nuclei).

Monocyte. A large white blood cell that is the immature circulating form of a macrophage.

Morula. A mass of cells, resulting from the early cleavage divisions of the zygote, that precedes the blastula in early embryonic development.

Motor End Plate (synonym: myoneural junction). A chemical synapse between a nerve and a striated muscle fiber.

Motor Neuron. A large neuron, with its cell body in the central nervous system, that sends an axon out to innervate an effector—usually a skeletal muscle fiber.

Mucopolysaccharide. A general term for large macromolecules that consist of a complex of protein(s) and polysaccharide(s) in which the polysaccharide component is often the major part. Example: mucus and cartilage matrix contain large amounts of mucopolysaccharides.

Mucosa (synonym: mucous membrane). The inner lining of many organs; consists of an epithelium, the lamina propria that supports the epithelium, and the muscularis mucosae.

Mucous Cells. Cells that produce mucus.

Mucous Membrane. See mucosa.

Mucous Neck Cells. Epithelial cells, found in the necks of the gastric glands, that secrete mucus.

Mucus (adjectival form: Mucous). A class of viscous, slippery secretion, rich in mucins, secreted by mucous membranes and mucous glands.

Müller Cells. Specialized neuroglial cells within the retina.

Multinucleate. Having more than one nucleus.

Muscle Fiber. A muscle cell.

Muscularis Externa. The thick layers of smooth muscle, situated between the submucosa and adventitia of the digestive tract, that provides the motive force for peristaltic movements of the gut.

Muscularis Mucosae. A loosely woven sheet of smooth muscle fibers located beneath (outside of) the lamina propria of the alimentary canal.

Myelin Sheath. A fatty sheath, composed of the concentrically wrapped cell membrane of a glial cell, that surrounds some axons of the central and peripheral nervous system. An effective electrical insulator, it permits the rapid "saltatory conduction" characteristic of myelinated nerves.

Myoblast. An embryonic cell that develops into a muscle fiber.

Myocardium. The middle layer of the heart, located between the endocardium and epicardium, that contains a large mass of cardiac muscle fibers.

Myoepithelial Cell. An epithelial cell, rich in myofilaments, that can contract. Example: myoepithelial cells surround secretory acini of salivary glands.

Myofibril. A long, slender, cylindric structural component of a muscle fiber. Each myofibril, which consists of a series of sarcomeres joined end to end, is surrounded by membranes of the sarcoplasmic reticulum. Many myofibrils, oriented parallel and side by side, fill the cytoplasm of a muscle fiber.

Myofilament. A small, filamentous component of the sarcomere in skeletal muscle. Myofilaments are classified as either thick filaments (made of myosin) or thin filaments (made of actin).

Myometrium. The muscular portion of the wall of the uterus.

Myoneural Junction. See Motor end plate.

Myosin. The major protein of the thick filaments of the sarcomeres of striated muscle.

Myotube. A stage in the formation of a skeletal muscle fiber from embryonic muscle cells (myoblasts); the myoblasts align end to end to form a myotube.

Nephron. The major structural and functional unit of the kidney.

Nerve Fiber Layer. A region of the retina, near the vitreous humor, containing axons of ganglion cells.

Neurofilaments. Slender, proteinaceous cytoplasmic filaments, found in axons and dendrites of nerve cells, whose small size (70 to 100 Å in diameter) makes electron microscopy necessary for their visualization. Thought to be cytoskeletal elements.

Neuroglia. A generic term for a variety of nonneuronal, supporting cells in the nervous system.

Neurohypophysis (synonym: pars nervosa). The posterior pituitary, which consists of axons (and their terminals) that extend down from cell bodies of neurosecretory cells in the hypothalamus.

Neuron. A nerve cell. Most neurons consist of a cell body (soma), an axon, and a group of dendrites.

Neurosecretory Cell. A neuron that makes, stores, and releases a substance that is eventually secreted from an axon terminal. Example: chromaffin cells of the adrenal medulla.

Neurotransmitter. A chemical, released from an axon terminal at a synapse, that usually exerts an effect on the ionic conductance of the membrane of the postsynaptic cell.

Neutrophil (synonyms: polymorphonuclear leukocyte; PMN). The most common of the white blood cells; classified as a granulocyte; phagocytic in function.

Nexus. See Gap junction.

Nissl Bodies. See Nissl substance.

Nissl Substance (synonym: Nissl bodies). A basophilic substance, prominent in the cytoplasm of nerve cell bodies, consisting of the rough endoplasmic reticulum and free ribosomes.

Node of Ranvier. Located along the length of a myelinated nerve fiber, nodes of Ranvier are "naked" areas of the axon between segments of the myelin sheath laid down by adjacent glial cells.

Nomarski Interference Microscopy. A technique using a specially modified light microscope that enables one to see unstained cells of sectioned material in great detail. The image produced seems set in relief, much like the head of a coin.

Norepinephrine. A hormone, classified as a catecholamine, produced by the adrenal medulla; also a neurotransmitter at many synapses in the sympathetic nervous system.

Nuclear Envelope. A double membrane that surrounds the nucleus, the nuclear envelope is a specialized, perinuclear cisterna of the endoplasmic reticulum.

Nuclear Pore. A tiny perforation, some 700 Å in diameter, in the nuclear envelope. Nuclear pores are numerous; they provide for exchange of materials between nucleus and cytoplasm.

Nucleolus. A small, darkly staining mass within the nucleus wherein ribonucleoprotein is produced.

Nucleus. A large, membrane-limited compartment within the cell that contains the genetic material, DNA, in the form of chromosomes.

Odontoblast. A large cell that lines the pulp cavity of the tooth and secretes dentin.

Olfactory Cilia. Small sensory cilia, projecting from the olfactory vesicle of the ciliated olfactory receptor neuron, thought to be a site of sensory transduction of olfactory stimuli.

Olfactory Nerve. A nerve (Cranial Nerve I) consisting of axons of the olfactory receptor neurons that travels from the olfactory mucosa to the brain.

Olfactory Vesicle. The swollen terminal of the dendrite of an olfactory receptor (which is a bipolar neuron) that bears the olfactory cilia.

Oligodendrocyte. A glial cell that makes the myelin sheaths that envelop the axons of many neurons in the central nervous system. (Note: Schwann cells myelinate axons in the peripheral nervous system.)

Oocyte. The immature ovum, or egg.

Optic Nerve. A major cranial nerve (Cranial Nerve II) that connects the retina with higher centers in the brain. It is made up of a bundle of axons from ganglion cells in the retina.

Organ of Corti. That region in the cochlea of the inner ear that contains the "hair cells"—mechanoreceptors sensitive to sound vibrations.

Organelle. A small, discrete, structural and functional unit within a cell. Example: the mitochondrion.

Osmosis. Movement of a solvent through a semipermeable membrane in the direction of the greater concentration of solute. Example: in a vial of sugar-water, capped with a semipermeable membrane and immersed in a beaker of water, water will move from the beaker across the membrane and into the vial.

Osteoblast. A cell that actively secretes unmineralized bone matrix, or osteoid. An immature osteocyte.

Osteoclast. A large, multinuclear, phagocytic cell that eats bone.

Osteocyte. A mature bone cell encased in mineralized bone matrix.

Osteoid. Newly secreted, unmineralized bone matrix, made largely of collagen, that provides a site for deposition of hydroxyapatite crystals during the mineralization process.

Osteon. See Haversian system.

Outer Nuclear Layer. A histologically distinct region of the retina containing nuclei of the rod and cone photoreceptors.

Outer Plexiform Layer. A histologically distinct region of the retina, located between the outer and inner nuclear layers, that contains nerve fibers and synapses.

Outer Segment. That part of a vertebrate rod or cone photoreceptor consisting of a stack of membranes containing the photosensitive pigment.

Ovary. One of the paired organs in the female reproductive system in which the egg matures and from which it is released at ovulation.

Oviduct. See Uterine tube.

Ovulation. The release of the egg from the ovary, preceded by rupture of the ovarian follicle.

Ovum. The unfertilized egg.

Oxyntic Cell. See Parietal cell.

Oxytocin. A hormone, produced in the hypothalamus and released from the neurohypophysis (posterior pituitary), that promotes milk letdown and contraction of uterine smooth muscle.

Pacinian Corpuscle. A large mechanoreceptor, found deep in the dermis of the skin and in other connective tissues, that is sensitive to deep pressure.

Pancreatic Duct. The duct that carries secretions of the exocrine pancreas (i.e., pancreatic juice) from the pancreas to the duodenum.

Pancreatic Juice. The collective secretions of the exocrine pancreas, including digestive enzymes and the buffer, bicarbonate.

Paneth Cells. Large cells, situated at the base of the intestinal glands of the small intestine, characterized by conspicuous eosinophilic cytoplasmic granules thought to contain the antibacterial enzyme, lysozyme. May be phagocytic.

Parafollicular Cells (synonyms: clear cells; C-cells). Light-staining cells, located at intervals beneath the follicular epithelium of the thyroid gland, that secrete the hormone calcitonin (which lowers blood calcium).

Parakeratinized. Refers to cells that are filled with keratin, yet retain their nuclei.

Parasympathetic Nervous System. A subdivision of the autonomic nervous system, consisting chiefly of cholinergic fibers, that tends to stimulate secretion, increases tone and contractility of smooth muscle, and causes vasodilation.

Parathyroid Gland. A gland located near the thyroid gland; its secretion, parathyroid hormone, activates osteoclasts and raises blood calcium levels.

Parathyroid Hormone. See Parathyroid gland.

Parietal Cells (synonym: oxyntic cells). Large, round, eosinophilic cells, found in the epithelium lining the gastric glands of the stomach, that secrete hydrochloric acid.

Parietal Layer. A general term relating to the cellular lining of the wall of a cavity. Example: the parietal layer lines the inner surface of the outer wall of Bowman's capsule.

Parotid Gland. One of a pair of large bilateral serous salivary glands located below and in front of the ear.

Pars Distalis. The anterior lobe of the pituitary gland; the largest subdivison of the pituitary gland.

Pars Intermedia. A thin strip of tissue sandwiched between the pars distalis and the pars nervosa of the pituitary gland.

Pars Nervosa. See Neurohypophysis.

Pars Tuberalis. A collar of cells that surrounds the infundibulum of the pituitary gland.

Pedicle. A foot-process of the podocytes that wrap around the capillaries of the glomerulus in Bowman's capsule of the nephron.

Pepsin and Pepsinogen. The proenzyme pepsinogen is secreted by chief cells of the stomach's gastric glands and, when released into the acidic stomach lumen, is cleaved to form the active proteolytic enzyme pepsin.

Perichondrium. A tough membrane of dense connective tissue that surrounds hyaline and elastic cartilage (except at joint surfaces); it contains immature cartilage cells, or chondroblasts, that secrete matrix and form mature chondrocytes during cartilage development.

Perikaryon. The cytoplasm surrounding the nucleus; usually used in reference to the cell bodies of nerve cells.

Perimetrium. The serosal covering of the uterus continuous with the peritoneal lining of the body cavity.

Perineurium. A sheath of connective tissue that surrounds a bundle of nerve fibers within a large nerve.

Periodontal Ligament. The ligament made of dense connective tissue that surrounds the root of the tooth and anchors the tooth to the walls of its bony socket.

Periosteum. A tough membrane of dense connective tissue that surrounds bones; it contains the osteoblasts that secrete bone matrix during bone growth.

Peripheral Nervous System. That part of the nervous system not enclosed within the skull or spinal column.

Peristalsis. The undulating, wavelike motion of the intestines, generated by rhythmic smooth-muscle contractions, that moves material during the digestive process.

Peyer's Patches. Large, conspicuous lymphatic nodules in the wall of the ileum of the small intestine.

Phagocytosis. The process by which one cell engulfs and frequently digests a bacterium, another cell, or other material.

Phalangeal Cells. Supporting cells located within the organ of Corti of the cochlea that, together with the pillar cells, hold the hair cells in place.

Pheromone. A chemical substance, secreted by the male or female of a species, that attracts members of the opposite sex; often airborne and detected by the chemosensory system.

Pigment Epithelium. The outermost layer of the retina; a layer of pigment cells that absorbs photons and often phagocytoses worn-out rod outer segments.

Pillar Cells. Supporting cells located within the organ of Corti of the cochlea that, together with the phalangeal cells, hold the hair cells in place.

Pinocytosis. The process by which a cell "drinks" small amounts of material by pinching off tiny vesicles of its plasma membrane that contain the material and taking them into its cytoplasm.

Pituicytes. Fusiform cells, similar to neuroglia, associated with neurosecretory axons in the neurohypophysis.

Placenta. The highly vascular organ attached to the interior of the uterus that joins mother and fetus during intrauterine life and provides for metabolic interchange.

Plasma. The noncellular, fluid phase of the blood in which the blood cells and platelets are suspended.

Plasma Cell. A type of cell in connective tissues that makes and secretes antibodies; a mature B-lymphocyte.

Plasma Membrane. See Cell membrane.

Plasmalemma. See Cell membrane.

Platelet. An anucleate fragment of the cytoplasm of a megakaryocyte, found in circulating blood, that functions in blood clot formation.

Plicae Circulares. Large folds of the intestinal wall that include the submucosa.

Pneumocyte Type II (synonyms: septal cell; greater alveolar cell). A cuboidal epithelial cell in the wall of the alveolus that secretes pulmonary surfactant, a substance that reduces surface tension and functions to prevent collapse of alveoli.

Podocyte. An epithelial cell, found in the visceral (inner) layer of Bowman's capsule of the nephron, endowed with elaborately branched foot processes that ensheath glomerular capillaries.

Poliomyelitis. A debilitating disease in which viruses infect and frequently kill spinal motor neurons, thereby causing paralysis and degeneration of the muscles innervated by those motor neurons.

Polymorphonuclear Leukocyte. See Neutrophil.

Polysaccharide. A carbohydrate that can be broken down into two or more monosaccharide molecules. Examples: glycogen, cellulose.

Portal Triad. A structural and functional unit of a liver lobule that contains a branch of the hepatic artery, portal vein, and bile duct.

Portal Vein. The vein that brings blood from the gut and spleen to the liver.

Predentin. Organic fibrillar matrix of dentin secreted by odontoblasts. Predentin becomes calcified and forms dentin.

Primary Follicle. An early stage in the development of the ovarian follicle in which the ovum is surrounded by a single layer of cuboidal (follicular) epithelial cells.

Primary Nodule. A region within lymphoid tissue that actively produces lymphocytes by mitotic division of stem cells in the germinal center of the primary nodule.

Primary Spermatocytes. Large cells derived from spermatogonia that undergo meiosis and give rise to secondary spermatocytes.

Primordial Follicle. A very early stage in the development of the ovarian follicle in which the ovum is surrounded by a single layer of squamous epithelial cells.

Principal Cell. A generic term referring to the most numerous cells within a gland or organ. Example: the principal cells of the thyroid gland secrete thyroid hormone.

Progesterone. A steroid hormone secreted by the corpus luteum of the ovary that prevents maturation of ovarian follicles and prepares the uterus for implantation of the fertilized egg.

Prolactin. A proteinaceous hormone secreted by the anterior pituitary that stimulates milk secretion.

Proliferative Phase. That phase of the menstrual cycle in which the functionalis of the endometrium lining the uterus is reconstructed.

Prostaglandins. A general term describing a variety of cyclic fatty acids that perform hormone-like functions, including modulation of smooth-muscle contraction and blood pressure.

Prostate Gland. A gland of the male reproductive system, located near the bladder, that secretes a viscous fluid that is a major component of the seminal fluid.

Prostatic Concretions. Hard, mineralized bodies found within the prostate gland of older males.

Prostatic Fluid. Fluid secreted by the prostate gland that is propelled into the urethra during ejaculation.

Protein. A macromolecule made up of long sequences of amino acids.

Proximal Convoluted Tubule. The first tubular portion of the nephron, directly connected to Bowman's capsule, into which glomerular filtrate flows. It transports useful materials such as salts, amino acids, and sugars from the glomerular filtrate back into the blood.

Pseudopodia. Extensions of a cell's plasma membrane and cytoplasm ("false feet") that often engulf material during the process of phagocytosis; they also participate in cellular locomotion.

Ptyalin. An amylase, found in saliva, that converts starches into sugars.

Pulmonary Alveolar Macrophage (synonym: dust cell). A wandering macrophage, found in the alveoli of the lung, that "sweeps" the lining of the lung of particulate matter and debris.

Pulp. The substance within the pulp cavity in the core of the tooth that contains connective tissue, nerves, and blood vessels.

Radial Spokes. Components of the ciliary axoneme that connect the central sheath that surrounds the central pair of microtubules with the nine outer microtubular doublets.

Red Pulp. Regions of the spleen that contain venous sinuses and associated cells.

Renal Corpuscle. That part of the nephron that includes Bowman's capsule and its contained glomerular capillaries.

Renal Pelvis. The connection between the kidney and the ureter; the funnel-shaped end of the ureter that receives urine from the kidney.

Residual Bodies. Membrane-limited cytoplasmic inclusions that contain material indigestible by the cell's lysosomes.

Reticular Fiber. A class of thin connective tissue fiber, based on the collagen molecule, that reacts with certain silver stains. Reticular fibers are commonly found in lymphatic organs such as the spleen and lymph nodes.

Reticulocyte. This term describes each of two dramatically different kinds of cells: a connective tissue cell, similar to the fibroblast, that secretes reticular fibers; and an immature, circulating erythrocyte, within whose cytoplasm wisps of rough endoplasmic reticulum persist.

Reticuloendothelial System. A diffuse system of cells, found in lymphoid organs and many connective tissues, that includes all of the body's phagocytic cells (with the exception of circulating leukocytes).

Ribonucleoprotein. A combination of protein and ribonucleic acid.

Ribosome. A small, dense, cytoplasmic inclusion that functions as the site of assembly of protein from its amino acid components.

RNA. Ribonucleic acid—an abundant class of nucleic acids associated, among other things, with the translation and transcription of genetic information.

Rod. The class of retinal photoreceptor that mediates vision in dim light; rods "see" black and white, but not color.

Romanovsky's Stain. A class of stains, commonly used on smears of blood and bone marrow, that include a basic dye such as methylene blue, an acid dye such as eosin, and alcohol, which fixes the cells. Example: Wright's stain.

Root. The portion of the tooth located below the gumline.

Rough Endoplasmic Reticulum (abbreviation: RER). A system of intracellular membranes, commonly associated with the synthesis of "protein for export," that appears in the cytoplasm of the cell as flattened sacs, or cisternae, whose membranes are heavily encrusted with ribosomes.

Sarcolemma. The cell membrane surrounding a skeletal or cardiac muscle fiber.

Sarcomere. A unit of structure and function within a myofibril of a skeletal or cardiac muscle fiber bordered by two adjacent Z bands.

Sarcoplasmic Reticulum. The modified smooth endoplasmic reticulum of a skeletal or cardiac muscle fiber that sequesters calcium and releases it under appropriate conditions of stimulation.

Schmidt-Lantermann Cleft. An irregularity in the myelin sheath of a nerve.

Schwann Cell. A class of neuroglial cell that functions in wrapping the myelin sheath around a peripheral nerve.

Sclera. The outermost layer of the eyeball, rich in connective tissue, that presents itself as the "whites" of the eyes.

Sebaceous Gland. A gland of the skin, usually associated with a hair, that secretes an oily substance called sebum.

Secondary Follicle. That stage in the development of the ovarian follicle in which the ovum is surrounded by several layers of cuboidal (follicular) epithelial cells.

Secondary Papillae. Projections of the papillary layer of the dermis upward into the basal layer of the epidermis.

Secondary Spermatocytes. Small cells, derived from primary spermatocytes that undergo meiosis, that give rise to spermatids.

Secretory Duct (synonym: striated duct). A medium-sized, intralobular duct within a salivary gland.

Secretory Granules (synonym: secretory vesicles). Membrane-limited packets of material within the cytoplasm—frequently found near the apical pole of the cell—destined to be released into the lumen of a gland, duct, or organ.

Secretory Phase. That phase of the menstrual cycle in which the endometrium of the uterus prepares for implantation.

Secretory Vesicles. See Secretory granules.

Semen. Material that contains seminal fluid and spermatozoa released from the penis of the male during ejaculation.

Seminal Fluid. The fluid component of semen in which spermatozoa are suspended.

Seminal Vesicle. An outpocketing of the vas deferens, lined by a secretory epithelium, that stores seminal fluid prior to ejaculation.

Seminiferous Tubule. One of several long, coiled tubules within the testis that contains the germinal epithelium.

Septal Cell. See Pneumocyte type II.

Septum (plural: septa). A generic term referring to a thin wall that divides two cavities or masses of soft tissue.

Serosa. The layer that forms the outer lining of organs, such as the duodenum, that consists of an extension of the inner wall of the body cavity.

Serous Cells. Cells that produce a watery secretion rich in proteins and glycoproteins. Example: cells of serous acini of the parotid gland.

Serous Demilune. A half-moon-shaped cap of serous cells fitted around a mucous acinus within a salivary gland.

Sertoli Cell (synonym: nurse cell). A larger cell within the seminiferous tubule to which spermatids attach during spermiogenesis.

Sinusoid. A class of large, leaky capillaries, such as those in the liver, that permit passage of large objects through their perforated walls.

Skeletal Muscle. A class of striated muscle whose large, multinucleate fibers, under control of motor neurons, generate the contractile forces responsible for voluntary movements.

Skeletal Muscle Cell. See Skeletal muscle fiber.

Skeletal Muscle Fiber. The contractile unit of skeletal muscle; a skeletal muscle cell; a large, multinucleate cell that is a syncytium.

Smooth Endoplasmic Reticulum (abbreviation: SER). A system of intracellular membranes in the cytoplasm of the cell. Devoid of ribosomes, the SER is organized as an anastomosing network of tubules and participates in a variety of cellular functions such as glycogen metabolism and steroid biosynthesis.

Smooth Muscle. A class of muscle whose small, fusiform, mononucleate fibers lack the striations characteristic of skeletal and cardiac muscle. Innervated by the autonomic nervous system, smooth muscles power involuntary movements such as intestinal peristalsis and constriction of airways and blood vessels.

Soma. A general term meaning "body" that often refers to the cell body of a neuron.

Somatotropes. Cells of the anterior pituitary that secrete somatrotrophic (growth) hormone.

Somatotrophic Hormone. See Growth hormone.

Somatotropin. See Growth hormone.

Spermatid. A haploid cell, derived from a secondary spermatocyte, that differentiates to form a spermatozoon in the process of spermatogenesis.

Spermatocyte. A cell in the germinal epithelium of the seminiferous tubule, classified as either a primary spermatocyte or a secondary spermatocyte. A primary spermatocyte, derived from a spermatogonial cell, divides to form two secondary spermatocytes; each secondary spermatocyte gives rise to two spermatids.

Spermatogenesis. The formation of a spermatozoon from a stem cell, the spermatogonium.

Spermatogenic Cells. A general term referring to cells in the spermatogenic series: spermatogonia, primary spermatocytes, secondary spermatocytes, and spermatids.

Spermatogonia. Stem cells located at the periphery of the germinal epithelium in the seminiferous tubule that undergo mitotic division and give rise to primary spermatocytes.

Spermatozoon. A mature sperm cell, equipped with a head and a tail, designed to fertilize the egg.

Spermiogenesis. The morphogenetic transformation of spermatids into spermatozoa.

Spicules. Small spikes that traverse the marrow spaces within spongy bone.

Splenic Cords (synonym: cords of Billroth). Dense regions of tissue within the red pulp of the spleen that contain venous sinuses and associated cells.

Spongy Bone (synonyms: cancellous bone; trabecular bone). A kind of bone, located within the marrow spaces of large bones, that consists of a network of spicules (spikes) and trabeculae (plates).

Squames. Flattened, scalelike, dead keratinized cells periodically shed from the surface of the skin.

Squamous Epithelium. An epithelium characterized by flat surface cells.

Stellate Reticulum. Loose connective tissue associated with the developing tooth.

Stereocilia. Long microvilli, such as those found extending from the surface of cells of the epididymis and hair cells of the cochlea. Stereocilia are in no way related to cilia.

Steroid. A large class of chemical substances, including many vitamins, hormones, drugs, and cellular components, based on a four-ring phenanthrene skeleton.

Stratified Squamous Epithelium. An epithelium consisting of several layers of cells; the uppermost layer contains flattened, or squamous, cells.

Stratum Basale (synonym: stratum germinativum). The lower layer of the epidermis containing mitotically active stem cells that supply cells for the upper layers of the skin.

Stratum Corneum. The superficial layer of the epidermis that consists of flattened, keratinized cells.

Stratum Germinativum. See Stratum basale.

Stratum Granulosum. A layer of cells in the epidermis, located above the stratum spinosum, that contains conspicuous keratohyalin granules.

Stratum Lucidum. A clear layer of epidermal cells located between the stratum corneum and stratum granulosoum of thick skin, such as the sole of the foot.

Stratum Spinosum (synonyms: spiny layer; prickle cell layer). A layer of cells in the epidermis, just above the stratum germinativum, characterized by a multitude of intercellular attachments called desmosomes.

Striated Border (synonym: brush border). A feltwork of closely packed, parallel microvilli that extend from the apical cell surface of epithelia such as those lining the intestine and the proximal convoluted tubule of the kidney.

Striated Duct. See Secretory duct.

Subcapsular Sinus (synonyms: cortical sinus; marginal sinus). The space beneath the capsule covering a lymph node, it receives incoming lymph from small afferent lymphatic vessels.

Sublingual Gland. One of a pair of bilateral salivary glands situated beneath the tongue; has both mucous and serous acini.

Submandibular Gland (synonym: submaxillary gland). One of a pair of large bilateral salivary glands located beneath the lower jaw, or mandible; has both mucous and serous acini.

Submaxillary Gland. See Submandibular gland.

Submucosa. A layer of dense irregular connective tissue found beneath the mucosa of many organs.

Supporting Cell (synonym: sustentacular cell). A generic term for a kind of cell, usually within an epithelium, that supports, or sustains, other cells.

Surface Mucous Cells. Epithelial cells found on the surface of the gastric mucosa that have a protective apical cap of mucus beneath the cell surface.

Surfactant. A wetting agent, secreted by the pneumocyte type II, that lowers surface tension and prevents collapse of the alveoli.

Sustentacular Cell. See Supporting cell.

Sympathetic Nervous System. A subdivision of the autonomic nervous system that contains mainly adrenergic fibers and frequently depresses secretion, decreases the contractility of smooth muscle, and causes vasoconstriction.

Synapse. A functional point of contact between two nerve cells or processes that permits the passage of an impulse.

Synaptic Cleft. The narrow intercellular (extracellular) space between the two adjacent nerve cell membranes in a synapse.

Synaptic Vesicle. A tiny, membrane-limited vesicle, located at the synapse, bearing the chemical that functions as a neurotransmitter that, when released from the presynaptic nerve terminal, excites (or inhibits) the postsynaptic neuron.

Syncytium. A large, multinucleate cell, derived from many cells, whose cell membranes have fused to form one common cellular boundary.

Synovial Fluid. The fluid within a joint, secreted by the epithelium that lines the joint capsule, that serves to lubricate the articulating surfaces within the joint.

Systole. The strong pulse generated by the contraction of the left ventricle of the heart.

T-Lymphocyte. A class of lymphocyte that matures in the thymus and participates in cell-mediated immunity.

T-System. A system of tubular invaginations of the cell membrane in skeletal and cardiac muscle fibers that carry electrical excitation inward to all the sarcomeres of the myofibrils. The transverse tubules of the T-system are usually closely associated with the sarcoplasmic reticulum.

Taste Bud. A teardrop-shaped cluster of cells associated with the epithelium of circumvallate, foliate, and some fungiform papillae of the tongue, containing chemoreceptors that mediate gustation.

Taste Pore. The opening at the apical surface of the taste bud.

Tectorial Membrane. A thin sheet of connective tissue in the organ of Corti of the cochlea that makes contact with the stereocilia of the mechanoreceptive hair cells.

Tendon. A strap of dense regular connective tissue that connects muscle to bone.

Terminal Cisternae. Dilated cisternae of the sarcoplasmic reticulum of skeletal and cardiac muscle fibers. Two terminal cisternae usually surround a single tubule of the T-system.

Tertiary Follicle (synonym: growing follicle). A large, well-developed ovarian follicle that contains a fluid-filled cavity, the antrum. A tertiary follicle can continue to grow to form a mature Graafian follicle.

Testicle. See Testis.

Testis (synonym: testicle). The organ of the male reproductive system in which spermatogenesis occurs.

Theca. An enclosing case or sheath.

Theca Externa. The outer, fibrous region of the theca folliculi of the ovarian follicle.

Theca Folliculi. A sheath of connective tissue that surrounds an ovarian follicle.

Theca Interna. The inner, highly cellular layer of the theca folliculi of the ovarian follicle.

Theca Lutein Cells. Progesterone-secreting cells of the corpus luteum.

Thymus. A glandular structure located in the chest and made of lymphoid tissue that participates in the function and development of the immune system.

Thyroglobulin. A glycoprotein macromolecule, contained within the colloid in the lumen of a follicle of the thyroid gland, that is complexed with thyroid hormone.

Thyroid Hormone (synonym: thyroxine). The hormone secreted by the thyroid gland that, among other functions, is important in the control of metabolic rate.

Thyrotrope. A cell (basophil) of the anterior pituitary that secretes thyroid-stimulating hormone (thyrotropin).

Thyrotropin. A hormone, secreted by the anterior pituitary, that stimulates secretion of thyroid hormone by the thyroid gland.

Thyrotropin-Releasing Factor. A hormone, secreted by the hypothalamus of the brain, that stimulates the anterior pituitary to secrete thyrotropin.

Thyroxine. See Thyroid hormone.

Tight Junction (synonym: zonula occludens). A type of intercellular junction, commonly found at the apical pole of epithelial cells, in which the closely apposed cell membranes prevent the flow of materials into the extracellular (intercellular) space between two neighboring cells.

Trabeculae. A generic term referring to thin plates of supporting material within a tissue or organ. Example: trabeculae of spongy bone.

Transcription. The process by which genetic information contained in DNA produces a complementary sequence of bases in an RNA chain.

Transfer Vesicles. Membrane-limited vesicles that transfer material from the rough endoplasmic reticulum to the Golgi apparatus.

Transitional Epithelium. A class of epithelium, several cell layers thick, that stretches or contracts (hence changes in appearance) when the container it lines is filled or emptied. Example: the epithelium lining the urinary bladder.

Trophic Hormone. A hormone secreted by one gland that stimulates secretion of a hormone by another gland. Example: thyroid-stimulating hormone (TSH), released by the anterior pituitary, stimulates secretion and release of thyroid hormone from the thyroid gland.

Trypsin. A digestive enzyme, secreted by the pancreas into the duodenum of the small intestine, that breaks down proteins (is proteolytic).

Tunica Adventitia. An envelope of loose connective tissue that surrounds blood vessels larger than arterioles or venules.

Tunica Albuginea. A tough capsule of dense connective tissue that envelops organs such as the testis.

Tunica Intima. The innermost layer of a blood vessel; lined by endothelium, the tunica intima is in contact with blood in the lumen.

Tunica Media. The thick middle layer of the wall of a blood vessel, rich in smooth muscle and, in the case of arteries, elastic tissue.

Unit Membrane. A term used to describe the trilaminar, "railroad-track" structure displayed by many biologic membranes when fixed in osmium tetroxide, cut in cross section, and viewed with the electron microscope.

Ureter. The tube that carries urine from the kidney to the bladder.

Urethra. The canal that carries urine from the bladder to outside the body.

Urinary Space. The space within Bowman's capsule of the nephron, continuous with the lumen of the proximal convoluted tubule, that receives the glomerular filtrate.

Uterine Tube (synonyms: fallopian tube; oviduct). The tube through which the egg, following ovulation, passes en route from ovary to uterus.

Uterus. The organ of the female reproductive system that contains the developing fetus prior to birth.

Vas Deferens (synonym: ductus deferens). A thick-walled tube that carries spermatozoa from the testis to the urethra.

Vasa Recta. A system of small, straight blood vessels, located in the medulla of the kidney, that are closely associated with tubules of the nephron.

Vasopressin (synonyms: antidiuretic hormone; ADH). A hormone made in the hypothalamus and released by the neurohypophysis that promotes water retention by the kidneys.

Venous Sinus. A large, very leaky capillary, such as those found in the liver and spleen.

Villus (plural: villi). A small infolding of the intestinal wall that projects into the lumen; the villus is lined by simple columnar epithelium and supported by the lamina propria.

Visceral Layer. The inner epithelial lining of Bowman's capsule of the nephron.

Vitreous Humor. The viscous, dense, jellylike material that fills the posterior chamber of the eyeball (behind the lens and ciliary body).

White Pulp. That part of the tissues of the spleen that consists of arterioles and surrounding clusters of lymphocytes.

Woven Bone. A kind of bone found in embryos, young children, and certain pathological states in which orderly lamellae of collagen fibers are not present.

Zona Fasciculata. A layer of the adrenal cortex, just internal to the zona glomerulosa, that secretes glucocorticoids such as cortisone.

Zona Glomerulosa. The outermost secretory layer of the adrenal cortex that secretes mineralocorticoids such as aldosterone.

Zona Pellucida. A dark-staining zone surrounding the egg within the developing ovarian follicle, consisting of cytoplasmic extensions of the oocyte and granulosa cells and the material in which they are embedded.

Zona Reticularis. The innermost layer of the adrenal cortex that secretes steroids similar to sex hormones.

Zonula Adherens. See Intermediate junction.

Zonula Occludens. See Tight junction.

Zygote. The fertilized egg.

Zymogen Granule. A secretory vesicle, usually found in the apical pole of a secretory cell, containing enzyme precursors.

Index